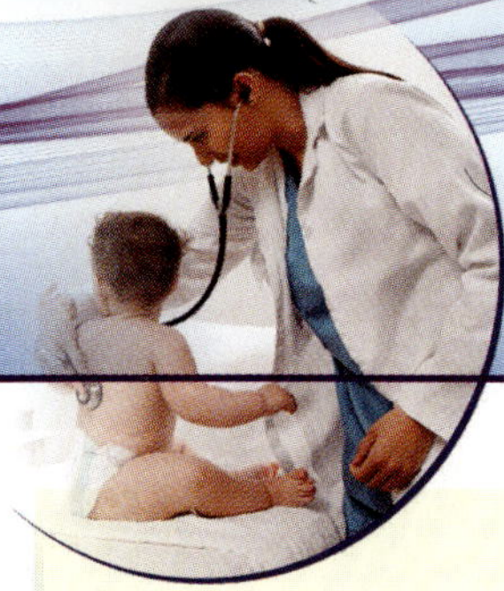

Fourth Edition

Manipal Manual of Clinical Paediatrics

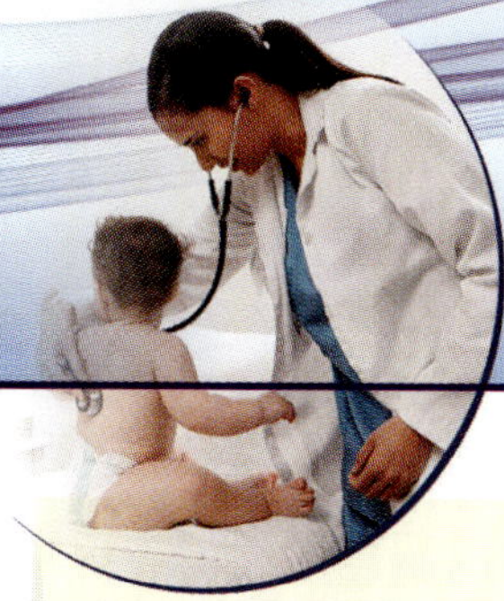

Fourth Edition

Manipal Manual of Clinical Paediatrics

Kafeel Khan

MBBS MD (Paediatrics) (KMC, Manipal)

Associate Professor
Department of Paediatrics
Kamineni Institute of Medical Sciences
Telangana

Formerly
Associate Professor and Head
IMCH, Tamil Nadu

Associate Professor
Jaipur National University, Rajasthan

Assistant Professor
BRD Medical College, Gorakhpur, Uttar Pradesh
SMIMS, Gangtok, Sikkim

CBSPD CBS

CBS Publishers & Distributors Pvt Ltd

New Delhi • Bengaluru • Chennai • Kochi • Kolkata • Lucknow • Mumbai
Hyderabad • Jharkhand • Nagpur • Patna • Pune • Uttarakhand

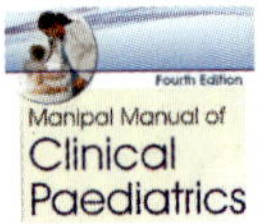

Disclaimer

Science and technology are constantly changing fields. New research and experience broaden the scope of information and knowledge. The author has tried his best in giving information available to him while preparing the material for this book. Although, all efforts have been made to ensure optimum accuracy of the material, yet it is quite possible some errors might have been left uncorrected. The publisher, the printer and the author will not be held responsible for any inadvertent errors, omissions or inaccuracies.

ISBN: 978-93-5466-787-9

Fourth Edition: 2025

First Edition: 2013
Second Edition: 2020
Third Edition: 2023

Published by Satish Kumar Jain and produced by Varun Jain for

CBS Publishers and Distributors Pvt Ltd

4819/XI Prahlad Street, 24 Ansari Road, Daryaganj, New Delhi 110 002, India
Ph: 011-23289259, 23266838 Website: www.cbspd.com
Fax: 011-23243014 e-mail: delhi@cbspd.com

Corporate Office: 204 FIE, Industrial Area, Patparganj, Delhi 110 092, India
Ph: 011-4934 4934
Fax: 011-4934 4935 e-mail: publishing@cbspd.com; publicity@cbspd.com

Branches

- **Bengaluru:** Seema House 2975, 17th Cross, KR Road, Banasankari 2nd Stage, Bengaluru 560 070, Karnataka, India
  Ph: +91-80-26771678/79 Fax: +91-80-26771680 e-mail: bangalore@cbspd.com
- **Chennai:** 7, Subbaraya Street, Shenoy Nagar, Chennai 600 030, Tamil Nadu, India
  Ph: +91-44-26680620, 26681266 Fax: +91-44-42032115 e-mail: chennai@cbspd.com
- **Kochi:** 42/1325, 36, Power House Road, Opposite KSEB, Kochi 682 018, Kerala, India
  Ph: +91-484-4059061-67 Fax: +91-484-4059065 e-mail: kochi@cbspd.com
- **Kolkata:** C/o Hind Ceramics Compound, 1st Floor, 147, Nilgunj Road, Belghoria, Kolkata 700 056, West Bengal, India
  Ph: +91-33-25633055/56 e-mail: kolkata@cbspd.com
- **Lucknow:** Basement, Khushnuma Complex, 7-Meerabai Marg (behind Jawahar Bhawan), Lucknow 226 001, Uttar Pradesh, India
  Ph: +91-522-4000032 e-mail: tiwari.lucknow@cbspd.com
- **Mumbai:** PWD Shed, Gala No. 25/26, Ramchandra Bhatt Marg, Next to JJ Hospital Gate No. 2, Opp Union Bank of India, Noorbaug, Mumbai 400 009, Maharashtra, India
  Ph: +91-22-66661880/89 e-mail: mumbai@cbspd.com

Representatives

- **Hyderabad** 0-9885175004
- **Jharkhand** 0-9811541605
- **Nagpur** 0-8692091830
- **Patna** 0-9334159340
- **Pune** 0-9664372571
- **Uttarakhand** 0-9716462459

Printed at: Sri Prints & Sales, Delhi, India

to

my loving families

Late Er Shakeel Khan, Mrs Nuzhat Perween
Mr Adeel Khan, Dr Ayesha Khan,
Dr Ahmar Uddin, Dr Farkhanda A,
Er. Kashif J Khan, Mrs Khalida K, Dr Fazeel Khan,
Mr Samar Khan, Mrs Zeenat Fatima,
and my lovely wife Dr Shabista Khan
for teaching me the value of hard work and for their
selfless love and support

all the kids who taught me milestones especially
Zara, Jasir, Rida, Abaan, Rahil, Zabrina
and to the new addition of our family
Oliver and Yusuf

all my friends, colleagues, and seniors
for their support, encouragement and never
letting me doubt my dreams

all my patients and their families and teachers
who continue to aid in my development as paediatrician

and my alma mater
KMC, Manipal

Foreword

It is with great pleasure and profound respect that I present the foreword for the fourth edition of the *Manipal Manual of Clinical Paediatrics.* This manual has evolved into an indispensable resource for medical students, residents, nurses, and paramedics across India and beyond. This edition epitomizes the relentless dedication of Dr Kafeel Khan and his team toward enhancing paediatric education and clinical care.

Dr Khan's efforts have culminated in the first paediatric manual tailored to the competency-based curriculum (CBME) outlined by the National Medical Council. This adaptation is pivotal, ensuring that the manual remains at the forefront of medical education, offering a practical guide that covers essential history-taking and examination skills. It encapsulates a wealth of knowledge through mnemonics, tables, charts, diagrams, and triads, alongside vivid illustrations of clinical signs. This approach not only facilitates quick revision but also ensures that critical information is easily retrievable, making it an indispensable companion for medical graduates.

Beyond his contributions to paediatric literature, Dr Khan's distinction in the field of paediatrics is unparalleled. His aptitude for diagnosing diseases, coupled with his excellence in teaching, reflects his comprehensive understanding of both the science and art of medicine. Moreover, Dr Khan is celebrated not only for his professional achievements but also for his humility and the profound humanity with which he approaches both his patients and students.

The *Manipal Manual of Clinical Pediatrics*, under Dr Khan's stewardship, has set a new standard for medical textbooks. It is a beacon for those navigating the complexities of pediatric care and education, embodying the spirit of innovation and compassion that is essential in the medical profession.

I believe and strongly recommend every medical graduate to make this manual your companion.

Dr Prasad Thanda
Professor and Head
Department of Paediatrics
Kamineni Institute of Medical Sciences, Telangana

Foreword

I am really proud to write this foreword for *Manipal Manual of Clinical Paediatrics* by Dr Kafeel Khan.

There are many changes bound to happened post-COVID either is history taking , examination, formulary and treatment protocols. It is very important to update this concise yet very informative paediatric book aimed to serve undergraduate medical students, nurses, paramedics and residents.

Some chapters that are exceptionally well written and highly recommended are growth and development, nutrition, immunization (including corona vaccine), neonatology, paediatric drugs, instruments, X-rays, poisoning, emergency paediatrics, musculo-skeletal disorders, rheumatology and COVID-19.

I hope this manual will serve its purpose and become a must-be companion for the readers during their posting in paediatric ward.

But this book definitely is not a substitute for the theory text-books on paediatrics.

I must finally congratulate Dr Kafeel Khan, and wish him great success in his future to continue his research and academic work.

Dr Vasanthamani Palanisamy
MD DGO MNAMS MBA
Dean
Indira Medical College and Hospital
Thiruvallur, Tamil Nadu

Foreword

"Children are heritage from the LORD,
Offspring a reward from him"

Manipal Manual of Clinical Paediatrics was first published in 2013 and I feel proud to write this foreword for the updated and revised version, what I call *"Pearl Book"* as this is an informative and well-written book touching upon most aspects of practical and clinical pediatric.

I have always emphasised to my students that diagnostic tools would never replace a good history and thorough clinical examination. Keeping this in mind and the modification made in this edition, I feel this book would be better readable and practically useful.

I must congratulate Dr Kafeel Khan, a bright student and now a famous successful paediatrician who worked with me for 10 years during his undergraduation and postgraduation for this excellent addition to the medical student's book shelf. I sincerely hope that this book will continue to be favorite book to carry in paediatric wards by undergraduates, postgraduates as well as paramedics.

I wish Dr Kafeel Khan a great success for his future projects aimed at betterment of health of children.

Dr Leslie Lewis
MBBS DCH DNB (Paediatrics)
Professor and Head
Department of Paediatrics
Kasturba Medical College, Manipal, Karnataka

Foreword

It gives me immense pleasure to write this foreword for the very informative and well-written pocket book for undergraduate students and residents. This is a concise book on paediatrics touching upon the most aspects of practical and clinical paediatrics. The illustrations/tables add to recall of appropriate basic science knowledge at the time of analysis of the clinical problems. This book definitely is not a substitute for the textbooks on paediatrics which a student has to read for learning paediatrics.

I must finally congratulate the author for this excellent addition to the medical student's book shelf which I am certain will be carried by students starting their clinical practice in the years to come. I am sure Dr Kafeel Khan will be motivated enough after this book to work hard for his future projects.

Dr Sudip Dutta
MBBS MD (Paediatrics)
Professor and Head
Department of Paediatrics
CRH, SMIMS
Gangtok, Sikkim

Preface to the Fourth Edition

Twelve years ago, as a final-year MD paediatrics student at KMC, Manipal, I embarked on a journey to distill my learning and experiences into a resource that could bridge the gap between extensive theoretical knowledge and practical clinical application. With immense support and encouragement, what began as a pocket-sized handbook in 2013, it has matured into a cornerstone clinical manual for a broad audience including undergraduates, nursing and paramedic staff, and residents.

Despite the plethora of clinical textbooks authored by esteemed professionals, a void existed for a succinct, yet all-encompassing, user-friendly manual tailored to the Competency-Based Medical Education (CBME) curriculum prescribed by the National Medical Council (NMC). It is with great pride that I present this fourth edition, a pioneering effort in aligning with CBME guidelines.

Significant expansions have been made in sections on growth and development, nutrition, immunization, neonatology, paediatric drugs, and X-rays, and added new chapters on ECG, the Objective Structured Clinical Examination (OSCE), and COVID-19.

I extend my heartfelt gratitude to Dr Fazeel Ahmad Khan (MBBS, and DNB orthopaedic), a senior clinical fellow at the University Hospital, Birmingham, UK, for his invaluable contribution to the musculoskeletal and rheumatology chapter.

This publication would not have been possible without the collective effort and dedication of my esteemed colleagues—Dr Shabista Khan, Dr Satish Reddy, Dr Banoth Balaram, Dr Suresh Thomas, Dr Satish Vadapalli, Dr Sariq Nawaz, Dr Azam N, Dr Jagdish Solanki and especially Assistant Professor Dr Chandini J and Dr Srikanth Vijjapu along with my diligent juniors.

I am thankful to my PMT days teacher/my Guru S Ahmad sir for helping me to prepare the manuscript.

For the prompt publication and global availability of the manual, I give credit to M/s CBS Publishers and Distributors.

For future enhancements, please share your thoughts at teamdrkafeel@gmail.com or drkafeelkhan@twitter.com.

Kafeel Khan

Preface to the First Edition

When I was doing my UG, I felt the need to have a pocket-sized clinical book to carry in the ward and refer it immediately in need. While we have many clinical books written by great authors we do not have a concise yet comprehensive easy to use manual. I wrote this book designed to serve the felt needs of undergraduates and residents and hope that the manual will serve this purpose. This manual gives you the quick revision of good history taking/ examination in a very simple manner. This Manual contains a number of mnemonics, tables, charts, diagrams, formulas and easy to remember tips which will enable easy registration and recall of the clinical aspect of paediatrics. It also provides the essential information on growth and development, nutrition, immunization, neonatology, common and essential used drugs, instruments, X-rays.

I am sure you will find this manual useful and informative and hope this manual becomes a good companion during your paediatrics posting.

Suggestion for further improvement of the manual would be welcomed and gratefully acknowledged.

This book would not have been possible without the effort of my colleagues Dr Ganga S, Dr Ashish P, Dr Satish V, Dr Subodh Shetty, Dr Aruna S, Dr Satish Reddy, Dr Narendra Rai, Dr Ankur Sinha specially Dr Tsultem Doma Bhutia and my juniors Dr Bhanu, Dr Bijya Jha, Dr Aditya K. Each of them selflessly dedicated his/her time and expertise to improve the quality and contents of this publication.

I am thankful to Mr Fakhruddin Ahmad for typing the manuscript. The credit for prompt publication of the manual goes to the publishers, Dr Rakesh Dubey and Rahul Singh.

Kafeel Khan

Hippocratic Oath

I swear by Apollo Physician, by Asclepius, by Hygieia, by Panacea, and by all the gods and goddesses, making them my witnesses, that I will carry out, according to my ability and judgment, this oath and this indenture.

To hold my teacher in this art equal to my own parents; to make him partner in my livelihood; when he is in need of money to share mine with him; to consider his family as my own brothers, and to teach them this art, if they want to learn it, without fee or indenture; to impart precept, oral instruction, and all other instruction to my own sons, the sons of my teacher, and to indentured pupils who have taken the physician's oath, but to nobody else.

I will use treatment to help the sick according to my ability and judgment, but never with a view to injury and wrong-doing. Neither will I administer a poison to anybody when asked to do so, nor will I suggest such a course. Similarly, I will not give to a woman a pessary to cause abortion, but I will keep pure and holy both my life and my art. I will not use the knife, not even, verily, on sufferers from stone, but I will give place to such as are craftsmen therein.

Into whatsoever houses I enter, I will enter to help the sick, and I will abstain from all intentional wrong-doing and harm, especially from abusing the bodies of man or woman, bond or free. And whatsoever I shall see or hear in the course of my profession, as well as outside my profession in my intercourse with men, if it be what should not be published abroad, I will never divulge, holding such things to be holy secrets.

Now if I carry out this oath, and break it not, may I gain for ever reputation among all men for my life and for my art; but if I break it and foreswear myself, may the opposite befall me.

Translated by

—WHS Jones

The Physician's Pledge (NMC)*

1. As a member of the medical profession,
2. I solemnly pledge to dedicate my life to the service of humanity;
3. The health and well-being of my patient will be my first consideration;
4. I will respect the autonomy and dignity of my patient;
5. I will maintain the utmost respect for human life;
6. I will not permit considerations of age, disease or disability, creed, ethnic origin, gender, nationality, political affiliation, race, sexual orientation, social standing, or any other factor to intervene between my duty and my patient;
7. I will respect the secrets that are confided in me, even after the patient has died;
8. I will practise my profescion with conscience and dignity and in accordance with good medical practice;
9. I will foster the honour and noble traditions of the medical profession;
10. I will give to my teachers, colleagues, and students the respect and gratitude that is their due;
11. I will share my medical knowledge for the benefit of the patient and the advancement of health care;
12. I will attend to my own health, well-being, and abilities in order to provide care of the highest standard;
13. I will not use my medical knowledge to violate human rights and civil liberties, even under threat;
14. I make these promises solemnly, freely, and upon my honour.

---

*NMC Act (the National Medical Commission Act), 2019 also known as National Medical Commission Registered Medical Practitioner (Professional Conduct) Regulations Act, 2022.

Contents

Foreword by Dr Prasad Thanda vii
Foreword by Dr Vasanthamani Palanisamy viii
Foreword by Dr Leslie Lewis ix
Foreword by Dr Sudip Dutta x
Preface to the Fourth Edition xi
Preface to the First Edition xii
Hippocratic Oath xiii
The Physician's Pledge (NMC) xiv
Index of Competency xvii
Abbreviations xxxi

1. **Paediatric Case Sheet** 1
2. **Development History** 6
3. **Dietic History** 13
4. **Immunization** 18
5. **Socioeconomic Status Scale** 35
6. **Vitals** 38
7. **Anthropometry** 44
8. **General Examination** 54
9. **Sexual Maturity Rating (SMR): Tanner Staging** 74
10. **Skin Diseases** 78
11. **Respiratory System** 81
12. **Coronavirus Disease** 94
13. **Cardiovascular System** 104
14. **Gastrointestinal System** 115
15. **Central Nervous System** 123
16 **Muscle, Bones, Joints and Rheumatic Disorders** 145

17. Neonatology 156
18. Drugs/Formulary 181
19. Emergency Paediatrics 195
20. OSCE and AETCOM 205
21. Procedure and Instruments 223
22. X-ray 233
23. Electrocardiogram (ECG or EKG) 241
24. Growth Charts 255
25. Miscellaneous 261

Index *269*

Index of Competency

Competency Based Undergraduate Curriculum for the Indian Medial Graduate

Code	Competency	Domain K/S/A/C	Level K/KH/SH/P	Teaching learning method	Page No.
PE1.4	Perform anthropometric measurements, document in growth charts and interpret	S	P	Small group discussion	44, 255
PE1.7	Perform developmental assessment and interpret	S	P	Bedside clinics, skills lab	6
PE 2.2	Assessment of a child with failing to thrive including eliciting an appropriate history and examination	S	SH	Bedside clinics	49
PE2.3	Counselling a parent with failing to thrive child	A/C	SH	OSPE	49, 206
PE2.5	Assessment of a child with short stature: Elicit history, perform examination, document and present	S	SH	Bedside clinics, skills lab	46
PE3.3	Assessment of a child with developmental delay—Elicit document and present history	S	SH	Bedside clinics, skills lab	11
PE3.4	Counsel a parent of a child with developmental delay	S	SH	DOAP session	10, 206
PE3.7	Visit a child developmental unit and observe its functioning	S	KH	Lecture, small group discussion	
PE4.6	Visit to the child guidance clinic	S	KH	Lecture, small group discussion	
PE6.9	Perform routine Adolescent Health check up including eliciting history, performing examination including SMR (Sexual Maturity Rating), growth assessments (using Growth charts) and systemic exam including thyroid and Breast exam and the HEADSS (Home, Education, Activities, Drugs Suicidality, and Sex) screening	S	SH	Bedside clinics	74, 259

Code	Competency	Domain K/S/A/C	Level K/KH/ SH/P	Teaching learning method	Page No.
PE6.11	Visit to the adolescent clinic	S	KH	DOAP session	
PE7.5	Observe the correct technique of breast feeding and distinguish right from wrong techniques	S	P	Bedside clinics, skills lab	175
PE7.7	Perform breast examination and identify common problems during lactation such as retracted nipples, cracked nipples, breast engorgement, breast abscess	S	SH	Bedside clinics skill lab	175
PE7.8	Educate mothers on ante natal breast care and prepare mothers for lactation	A/C	SH	DOAP session	175, 176
PE7.9	Educate and counsel mothers for best practices in breast feeding	A/C	SH	DOAP session	174
PE7.10	Respects patient privacy	A	SH	DOAP session	
PE7.11	Participate in breast feeding week celebration	A	SH	DOAP	177
PE8.4	Elicit history on the complementary feeding habits	S	SH	Bedside clinics, skills lab	16
PE8.5	Counsel and educate mothers on the best practices in complimentary feeding	A/C	SH	DOAP session	16, 17
PE9.4	Elicit document and present an appropriate nutritional history and perform dietary recall	S	SH	Bedside clinics, Skills lab	14
PE9.5	Calculate the age related calorie requirement in health and disease and identify gap	S	SH	Bedside clinics, small group discussion	13
PE9.6	Assess and classify the nutrition status of infants, children and adolescents and recognize deviations	S	SH	Bedside clinics, Small group discussion	45
PE9.7	Plan an appropriate diet in health and disease	S	SH	Bedside clinic, small group discussion	13

Code	Competency	Domain K/S/A/C	Level K/KH/ SH/P	Teaching learning method	Page No.
PE10.3	Assessment of a patient with SAM and MAM, diagnosis, classification and planning management including hospital and community based intervention, rehabilitation and prevention	S	SH	Bedside clinics, skills lab	45, 48
PE10.4	Identify children with under nutrition as per IMNCI criteria and plan referral	S	SH	DOAP session	210
PE10.5	Counsel parents of children with SAM and MAM	S	SH	Bedside clinic, Skills station	45, 206
PE11.3	Assessment of a child with obesity with regard to eliciting history including physical activity, charting and dietary recall	S	SH	Bedside clinics, Standardized patients	51, 259
PE11.4	Examination including calculation of BMI, measurement of waist hip ratio, identifying external markers like acanthosis, striae, pseudogynaecomastia, etc	S	SH	Bedside clinics, Standardized patients, and videos	51, 77
PE11.5	Calculate BMI, document in BMI chart and interpret	S	P	Bedside clinics, small group discussion	51, 259
PE12.3	Identify the clinical features of dietary deficiency/excess of Vitamin A	S	SH	Bedside clinics, small group discussion	63, 64
PE12.4	Diagnose patients with Vitamin A deficiency, classify and plan management	S	SH	Bedside clinics, skill station	32, 63
PE12.8	Identify the clinical features of dietary deficiency of Vitamin D	S	SH	Bedside clinics, skills station	63, 154
PE12.9	Assess patients with Vitamin D deficiency, diagnose, classify and plan management	S	SH	Bedside clinics	154
PE12.17	Identify the clinical features of vitamin B complex deficiency	S	SH	Bedside clinics, skills lab	62

Code	Competency	Domain K/S/A/C	Level K/KH/ SH/P	Teaching learning method	Page No.
PE12.18	Diagnose patients with Vitamin B complex deficiency and plan management	B	SH	Bedside clinics, skills lab	62
PE12.21	Identify the clinical features of vitamin C deficiency	S	SH	Bedside clinics, skills lab	62
PE13.3	Identify the clinical features of dietary deficiency of Iron and make a diagnosis	S	SH	Bedside clinics, skills lab	63, 217
PE13.4	Interpret haemogram and iron panel	S	SH	Bedside clinics, small group discussion	217
PE13.5	Propose a management plan for Fe deficiency anaemia	S	SH	Bedside clinics, skills lab	218
PE15.3	Calculate the fluid and electrolyte requirement in health	S	SH	Bedside clinics, small group discussion	194
PE15.4	Interpret electrolyte report	S	SH	Bedside clinics, small group discussion	261
PE15.5	Calculate fluid and electrolyte imbalance	S	SH	Bedside clinics, small group discussion	194
PE15.6	Demonstrate the steps of inserting an IV cannula in a model	S	SH	Skills lab	
PE15.7	Demonstrate the steps of inserting an interosseous line in a mannequin	S	SH	Skills lab	
PE16.2	Assess children <2 months using IMNCI Guidelines	S	SH	DOAP session	210
PE16.3	Assess children >2 to 5 years using IMNCI guidelines and Stratify Risk	S	SH	DOAP session	210
PE18.6	Perform postnatal assessment of newborn and mother, provide advice on breast feeding, weaning and on family planning	S	SH	Bed side clinics, skill lab	16, 157, 175

Code	Competency	Domain K/S/A/C	Level K/KH/ SH/P	Teaching learning method	Page No.
PE18.7	Educate and counsel caregivers of children	A	SH	Postnatal ward, standardized patient	10, 16, 32, 173
PE18.8	Observe the implementation of the program by visiting the Rural Health Centre	S	KH	Bed side clinics, skill lab	214
PE19.6	Assess patient for fitness for immunisation and prescribe an age appropriate immunization schedule	S	P	Outpatient clinics, skills lab	31
PE19.7	Educate and counsel a patient for immunization	A/C	SH	DOAP session	18
PE19.8	Demonstrate willingness to participate in the national and sub national immunisation days	A	SH	Lecture, small group discussion	31
PE19.11	Document immunization in an immunization record	S	SH	Outpatient clinics, skills lab	32
PE19.12	Observe the administration of UIP vaccines	S	SH	DOAP session	31
PE19.13	Demonstrate the correct administration of different vaccines in a mannequin	S	SH	DOAP session	19
PE19.14	Practice infection control measures and appropriate handling of the sharps	S	SH	DOAP session	215
PE20.3	Perform neonatal resuscitation in a mannequin	S	SH	DOAP session	159
PE20.4	Assessment of a normal neonate	S	SH	Bedside clinics, skills lab	157
PE20.5	Counsel/educate mothers on the care of neonates	A/C	SH	DOAP session	173, 175
PE20.6	Explain the follow up care for neonates including breast feeding, temperature maintenance, immunisation, importance of growth monitoring and red flags	S	SH	DOAP session	31, 173, 175, 255

Code	Competency	Domain K/S/A/C	Level K/KH/ SH/P	Teaching learning method	Page No.
PE20.18	Identify and stratify risk in a sick neonate using IMNCI guidelines	S	SH	DOAP session	173, 210
PE21.8	Elicit, document and present a history pertaining to diseases of the genitourinary tract	S	SH	Bedside clinics, skills lab	220
PE21.9	Identify external markers for kidney diseases like failing to thrive, hypertension, pallor, ichthyosis, anasarca	S	SH	Bedside clinics, skills lab	220
PE21.10	Analyse symptom and interpret the physical finding and arrive at an appropriate provisional/differential diagnosis	S	SH	Bedside clinics, skills lab	54, 220
PE21.11	Perform and interpret the common analytes in a urine examination	S	SH	Bedside clinics, skills lab	220
PE21.12	Interpret report of plain X-ray of KUB	S	SH	Bedside clinics, skills lab	209, 220, 233
PE21.13	Enumerate the indications for and interpret the written report of ultrasonogram of KUB	S	SH	Bedside clinics, skills lab	220
PE21.16	Counsel/educate a patient for referral appropriately	A/C	SH	DOAP session	222
PE22.2	Counsel a patient with chronic illness	S	SH	Bedside clinics, skills lab	206
PE23.7	Elicit appropriate history for a cardiac disease, analyse the symptoms e.g. breathlessness, chest pain, tachycardia, feeding difficulty, failing to thrive, reduced urinary output, swelling, syncope, cyanotic spells, suck rest cycle, frontal swelling in infants	S	SH	Bedside clinics, skills lab	104, 264
PE23.8	Identify external markers of a cardiac disease, e.g. cyanosis, clubbing, dependent edema, dental caries, arthritis, erythema rash, chorea, subcutaneous nodules, Osler's node, Janeway lesions and document	S	SH	Bedside clinics, skills lab	54, 104

Code	Competency	Domain K/S/A/C	Level K/KH/SH/P	Teaching learning method	Page No.
PE23.9	Record pulse, blood pressure, temperature and respiratory rate and interpret as per the age	S	SH	Bedside clinics, skills lab	38
PE23.10	Perform independently examination of the cardio-vascular system -look for precordial bulge, pulsations in the precordium, JVP and its significance in children and infants, relevance of percussion in pediatric examination, auscultation and other system examination and document	S	SH	Bedside clinics, skills lab	104
PE23.11	Develop a treatment plan and prescribe appropriate drugs including fluids in cardiac diseases, anti-failure drugs, and inotropic agents	S	SH	Bedside clinics, skills lab	198, 263
PE23.12	Interpret a chest X-ray and recognize cardiomegaly	S	SH	Bedside clinics, skills lab	234
PE23.13	Choose and interpret blood reports in cardiac illness	S	P	Bedside clinics, small group discussion	261
PE23.14	Interpret pediatric ECG	S	SH	Bedside clinics, skills lab	241
PE23.15	Use the ECHO reports in management of cases	S	SH	Bedside clinics, skills lab	
PE23.18	Demonstrate empathy while dealing with children with cardiac diseases in every patient encounter	A	SH	Small group discussion	206
PE24.9	Elicit, document and present history pertaining to diarrheal diseases	S	SH	Bedside clinics, skills lab	59
PE24.10	Assess for signs of dehydration, document and present	S	SH	Bedside clinics, skills lab	59
PE24.11	Apply the IMNCI guidelines in risk stratification of children with diarrheal dehydration and refer	S	SH	Bedside clinics, skills lab	59, 210

Code	Competency	Domain K/S/A/C	Level K/KH/ SH/P	Teaching learning method	Page No.
PE24.12	Perform and interpret stool examination including hanging drop	S	SH	Bedside clinics, skills lab	
PE24.13	Interpret RFT and electrolyte report	S	SH	Bedside clinics, small group discussion	261
PE24.14	Plan fluid management as per the WHO criteria	S	SH	Bedside clinics, small group activity	194
PE24.15	Perform NG tube insertion in a manikin	S	P	DOAP session	225
PE24.16	Perform IV cannulation in a model	S	P	DOAP session	
PE24.17	Perform interosseous insertion model	S	P	DOAP session	
PE26.5	Elicit document and present the history related to diseases of gastrointestinal system	S	SH	Bedside clinics, skills lab	1, 115
PE26.6	Identify external markers for GI and liver disorders, e.g. jaundice, pallor, gynaecomastia, spider angioma, palmar erythema, ichthyosis, caput medusa, clubbing, failing to thrive, Vitamin A and D deficiency	S	SH	Bedside clinics, skills lab	54, 62, 117
PE26.7	Perform examination of the abdomen, demonstrate organomegaly, ascites, etc.	S	SH	Bedside clinics, skills lab	116
PE26.8	Analyse symptoms and interpret physical signs to make a provisional/ differential diagnosis	S	SH	Bedside clinics, skills lab	54, 115
PE26.9	Interpret liver function tests, viral markers, ultrasonogram report	S	SH	Bedside clinics, skills lab	261
PE26.10	Demonstrate the technique of liver biopsy in a perform liver biopsy in a simulated environment	S	SH	DOAP session	226
PE26.13	Counsel and educate patients and their family appropriately on liver diseases	A/C	P	Bedside clinics, skills lab	206

Code	Competency	Domain K/S/A/C	Level K/KH/ SH/P	Teaching learning method	Page No.
PE27.10	Observe the various methods of administering oxygen	S	KH	Demonstration	163
PE27.14	Assess emergency signs and prioritize	S	SH	DOAP session skills lab	195
PE27.15	Assess airway and breathing: recognise signs of severe respiratory distress. Check for cyanosis, severe chest indrawing, grunting	S	P	DOAP session, skills lab	92 159, 173
PE27.16	Assess airway and breathing. Demonstrate the method of positioning of an infant and child to open airway in a simulated environment	S	P	DOAP session, skills lab	161
PE27.17	Assess airway and breathing: administer oxygen using correct technique and appropriate flow rate	S	P	DOAP session, skills lab	161, 163
PE27.18	Assess airway and breathing: perform assisted ventilation by Bag and mask in a simulated environment lab	S	P	DOAP session, skills lab	161, 163
PE27.19	Check for signs of shock i.e. pulse, blood pressure, CRT	S	P	DOAP session, skills lab	38, 194
PE27.20	Secure an IV access in a simulated environment	S	P	DOAP session, skills lab	
PE27.21	Choose the type of fluid and calculate the fluid requirement in shock	S	P	DOAP session, skills lab	194
PE27.22	Assess level of consciousness and provide emergency treatment to a child with convulsions/coma – Position an unconscious child – Position a child with suspected trauma – Administer IV/per rectal Diazepam for a convulsing child in a simulated environment	S	P	DOAP session, skills lab	124, 142, 199
PE27.23	Assess for signs of severe dehydration	S	S	Bedside clinics, skills lab	59

Code	Competency	Domain K/S/A/C	Level K/KH/ SH/P	Teaching learning method	Page No.
PE27.27	Assess for hypothermia and maintain temperature	S	SH	Skills lab	38, 181
PE27.28	Provide BLS for children in manikin	S	P	Skills lab	196
PE27.30	Demonstrate confidentiality with regard to abuse	A	SH	Skills lab, standardized patients	221
PE27.31	Assess child for signs of abuse	S	SH	DOAP session, skills lab	222
PE27.32	Counsel parents of dangerously ill/terminally ill child to break a bad news	S	SH	DOAP session	206
PE27.33	Obtain informed consent	S	SH	DOAP session	211
PE27.34	Willing to be a part of the ER team	A	SH	DOAP session	
PE27.35	Attends to emergency calls promptly	A	SH	Bedside clinics, skill lab	
PE28.9	Elicit, document and present age appropriate history of a child with upper respiratory problem including stridor	S	SH	Bedside clinics, skill lab	81
PE28.10	Perform otoscopic examination of the ear	S	SH	DOAP session	82
PE28.11	Perform throat examination using tongue depressor	S	SH	DOAP session	232
PE28.12	Perform examination of the nose	S	SH	DOAP session	81
PE28.13	Analyse the clinical symptoms and interpret physical findings and make a provisional/ differential diagnosis in a child with ENT symptoms	S	SH	Bedside clinics	81
PE28.14	Develop a treatment plan and document appropriately in a child with upper respiratory symptoms	S	SH	Bedside clinics	90
PE28.15	Stratify risk in children with stridor using IMNCI guidelines	S	SH	Bedside clinics	88, 90, 210

Code	Competency	Domain K/S/A/C	Level K/KH/ SH/P	Teaching learning method	Page No.
PE28.16	Interpret blood tests relevant to upper respiratory problems	S	SH	Bedside clinics, small group discussion	261
PE28.17	Interpret X-ray of the paranasal sinuses and mastoid; and/or use written report in case of management interpret CXR in foreign body aspiration and lower respiratory tract infection, understand the significance of thymic shadow in pediatric chest X-rays	S	SH	Bedside clinics, small	81, 237
PE28.20	Counsel the child with asthma on the correct use of inhalers in a simulated environment	S/A/C	SH	DOAP	229
PE29.10	Elicit, document and present the history related to hematology	S	SH	Bedside clinics, skills lab	217
PE29.11	Identify external markers for hematological disorders, e.g. jaundice, pallor, petechiae purpura, ecchymosis, Lymphadenopathy, bone tenderness, loss of weight, mucosal and large joint bleed	S	SH	Bedside clinics, skills lab	54, 78,
PE29.12	Perform examination of the abdomen, demonstrate organomegaly	S	SH	Bedside clinics, skills lab	117
PE29.13	Analyse symptoms and interpret physical signs to make a provisional/ differential diagnosis	S	SH	Bedside clinics, skills lab	54, 114
PE29.14	Interpret CBC, LFT	S	SH	Bedside clinics, skills lab	261
PE29.15	Perform and interpret peripheral smear	S	SH	DOAP session	217
PE29.16	Discuss the indications for Hemoglobin electrophoresis and interpret report	K	K	Small group discussion	218
PE29.17	Demonstrate performance of bone marrow aspiration in manikin	S	SH	Skills lab	227

Code	Competency	Domain K/S/A/C	Level K/KH/ SH/P	Teaching learning method	Page No.
PE29.19	Counsel and educate patients about prevention and treatment of anemia	A/C	SH	Bedside clinics, skills lab	218
PE30.17	Elicit document and present an age appropriate history pertaining to the CNS	S	SH	Bedside clinics, skills lab	123
PE30.18	Demonstrate the correct method for physical examination of CNS including identification of external markers. Document and present clinical findings	S	SH	Bedside clinics, skills lab	124
PE30.19	Analyse symptoms and interpret physical findings and propose a provisional/ differential diagnosis	S	SH	Bedside clinics, skills lab	123, 141
PE30.20	Interpret and explain the findings in a CSF analysis	S	SH	Small group discussion	225
PE30.21	Enumerate the indication and discuss the limitations of EEG, CT, MRI	K	K	Bedside clinics	144
PE30.22	Interpret the reports of EEG, CT, MRI	S	SH	Bedside clinics, skills lab	144
PE30.23	Perform in a mannequin lumbar puncture. Discuss the indications, contraindication of the procedure	S	SH	Bedside clinics, skills lab	223
PE31.2	Recognize the clinical signs of allergic rhinitis	S	SH	Bedside clinics, skills lab	267
PE31.4	Identify atopic dermatitis and manage	S	SH	Bedside clinics, skills lab	267
PE31.6	Recognise symptoms and signs of asthma	S	SH	Bedside clinics, small group activity	90
PE31.7	Develop a treatment plan for asthma appropriate to clinical presentation and severity	S	SH	Bedside clinics, small group activity	91
PE31.9	Interpret CBC and CX ray in asthma	S	SH	Bedside clinics, small group activity	91
PE31.11	Observe administration of nebulisation	S	SH	DOAP session	228

Code	Competency	Domain K/S/A/C	Level K/KH/ SH/P	Teaching learning method	Page No.
PE32.2	Identify the clinical features of down's syndrome	S	SH	Bedside clinics, skills lab	72
PE32.3	Interpret normal karyotype and recognize trisomy 21	S	SH	Bedside clinics, skills lab	72
PE32.5	Counsel parents regarding 1. Present child 2. Risk in the next pregnancy	A/C	SH	Bedside clinics, skills lab	72, 206
PE32.7	Identify the clinical features of Turner's syndrome	S	SH	Bedside clinics, skills lab	73
PE32.8	Interpret normal karyotype and recognize the turner karyotype	S	SH	Bedside clinics, skills lab	71, 73
PE32.12	Identify the clinical features of Klineferlter's syndrome	S	SH	Bedside clinics, skills lab	73
PE32.13	Interpret normal karyotype and recognize the Klineferlter's karyotype	S	SH	Bedside clinics, skills lab	71, 73
PE33.2	Recognize the clinical signs of hypothyroidism and refer appropriately	S	SH	Bedside clinics, skills lab	180
PE33.3	Interpret and explain neonatal thyroid screening report	S	SH	Bedside clinics, small group discussion	180
PE33.5	Interpret blood sugar reports and explain the diagnostic criteria for type 1 diabetes	S	SH	Bedside clinics, small group activity	199
PE33.6	Perform and interpret urine dip stick for sugar	S	P	DOAP session	220
PE33.7	Perform genital examination and recognize ambiguous genitalia and refer appropriately	S	SH	Bedside clinics, skills lab	77
PE33.9	Perform Sexual Maturity Rating (SMR) and interpret	S	SH	Bedside clinics, skills lab	74
PE33.10	Recognize precocious and delayed Puberty and refer	S	SH	Bedside clinics, skills lab	77
PE33.11	Identify deviations in growth and plan appropriate referral	S	P	Bedside clinics, skills lab	44, 255

Code	Competency	Domain K/S/A/C	Level K/KH/SH/P	Teaching learning method	Page No.
PE34.5	Able to elicit, document and present history of contact with tuberculosis in every patient encounter	S	SH	Bedside clinics, skills lab	93
PE34.6	Identify a BCG scar	S	P	Bedside clinics, skills lab	21
PE34.7	Interpret a Mantoux test	S	P	Bedside clinics, skills lab	232
PE34.8	Interpret a chest radiograph	S	SH	Bedside clinics, skills lab	233
PE34.9	Interpret blood tests in the context of laboratory evidence for tuberculosis	S	SH	Bedside clinics, small group discussion	93
PE34.11	Perform AFB staining	S	P	DOAP	
PE35.1	Identify, discuss and defend medico-legal, socio-cultural and ethical issues as they pertain to health care in children (including parental rights and right to refuse treatment)	K	KH	DOAP	211

DOAP session → Demonstrate Observe Assess Perform
K/KH/SH/P → Knows/Knows how/Shows how/Performs
K/S/A/C → Knowledge/Skills/Attitude/Communication
OSPE → Objective Structured Practical Examination
OSCE → Objective Structured Clinical Examination
SDL → Self Directed Learning
SGD → Small Group Discussion

Abbreviations

–: Absent
+: Present
ABG: Arterial blood gas
AF: Anterior fontanelle
AGA: Appropriate for gestational age
AGN: Acute glomerulonephritis
ALF: Acute liver failure
ALT: Alanine transferase
AP: Antero-posterior
AR: Aortic regurgitation
ARC: AIDS-related complex
ARF: Acute renal failure
ARhF: Acute rheumatic fever
AS: Aortic stenosis
ASD: Atrial septal defect
ASO: Anti-streptolysin O titre
AST/SGOT: Aspartate transaminase/serum glutamic oxaloacetic transaminase
A-V fistula: Arteriovenous fistula
B/L: Bilateral
BA: Bronchial asthma
BAL: British anti-Lewisite or dimercaprol
BD/bid: Twice a day
Bkd: Backward
BP: Blood pressure
C/F: Clinical features
CAH: Congenital adrenal hyperplasia
Cal: Calorie
CBC: Complete blood count
CCF: Congestive cardiac failure
CFT: Capillary filling time
cm: Centimeter
CML: Chronic myelogenous leukaemia
COA: Coarctation of aorta
CT: Computed tomography
DM: Diabetes mellitus
DMARDs: Disease modifying anti-rheumatic drugs
DMD: Duchenne muscular dystrophy
DNS: Deviated nasal septum
DOA: Date of admission
DOE: Date of examination
e.g.: For example
ECG/EKG: Electrocardiography
ECHO: Echocardiography
EDTA: Ethylene-diamine-tetra-acetic acid
EEG: Electroencephalogram
ELBW: Extremely low birth weight
EMG: Electromyography
Fr: French scale
Fwd: Forward
GA: Gestational age
GBS: Guillain-Barre syndrome
GDM: Gestational diabetes mellitus
GH: Growth hormone
h/o: history of
Hb: Haemoglobin
Hg: Mercury
HR: Heart rate
Ht: Height
HTN: Hypertension
I/D: Intradermal
ICS: Intercostal space
ICT: Intracranial tension
IE: Infective endocarditis
IM: Intramuscular
IO: Intraosseous
IPD: In-patient department
ITP: Immune thrombocytopenic or thrombotic thrombocytopenic purpura
IUGR: Intrauterine growth retardation
IV line: Intravenous line

IV: Intravenous
JVP: Jugular venous pressure
KFT: Kidney function test
kg: Kilogram
L/N: Lymph nodes
LBW: Low birth weight
LCM: Left costal margin
Let: Lateral
Lf: Flocculation unit
LFT: Liver function test
LGA: Large for gestational age
LL: Lower limb
LS: Lower segment
Lt: Left
MG: Myasthenia gravis
mic/mcg: Microgram
ml: Millimeter
mm^3: Cubic millimeter
mmol/L: Millimols per liter
MODS: Multiple organ dysfunction syndrome
MR: Mitral regurgitation
MRI: Magnetic resonance imaging
MS: Mitral stenosis
NAD: No abnormality detected
NB: Newborn
NCV: Nerve conduction velocity
NEC: Necrotizing enterocolitis
NRP: Neonatal resuscitation programme
NS: Normal saline
NSAIDs: Nonsteroidal anti-inflammatory drugs
OD: Once a day
OPD: Out-patient department
ORS: Oral rehydration solution
PA view: Posterior-anterior view
$PaCO_2$: Partial pressure of carbon dioxide in arterial blood
PaO_2: Partial pressure of oxygen in arterial blood
PDA: Patent ductus arteriosus
PEM: Protein energy malnutrition
PET: Positron emission tomography
PIH: Pregnancy-induced hypertension
PO: Per oral
PPV: Positive pressure ventilation
PR: Pulse rate
PS: Pulmonary stenosis
qid: Four times a day
r/o: Rule out
RBC: Red blood cells
RCM: Right costal margin
RF factor: Rheumatoid factor
RL: Ringer's lactate
RR: Respiratory rate
Rt: Right
RVH: Right ventricular hypertrophy
S/C: Subcutaneous
SD: Standard deviation
SGPT: Serum glutamate pyruvate transaminase
SGA: Small for gestational age
SpO_2: Peripheral capillary oxygen saturation
T diameter: Transverse diameter
TA: Tricuspid atresia
TAPVC: Total anomalous pulmonary venous connection
TB: Tuberculosis
TDS/TID: Three times a day
Temp: Temperature
TGA: Transposition of great arteries
TOF: Tetralogy of Fallot
TR: Tricuspid regurgitation
TS: Tricuspid stenosis
tsp: Tablespoon
U/L: Unilateral
UL: Upper limb
US: Upper segment
USG: Ultrasonography
VLBW: Very low birth weight
VSD: Ventricular septal defect
WBC: White blood cells
Wt: Weight

NMC Guideline for Final MBBS Part—II Parctical Marks Distribution (Paediatrics)

<table>
<tr><th colspan="9">Total Marks = 100</th></tr>
<tr><td rowspan="2">Long Case</td><td rowspan="2">Short Case</td><td rowspan="2">Short Case (Neonate)</td><td rowspan="2">OSCE/ AETCOM</td><td colspan="4">VIVA</td><td rowspan="2">Total</td></tr>
<tr><td>Instru-ment</td><td>Nutrition</td><td>Drugs/ Vaccine</td><td>X-ray/ ECG</td></tr>
<tr><td>40</td><td>10</td><td>10</td><td>20</td><td>5</td><td>5</td><td>5</td><td>5</td><td>100</td></tr>
</table>

Practical/clinical internal assessment can include: Practical/ clinical tests, objective structured clinical examination (OSCE)/ objective structured practical examination (OSPE), directly observed procedural skills (DOPS), mini clinical evaluation exercise (mini-CEX), records maintenance and attitudinal assessment.

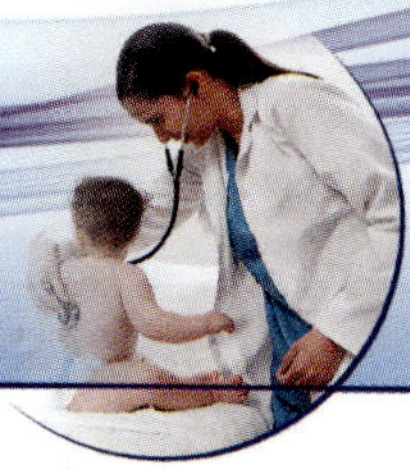

CHAPTER

1

Paediatric Case Sheet

1. **Personal data**

   Name______________________

   Age/Sex______________________ Date of Birth__________

   Address______________________

   Informant______________ Reliability______________

   DO Admission______ Date of Examination___________

2. **Chief complaints:** According to chronological order
3. **History of presenting illness:** Onset/duration/progress (OPD)/episodes/aggravating and relieving factors/variation (DSP-Diurnal/seasonal/postural)/associated symptom (SOCRATES)

   Negative history

   Growth of the child before the illness

   Bowel and bladder habits.

4. **Treatment history:** Treated outside at___OPD/IPD___basis prior to admission to this hospital. Since hospitalization at this centre child has been subjected to___blood/sputum/LP /X-ray and other investigation (report not known). Child is on ___IV fluids/oral medication___(nature not known)
5. **Past history:** No h/o measles/chickenpox/BA/TB/similar complaints/hospitalization in the past/surgical condition/ any drug allergy/h/o transfusion/h/o any chronic illness
6. **Birth history**

   Prenatal: 1st trimester

   2nd trimester

   3rd trimester

Natal: Gestational age/mode of delivery/cried immediately or not/when breast feeding started, birth weight_____ gram
Neonatal: Hospital stay/h/o jaundice/respiratory difficulties/feeding practices/any special care__________

7. **Development history:** GM/FM/PS/language/vision/hearing
8. **Dietic history:** Vegetarian/mixed/any food allergies

	Calorie	Protein
Appropriate content		
Expected		
Deficit in		

9. **Immunisation history:** BCG scar +/–,
   Last vaccine taken__________
   Next vaccine due___________
   Optional vaccine taken________
10. **Family history:**
    Pedigree chart up to 3 generations
    Consanguineous/nonconsanguineous
    H/o contact/DM/heart disease
    H/o similar illness/major illness/allergy/transfusion
11. **Socioeconomic history:** Modified Kuppuswamy's scale
12. **Summary:** Respected sir/madam I am presenting a suspected case of____name________years old male/female, resident of________address_____________. The informant is________ mother/father________and history seems to be reliable. Child was brought to________casualty/OPD________days back with chief complaints of__________, past history/birth history/family history________ significant/not significant with normal development and growth, immunized for age (optional vaccine________) is suspected to have.

    ____
13. **General examination**
    a. **General comment/observation**
       Posture/attitude of limb
       Alert/conscious/cooperative/sick looking/drowsy
       Well built/obese/thin/emaciated
       Dyspnoeic/cyanosed
       IV line/oxygen mask

b. **Vitals**

Temp: Afebrile/febrile________°F (axillary)

PR: Rate/rhythm/volume/character/radio-femoral delay/peripheral pulses B/L

RR: Rate/rhythm/type____abdominal/abdomino-thoracic/thoraco-abdominal, retraction/head bobbing/nasal flaring

BP: ____ mm Hg right arm supine position

CFT: <3 seconds

Jugular venous pressure **(JVP)** ____ cm above the sternal angle

SpO_2: ____%

c. **Anthropometry**

Birth weight:

	Observed	Expected	SD
Weight			
Height			
Weight for height			
HC			
MUAC			

Chest circumference/arm span/US: LS ratio (if indicated) interpretation____________________________

d. Pallor/icterus/cyanosis/clubbing/lymphadenopathy/oedema (PICCLE)

e. **Head-to-toe examination**

Breath/body odour

Skull: Shape/symmetrical/asymmetrical

Crack pot sign (also k/a Macewen's sign, e.g. hydrocephalus)/transillumination/bruit (heard on the side opposite the occulsion of internal carotid artery)

Hairs: Normal/hypopigmented/sparse

Anterior fontanelle: Closed (normally closed by 9–18 months)/open (0.6 cm – 3.6 cm, <0.6 cm small >3.6 cm large)

Pulsatile/non-pulsatile

Normal/depressed/bulging

Posterior Fontanelle closes by 2 months

Facies: Normal/dysmorphism

Sinus tenderness: B/L maxillary/frontal/ethmoid

Eyes: NAD/ptosis/hypertelorism/hypotelorism/cataract/nystagmus/strabismus

Evidence of vitamins deficiency.

Ears: NAD/low set ears/preauricular tag/discharge

Mouth and throat: Cleft lip/palate/philtrum

Oral hygiene/dentition/caries

Gum/tongue/throat/tonsils/post-pharynx

Nose: Flat nasal bridge/DNS/turbinate

Neck: Short neck/thyroid/vessels/hair line/webbing

Chest: Pectus excavatum (rickets/Marfan's syndrome)

Pectus carinatum (rickets)

Costochondral beading/wide-spaced nipple

Skin: Rash/haemangioma/petechiae/purpura/mongoloid spots

Limbs: Cubitus-valgus/varus, genu-valgum/varus clinodactyly/polydactyly/syndactyly

Spine: Kyphosis (forward-bending)/lordosis (backward bending)/scoliosis (lateral bending)

SMR stage

Evidence of vitamins deficiency/PEM

Look for general signs specific to systemic case

CNS: Look for neurocutaneous markers (cafe-au-lait spots, adenoma sebaceum, Ash leaf macule) [Neurofibromatosis (hyperpigmentation), tuberous sclerosis (hypopigmentation)]

Primitive/neonatal reflexes____________

CVS: Signs of IE/CCF/acute rheumatic fever

GI: Signs of dehydration/liver failure

RS:________________________

f. **Development-assessment:** GM/FM/PS/language/vision/hearing
Normal/global developmental delay/retarded in specific field
Currently functioning at_______,
Development quotient (DQ)_____

14. **Systemic examination**
CVS/RS/GIT/CNS/MSK
15. Summary: Child suspected to have____________________ with_______development and growth, immunized for age.
16. Provisional diagnosis
17. Differential diagnosis
18. Investigation planned
19. Treatment
20. Prevention

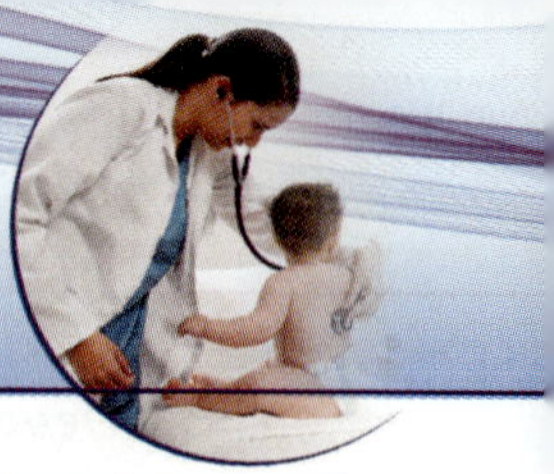

CHAPTER

2

Development History

Growth is quantitative and development is qualitative change in the body.

RULES/LAWS OF DEVELOPMENT

1. Continuous process
2. Cephalocaudal (head control developed first)
3. Proximal to distal (arm control first, fingers later)
4. Parallelism—sequence is same in all race/ethnic groups
5. Dissociation—rate may be different
6. Mass activity has to change into specific response
7. Primitive reflexes has to disappear
8. CNS maturation and environment factors both affect the development

$$\text{Developmental quotient (DQ)} = \frac{\text{Developmental age (DA)} \times 100}{\text{Chronological age (CA)}}$$

GROSS MOTOR

3 months	Neck holding/head control
5–6 months	Roll over
6 months	Sit with support
8 months	Sit without support
9 months	Stand with support/crawls/cruising around furniture
12 months	Stand without support

Contd.

15 months	Walks
18 months	Runs
2 years	Walks upstairs with 2 feet each step/walk backwards
3 years	Walks upstairs with 1 feet each step but coming down 2 feet each step/rides tricycle/*jumps*
4 years	Walks upstairs/downstairs with 1 feet each step/*hop*
5 years	*Skips*

FINE MOTORS

4 months	Bidextrous grasp		Hand regard
6 months	Unidextrous grasp	Transfer of objects	Mouthing
9 months	Immature pincer grasp		
12 months	Mature pincer grasp		
15 months	Imitates scribbling	Towers of 2	
18 months	Scribbling	Towers of 4	Feed with spoon without spillage
2 years	Vertical and circular strokes	Towers of 6	Undress completely
3 years	Draw circle	Towers of 9	Buttoning/unbuttoning
4 years	Draw square	Build bridge	Handedness
5 years	Draw triangle	Steps	Ties the shoelace

PERSONAL SOCIAL

Newborn	Spontaneous smile	
2 months	Social smile	
3 months	Recognises mother	
6 months	Stranger anxiety	
9 months	Waves bye/bye	Casting/object permanence (constancy)
12 months	Obeys simple command	

Contd.

15 months	Pointing	Kiss pictures
18 months	Mimicking	
2 years	Toilet training	Indicates 6 body parts
3 years	Knows name/age/gender	Knows 2 colours/dry by day
4 years	Plays with several children	Role playing /knows 4 colours
5 years	Understands opposites (e.g. fat and thin)	Dry by night

LANGUAGE–RECEPTIVE/EXPRESSIVE

3 months	Cooing
4 months	Squeals/laugh loud
6 months	Monosyllables
9 months	Bisyllables
12 months	1–2 words with meaning
18 months	10–20 words with meaning
2 years	100 words/can join two words/I/Me/you
3 years	Sing rhymes/speak in small sentences
4 years	Tell stories
5 years	Ask meaning of words/questions

Note: If child has ability to follow command (receptive language) and other component of milestones are normal, child may start speaking later. **Speech delay need not be a language delay**.

Tongue tie or exposure to multiple languages will not cause language delay.

HEARING

Newborn	Startle reaction, facial grimace, change in HR
4 months	Turns head towards the source of sound
6 months	Can imitate sounds
8 months	Can respond to name
10 months	Turn the head diagonally, directly towards the source of sound
1 year	Localise the sound source like adults

VISION

Newborn	Monocular fixation in response to visual stimulus
1 month	Can follow an object up to 60°
2 months	Follow the objects/mother
3 months	Can follow an object up to 180°
4 months	Binocular vision well established.
6 months	True coordination of the eyes and hands.
3 years	Can identify basic colours. Vision screening using an illiterate "E" chart
>7 years	Titmus fly test for stereo-acuity

Note: Allowance for preterm babies may be allowed up to 2 years of age

Say________years old child with global development delay/ dissociative delay (delay in_______field) his DQ is_______ functional age comes to________years

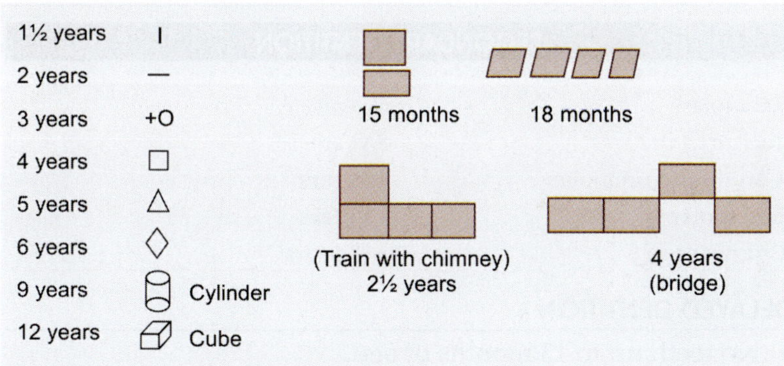

MNEMONIC—LOCSTD: 1½ years Line, 2 years Oval, 3 years Circle, 4 years Square, 5 years Triangle, 6 years Diamond

REMEMBER

At 6 months—**T**urning over, **T**ransfer of object
At 10 months—**C**rawling/**C**reeping/**C**ruising /**C**asting and **P**ivoting/**P**incer grasp/**P**ermanence (constancy)

9-months-old child standing, holding finger of his/her Mom with two fingers saying MAMA bye bye (**9 months GM**—standing with support, **FM**—immature pincer grasp, **Lang**—bisyllables, **PS**—waving bye bye)

3-year-old child came down from the stairs, jumped, start riding a tricycle, making a circle, singing rhymes, removed his shirt and said Hi to a girl
GM: Coming down 2 feet each step/rides tricycle/jumps.
FM: Draw circle/buttoning/unbuttoning
Lang: Sing rhymes/speak in small sentences
PS: Knows name/age/gender

Red Flag Signs

If vision and hearing is normal

Milestones	Not achieved by
Social smile	2 months
Head control	4 months
Sit without support	8 months
Stand without support	12 months

PRIMARY DENTITION HAS 20 TEETH

SECONDARY DENTITION	
1st molar	6 years
Incisors	8 years
Canine and premolar	10 years
2nd molar	12 years
3rd molar	>18 years

DELAYED DENTITION

- No teeth up to 13 months of age.
- Seen in constitutional delay/hypothyroidism/hypopituitarism/rickets/PEM
- Teeth are absent in ectodermal dysplasia

PERIOD OF GROWTH

Terminology	Period
Ovum	<14 days
Embryo	2–9 weeks
Foetus	9 weeks of gestation to birth

Contd.

Terminology	Period
Perinatal period	22 weeks of gestation to 7 days after birth
Newborn	First 28 days of life
Infancy	First year
Toddler	1–3 years
Preschool	3–6 years
School age	6–12 years
Adolescent	10–19 years (female) 12–20 years (male)

Test for Screening of Development

1. Denver Development Screening Test (DDST II)
2. Bayley's Scale of Infant Development (BSID)
3. Development Observation Chart (DOC)
4. Trivandrum Development Screening Chart (TDSC)

Test for Assessment of Intelligence

1. Draw a MAN test

INTEELLECTUAL DISABILITY

Intelligence quotient—**measure of child ability to perform cognitive tasks.**

IQ = (Mental age/chronological age) × 100

Grading	IQ
Intelligent	>110
Normal	90–109
Borderline	70–89
Mild intellectual disability	51–69
Moderate	36–50
Severe	20–35
Profound	<20

PICA: Repeated and chronic ingestion of non-nutritive substances for >1 month.

Trichotillomania: Hair pulling

Bruxism: Teeth grinding

ADHD (attention deficit hyperactive disorder): Inattention, hyperactivity, impulsivity

ASDs (Autism): Impaired socialization, impaired communication, stereotypic behaviour

Enuresis: Urinary incontinence >4 years of age in day time and >6 years of age in night time. Treatment is rarely initiated if a child is less than 7 years old.

Encopresis: Faecal incontinence above 4 years of age in the absence of organic pathology.

Specific Learning Disorders (SLD)

- Significant unexpected, specific, persistent difficulties in the acquisition and use of efficient________
  - Reading (dyslexia)
  - Writing (dysgraphia)
  - Mathematical (dyscalculia).

Breath Holding Spells

- Paroxysmal self limiting events
- Follow sequence = provocation → crying → holding breath (noiselessness) → change in colour (blue) → loss of consciousness (with or without change in body tone
- Occurs in 10% healthy children
- 6 months to 6 years
- Parent education, iron therapy helps.

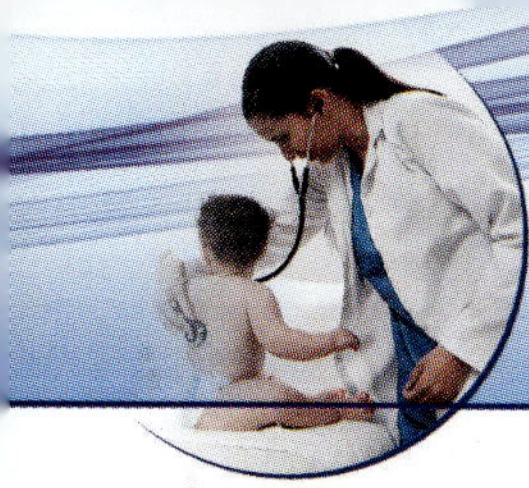

CHAPTER

3

Dietic History

EXPECTED CALORIE REQUIREMENT

Simple bedside calculation is:

Up to 1 year	100 cal/kg
>1 year	1000 + 100 cal for each year

Example for 8 years old child it is 1000 + 700 = 1700 cal

OR

Holliday and Segar formula

1st 10 kg	100 cal/kg/day
11–20 kg	1000 + (50 cal/kg/day)
>20 kg	1500 + (20 cal/kg/day)

Example: An 8-year-old child expected weight would be 24 kg

So

1st 10 kg	100 × 10 = 1000
11–20 kg	50 × 10 = 500
21–24 kg	20 × 4 = 80
Total	1580 cal

Protein requirements

<1 year	2 g/kg
1–9 years	1.5 g/kg
> 9 years	1.2 g/kg

Food item	Quantity	Calorie	Protein (g)
Cow's milk	100 ml	67	3
Cooked rice	1 cup (150 cc)	175	4
Cooked dal	1 big spoon (50 ml)	10	1
Uncooked dal	100 g	320	22
Chapatti	1	70	2
Paratha	1 (50 g)	150	4
Puri	1 (25 g)	80	2
Potato	100 g	100	1.6
Idli	1	50	1
Dosa	1	70	2
Sugar	1 small tsp	20	—
Ghee/butter	1 small tsp	36	—
Bread slice	1 (20 g)	50	1.7
Banana	1	100	1
Mango	1	50–100	—
Apple	1	50–100	—
Orange	1	50	0.5
Dry dates	100 g	300	2.5
Biscuit	1	15	0.25
Cream biscuit	1	25	0.25
Leafy vegetables	One serving	65	2–4
Coffee	1 cup	80	1.8
Tea	1 cup	60	1
Cold drinks	200 ml	150	—
Mashed potato	One serving	40	—
Curd	100 g	60	3.1
Cerelac/ragi/Nestum	6 tsp	100	2
Formula milk	30 ml	20	0.5
Ground nuts	100 g	560	25

Contd.

Food item	Quantity	Calorie	Protein (g)
Almonds	100 g	655	20
Cashew nuts	100 g	600	20
Boiled egg	1	86	6
Omelette	1	155	6
Fish	100 g	100	20
Chicken	100 g	110	25
Mutton	100 g	200	20
Pork	100 g	110	20
Beef	100 g	400	8
Veg momo	1 piece	40	0.5
Chicken momo	1 piece	60	3

POINTS TO REMEMBER

1. Uncooked cereals/100 g—rice and ragi (cal—350, protein—7 g), wheat/maize (cal—350, protein—11 g).
2. Uncooked pulses/100 g—350 cal, protein—20 g except soybeans (450 cal, protein—43 g).
3. All green leafy vegetables have negligible cal and proteins but are rich sources of iron, calcium and fibre.
4. All fruits have negligible protein and around 50 cal except banana and jack-fruit.
   Fruits with yellow/red colour (apricot, watermelon, grapes papaya, mango, orange) are rich in beta carotene, which can be converted to vitamin A.
5. **All meats (fish/chicken/mutton/beef)/100 g have 20–25 g protein**
6. When pulses are cooked it becomes 2 times of dry weight, rice 3 times and wheat 4 times .
7. **Essential fatty acids** are: Linoleic acid/linolenic acid/arachidonic acid
8. **Essential amino acid: MAT HILL PVT**
   (Methionine/Arginine/Threonine/Histidine/Isoleucine Leucine/Lysine/Phenylalanine/Valine/Tryptophan)
   Note: Semi-essential AA—Arginine and Histidine

9. Teaspoon 5 ml , tablespoon 15 ml, *Katori*/Cup 150 ml, glass 250 ml
10. The energy is derived from 3 sources

Substance	Energy	Balanced diet
Fat	9 kcal/gram	30% calories
Protein	4 kcal/gram	15%
Carbohydrate	4 kcal/gram	55%

11. If child is on breastfeeding say—child is consuming________ cal and________gram protein from complementary feeding with breastfeeding for________times a day.

12. Egg contains all the essential AA: a complete protein

WEANING/COMPLEMENTARY FEEDING

Weaning is the gradual systemic introduction of the food (in addition to breastfeeding) to meet the nutritional requirement of the infant .

Ideal age: 4–6 months of age.

6 months: Semi-solid

>9 months: Solid

>1 year: Should contain all 4 groups of food—milk, cereal/pulses, vegetables/fruits and meat/egg/fish. Egg white can be given , milk intake reduce to less than 500 ml/day, continue breastfeeding till 2 years of age.

Note: At starting of weaning, baby often tends to spit the food out, it is not because baby did not like that food. It is just drinking is different from eating and child had to learn that tongue movement.

FEEDING TODDLER

1. Self feeding is the mantra. Any child not self-feeding beyond 2 years of age means weaning training was a failure.
2. No force feeding. No extra attention.
3. Let him sit on the dinner table or a mat preferably with other family members.

4. No watching TV or playing on mobile while feeding.
5. Let him/her take his/her time to feed.
6. No snacks at meal time.
7. No comments on his/her appetite in front of others. No comparison with other kids.
8. Variety of meals to be served each day.
9. If he/she does not want to drink milk, could be given milk products instead.
10. Monitor weight/height every month.

FOOD MIX TO PREPARE AT HOME

Take
100 g Bengal gram (*Chana-sattu*)
100 g Wheat or jowar (Sorghum)
100 g Groundnut/Peanut
100 g Red gram/Pigeon pea (Arhar dal/yellow lentil)
Roast, grind and store in airtight containers.

For feeding >6 months

- Take 2–3 tablespoons of food mix
- Mix with boiled hot water or milk
- cook for 2–3 minutes
- Add sugar, cooked and mashed vegetables, mashed fruits and oil/ghee to the porridge and feed
- Feed 3–6 times a day

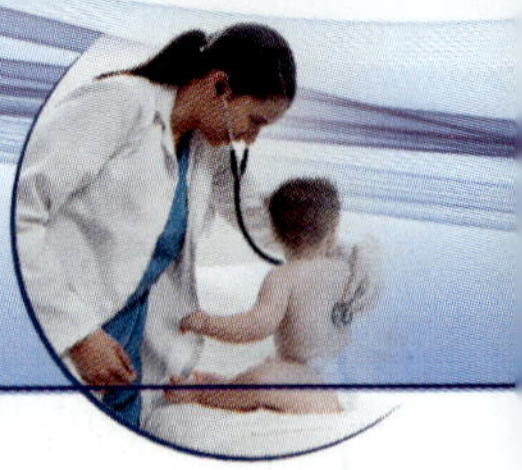

CHAPTER

4

Immunization

A vaccine uses the body's natural defenses to build resistance to specific infections by training the immune system to create antibodies, just as it does when it is exposed to a disease.

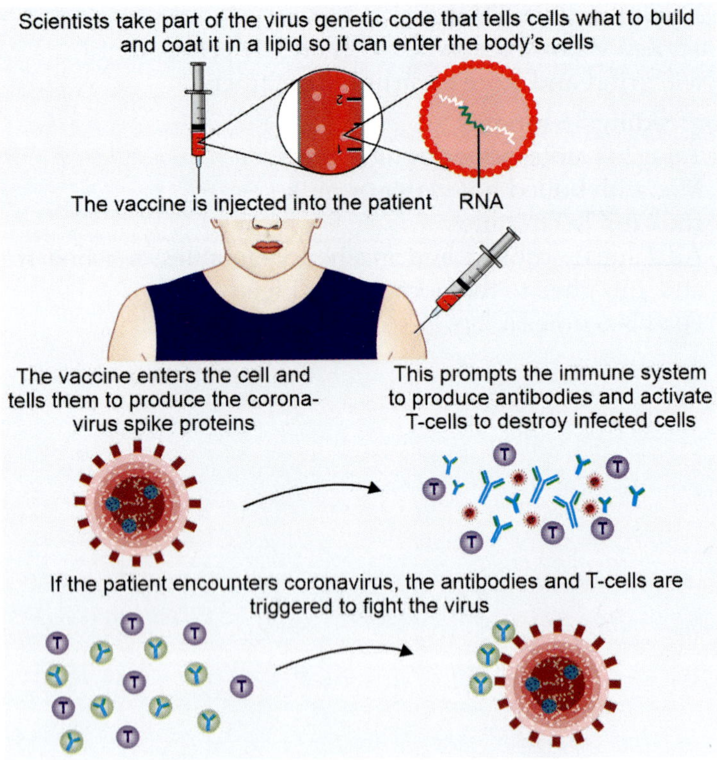

Immunization to fight from corona viruses

However, because vaccines contain only killed or weakened forms of germs they do not cause the disease or put one at risk of its complications. The immune system remembers the disease and if a vaccinated person is exposed to the germ in the future, it can quickly destroy it before the person become unwell.

CLASSIFICATION OF VACCINES

Type of vaccine	Vaccine	Route
Toxin based	Diphtheria and tetanus toxoid	IM
Live attenuated bacterial	• BCG	I/D
Live attenuated viral	• OPV, rotavirus	Oral
	• Measles, MMR, varicella, yellow fever, JE (SA-14-14-2) Hep A (biovac)	S/C
Killed bacterial	• Cholera • Pertusis (whole cell), plague	Oral IM
Killed viral	• Hep A, rabies, IPV, JE (JEEV and JENVAC) • Covaxin, Sputnik V	IM
Subunit (Recombinant)	• Hep B, pertusis (acellular), influenza, HPV, anthrax • **Covishield,** Corbevax	IM
Polysaccharides (unconjugated) for >2 years only	Pneumococcal 23, Meningococcal, typhoid	IM
Conjugated	Pneumococcal 13, Hib, typhoid (TCV), PNEUMOSIL-10	IM
mRNA based	Pfizer—BNT162b2, **Moderna**—mRNA-1273 Gemcovac (Indian)	IM
DNA based	ZyCoV-D Corona vaccine	I/D

POINTS TO REMEMBER

- All vaccines doses are 0.5 ml except
  1. BCG/fIPV/ZyCoV-D 0.1 ml (I/D)
  2. Hep A and Hep B after 19 years 1 ml, rabies 1 ml (IM)
  3. OPV two drops, rotavirus 1 or 2 ml (oral).

- There is no harm done if S/C vaccines are given IM. However, vaccines designated to be given IM should not be given S/C due to risk of side effects (as seen with aluminium adjuvant vaccines) or reduced efficacy (due to reduced blood supply in S/C tissue and hence reduced immunogenicity).
- The gluteal region should never be used for administration of IM injections due to risk of sciatic nerve injury and reduced efficacy (**rabies and hepatitis B vaccines**).
- **BCG** elicits cellular immune response.
- **All live vaccines to be reconstituted with sterile water except BCG which is reconstituted with normal saline.**
- The preferred site for injection is anterolateral thigh in newborns and infants and deltoid in older children.
- If multiple vaccines are administered at a single visit, administration of each preparation at a different anatomic site is desirable.
- Most commonly used adjuvant is **aluminium salt.**
- Keep all vaccines at **+2°C to + 8°C.**
- Do not freeze DTP/DT/TT/Tdap/Td/HepB/Hib/Hep A and diluents (easy **to remember is all T and Hep vaccines**) only live vaccine, e.g. OPV can be kept in freezer compartment.
- Two live vaccines can be given together or after 4 weeks gap.

Note: **After corona vaccination it is advisable to wait for 2 weeks for other vaccine.**

- Two or more killed antigens may be administered simultaneously or any interval between the doses (except **cholera and yellow fever**)
- Mixing of vaccines in the same syringe is not recommended.
- URTI/diarrhoea/mild fever/allergy to penicillin/ malnutrition/current therapy with antibiotic, i.e. in short minor illnesses are not a contraindication for vaccination.
- Live vaccines should be avoided in any immunodifficiency state (like on high dose of steroid/symptomatic HIV).
- If part of an oral vaccine (rotavirus) was spit out or person sneezes after intranasal vaccine—count as valid.

- Pressed injection site should be firmly for few seconds with dry cotton—do not rub.
- Cold chain contains—WIFs, WICs, DFs, ILR, cold boxes, vaccine carriers, refrigerator.
- **Hep B, tetanus and rabies vaccine** can be administered concurrently with their corresponding immunoglobulin (i.e. both active and passive immunization).
- If the mother is HBsAg positive/status unknown give HBIG and HepB vaccine within 12 hours together using different sites.
- Adolescent should receive **Tdap /Td, MMR, HepB, typhoid, HPV, Hep A, varicella and corona** vaccine if not previously immunized.

Note: Immunization of premature babies should be started at the same chronological age as for term babies.

  - A delay in the schedule dose does not mean restarting of the schedule , even for long gap—as memory B cell continues to persist. So start from where you have left.
  - After bone marrow transplant and after completion of successful chemotherapy, revaccination has to be started.

SALIENT POINTS ABOUT INDIVIDUAL VACCINE

BACILLUS-CALMETTE GUERIN (BCG) VACCINE

- Live attenuated Danish 1331 strain produced in Tamil Nadu.
- World TB day—March 24.
- At birth, **I/D** (intradermal), left shoulder at level of deltoid insertion

Diluents—**Normal saline** with **26 G** tuberculin syringe. 0.1 ml (0.05 ml in <4 weeks infant)

- Catch up may be given up to 5 years.
- Reconstituted vaccine should be used **within 4 hours**.
- Efficacy against miliary TB and tubercular meningitis around 80% but against pulmonary TB its around 50%.
- Should develop **4–8 mm scar in 8–12 weeks.** No treatment is required for this condition. If no scar after 3 months, no need to vaccinate with BCG a second time.

Rarely, a swelling may occur in the left armpit which is an enlargement of the axillary lymph nodes due to BCG vaccination. Usually, it lasts for a few months and disappears without any treatment.

- Child becomes **Mantoux positive** after 4 weeks.
- C/I–Symptomatic ARC, generalized eczema, hypogammaglobulinaemia.

BCG vaccination is not recommended during pregnancy

If HIV-infected individuals, including children, are receiving ART, are clinically well and immunologically stable (CD4% >25% for children aged 5 years), they should be vaccinated with BCG.

- Neonates born to women of unknown HIV status should be vaccinated as the benefits of BCG vaccination outweigh the risks.
- Neonates of unknown HIV status born to HIV infected women should be vaccinated if they have no clinical evidence suggestive of HIV infection, regardless of whether the mother is receiving ART.
- Neonates with HIV infection confirmed by early virological testing, BCG vaccination should be delayed until ART has been started and the infant confirmed to be immunologically stable (CD4 >25%).

POLIO VACCINE

- Live attenuated containing type bOPV **1 and 3 Polio virus.**
- At birth (zero dose), 6, 10, 14 weeks, 1st booster at 18–24 ms and 2nd booster at 5 years.
- Oral—***do boond zindagi ke.***
- Do not give hot liquid for half an hour. Can breastfeed.
- VVM (vaccine vial monitor)–discard the vaccine if inner white square changes colour like outer blue circle.
- Shed in stool for up to 6 weeks following vaccination—**Herd immunity.**
- IPV (contain 40, 8 and 32 D antigen units of type 1 and 3, respectively) and bOPV can be given together.

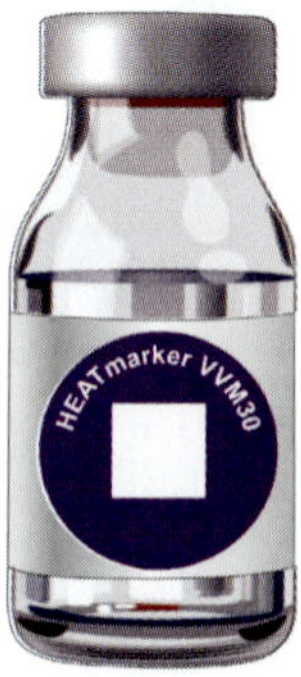

- Ideally IPV should replace OPV as early as possible.
  - *Note:* 3 doses of intradermal fractional doses of IPV (fIPV) (0.1 ml) recommended in mass immunization.
- Four doses of intramuscular/IPV in primary series is the best option (6 weeks, 14 weeks and booster at 16–18 months and 4–5 years)
- In case IPV is not available or feasible, the child should be offered three doses of bOPV. In such cases, the child should be referred for three fractional doses of IPV at a government facility at 6 and 14 weeks and a booster dose at 9 ms or at least one dose of intramuscular IPV, either standalone or as a combination vaccine, at 14 weeks of age.
- Use of OPV during national and subnational pulse polio days for all children.
- Globally only two countries are still endemic for polio are Pakistan and Afghanistan.
- In 2014, India was officially declared "Polio Free" by the WHO

DPT VACCINE

- Combination of diphtheria toxoid, tetanus toxoid and pertussis (whole cell or acellular) adsorbed on aluminium salt.
- 0.5 ml, deep IM, anterolateral aspect of thigh.
- 6, 10, 14 weeks and 1st booster at 18–24 months, 2nd booster at 5 years
- DTwP/DTaP (25 Lf units of diphtheria toxoid and tetanus toxoid) till 7 years.
- >7 years Td or Tdap (2.5 Lf units of diphtheria toxoid, 5 Lf of tetanus toxoid).
- Td to be repeated every 10 years after that
- Progressive neurological disease or h/o seizure with previous dose, persistent screaming episode (>3 hours)—whole cell pertussis (wP) is contraindicated. Give acellular pertussis vaccine (aP).
- **Mild fever/febrile seizure/cerebral palsy are not contra-indications.**
- Keep all vaccines at +2°C to + 8°C, do not freeze.
- TT contains 5 Lf of toxoid.

- Td vaccine is also used for tetanus prophylaxis after skin breaching injuries/trauma.
- TT has been replaced with Td in pregnant women.
- Give paracetamol 15 mg/kg if fever occurs after DPT immunization.

INACTIVATED INFLUENZA VACCINES

- Inactivated influenza vaccines (either trivalent or quadrivalent) (15 μg/0.5 ml) for all children older than 6 months.
- 0.5 ml, IM, 2 doses 4 weeks apart (>8 years single dose) and booster yearly.
- Usually in the pre-monsoon period (April)
- Annual influenza vaccination should be continued, for all, till 5 years of age; after the age of 5 years, this vaccine is recommended in the high-risk group only.

MEASLES VACCINE

- Live attenuated Edmonston-Zagreb measles strain.
- 0.5 ml, S/C at 9 months of age.
- Reconstituted vaccine should be used within 4 hours, **Diluents-sterile water.**
- Give vaccine within 72 hours of exposure for post-exposure prophylaxis.
- Measles vaccine has been replaced with MR (Measles + Rubella)

MMR (MEASLES/MUMPS/RUBELLA) VACCINE

- Live attenuated viral-freeze dried powder. **Diluent-sterile water.**
- 0.5 ml, S/C at 9 months of age. 2nd dose 15 months of age, 3rd dose at 5 years of age
- Reconstituted vaccine should be used within 4 hours.
- **MR vaccine as part of the national campaign is to be administered irrespective of previous vaccination.**

HEPATITIS-B VACCINE

- Inactivated subunit viral vaccine (rDNA techniques).
- At birth, 6, 10 and 14 weeks or 0, 1, 6 months.

- 0.5 ml but >19 years 1 ml IM.
- In case of use of a combination vaccines a total of four doses of hepatitis B vaccine are justified
- If the mother is HBsAg positive /status unknown give HBIG and HepB vaccine within 12 hours together using different sites

HEMOPHILUS INFLUENZAE TYPE B (HIB CONJUGATED VACCINES)

Haemophilus influenzae type b (Hib) is an important invasive bacteria causing diseases such as meningitis, bacteraemia, pneumonia, otitis media, osteomyelitis, septic arthritis and epiglottitis.

- Conjugated vaccines—Hib capsular polysaccharide
- 0.5 ml deep IM lateral aspect of thigh. 6, 10, 14 weeks and booster at 15–18 months.

- **>6 months** of age 2 doses at 4 weeks apart booster at 15–18 months.
- **>12 months** of age 2 doses at 4 weeks apart.
- **>15 months** one dose is enough.

PNEUMOCOCCAL VACCINE

Protects from pneumococcal meningitis, pneumonia.

There are 5 types of vaccines available:

1. Prevenar — PCV 13
2. Synflorix — PCV 10
3. Pneumosil — PCV 10
4. Pneumococcal polysaccharide vaccine (PPSV23)
5. Pneubevax 14

PCV 10 and PCV 13 not interchangeable for subsequent vaccination.

The PCVs (pneumococcal conjugate vaccines) are preferred for the initial immunization at all ages.

- 0.5 ml S/C or IM. 3 doses (6, 10, 14 weeks) and booster at 12–15 months.

- **>6 months** of age, 2 doses at 4 weeks apart, booster at 12–15 months.
- **>12 months** of age, 2 doses at 4 weeks apart.
- **>23 months** one dose is enough.

- **Unconjugated pneumococcal polysaccharide vaccine** is a 23 valent vaccine (PPSV 23) for >2 years only, 0.5 ml S/C or IM one dose is enough, 2nd dose recommended in high risk group only.

TYPHOID VACCINE

- Single dose of any of typhoid conjugate vaccine (TCV 25 μg) is recommended from 6 months onwards and can be administered with MMR also.
  - Booster dose of typhoid conjugate vaccine not recommended in subsequent years.
- Vi PS-capsular polysaccharide unconjugated vaccine 0.5 ml IM, >2 years of age, repeat every 3 years.

JAPANESE B ENCEPHALITIS VACCINE

Japanese encephalitis (JE) is a viral infection which is spread by bites of an infected Culex mosquito.

Three Vaccines are available in India

1. **SA 14-14-2 vaccine**
   - Cell culture derived live vaccine based on stable neuro-attenuated strain of JE virus: SA-14-14-2.
   - Efficacy of 99% with a single dose, 0.5 ml, S/C
   - This vaccine is available only in the national immunization schedule of the Government of India. It is administered as a 2-dose schedule at 9 months and 16–24 months
2. **JEEV:** Killed virus
3. **JENVAC:** Killed virus

   0.5 ml, IM, 2 doses 4 weeks apart, >1 year of age

   Note: At present, there is no recommendation for booster doses.

ROTAVIRUS VACCINE

Almost one-third to half of all diarrhoeal hospitalizations in India, is caused by the rotavirus.

Currently 4 Live Oral Vaccines are available

1. Single, attenuated human rotavirus strain **(Rotarix) 1 ml (Freezed dried)**

2. Pentavalent human bovine reassortant rotaviruses **(Rotateq) 2 ml (Liquid)**
3. Single, attenuated human rotavirus strain (Indian strain) **(Rotavac) 0.5 ml (Liquid)**
4. Human bovine pentavalent reassortant rotaviruses **(Rotasil) 2 ml (Liquid)**

Rotarix 2 doses, 4 weeks apart. Rest 3 doses, 4 weeks apart or 2, 4, 6 months of age.

- First dose should be given before 12 months of age.
- Past h/o **intussusceptions** is a absolute contraindication.
- Interchange between vaccine brands should be avoided.

VARICELLA/CHICKENPOX VACCINE

- Live attenuated vaccine from the **Oka strain.**
- >1 years of age, 0. 5 ml S/C, 2 doses at 3–6 months apart.
- Give at or after 15 months preferably (with MMR)
- It should be protected from light and needs to be used within 30 minutes of its reconstitution.
  Diluent—sterile water.
- For those >12 years, 2 doses are administered at an interval not less than 4 weeks

Vaccination should be postponed in those who:

Have recently had a blood transfusion, received certain other vaccines in the past 4 weeks, taking salicylates (such as aspirin).

HEPATITIS-A VACCINE

Two Types of Vaccines are available

1. Inactivated (killed) viral (Havrix) with aluminium hydroxide adjuvant.
   - >1 year of age, 0.5 ml IM at deltoid, 2 doses at 6–12 months apart.
2. Live attenuated vaccine (BIOVAC-A), single dose >1 year, IM

Note: No need to give if there is a past h/o Hep A infection.

CHOLERA VACCINE (SHANCHOL)

- Made from killed cholera germs.
- Orally, >1 year of age, 2 doses, 2 weeks apart

- It is given to residents of highly endemic areas and in areas where there is risk of an outbreak such as during pilgrimages like *Kumbh mela*, etc.
- Where there is a continued risk of *V. cholera* infection, revaccination is recommended after 3 years.

MENINGOCOCCAL VACCINES

- For high risk group only
- Menactra 0.5 ml, IM, >9 ms, 2 doses 3 ms apart.

HUMAN PAPILLOMAVIRUS (HPV) VACCINES

Four Vaccines are available

1. Quadri-valent (6, 11, 16, 18) **(GARDASIL)**
2. Bivalent vaccine (16, 18) **(CERVARIX) [withdrawn from India]**
3. Nonavalent (6, 11, 16, 18, 31, 33, 45, 52, 58) **(GARDASIL-9)**
4. **Cervavac,** India's first locally made quadrivalent (6, 11, 16, 18) HPV vaccine is developed by Serum Institute of India (SII) and Department of Biotechnology (DBT)

- All are manufactured by recombinant DNA technology that produces non-infectious virus like particles (VLP).
- Recommended target population for the prevention of cervical cancer in females aged 9–14 years, prior to becoming sexually active.
- A 2-dose schedule with a 6-month interval between doses is recommended for individuals receiving the first dose before 15 years of age.
- A 3-dose schedule should be used for all vaccinations initiated ≥15 years of age, including in those younger than 15 years known to be immunocompromised and/or HIV infected (regardless of whether they are receiving antiretroviral therapy)
- Data on the safety of HPV vaccination in pregnancy are limited, and HPV vaccination of pregnant women should be avoided.
- **0.5 ml, IM at deltoid.**
- IAP recommend, 9vHPV for boys 9–14 year, 2 doses.

RABIES VACCINES

Rabies can be transmitted to humans by mammalian bites. Over 90% are caused by dog bites, followed by cat bites and bites by camel, sheep, pigs, goat, donkey, monkeys, horses, cows and other large mammals.

- Domestic rodent (rat) bites and bites by small mammals, (e.g. rabbits, squirrels) usually do not cause rabies and do not warrant rabies vaccination.
- Any bites by known or unknown animals in the wild can cause rabies.
- In India, exposure to bats have not been reported to cause rabies.
- If pet dog is vaccinated yearly against rabies and the efficacy of the vaccine is confirmed by laboratory evidence, PEP is not required.

MANAGEMENT OF RABID ANIMAL BITE

1. Clean the wound under running tap water, with soap, for at least 15 minutes.
2. After wound washing, apply ointment that can kill viruses, e.g. povidone iodine.
3. The wound should not be covered with any bandage, unless profusely bleeding.

Category	PEP measure
1. Touching or feeding animals, animal licks on intact skin (*no exposure*)	Washing of exposed skin surfaces, *no PEP*
2. Nibbling of uncovered skin, minor scratches or abrasions without bleeding (*exposure*)	Wound washing and *immediate vaccination*
3. Single or multiple transdermal bites or scratches, contamination of mucous membrane or broken skin with saliva from animal licks (*severe exposure*)	Wound washing, anti rabies *vaccine* and the *rabies immunoglobulin/ monoclonal antibody* preparations, more than half the dose must be infiltrated locally into the wound, rest should be given IM on the opposite limb.

- Inactivated tissue culture vaccine
  - Purified chick embryo cell (PCEC) vaccine—Rabipur
  - Human diploid cell vaccine (HDCV)—Rabivax
  - Purified vero cell vaccine (PVRV)—Verorab.

- Post-exposure 1 ml, IM, 5 doses 0, 3, 7, 14 and 28 days
- IAP recommend 4 dose schedule 0–3–7–14 to 28 days.
- Prophylaxis 1ml, IM, 3 doses 0, 7, 28 days, Booster at 1 year and then every 5 years
- Sterile water as diluents, should be used within 6 hours of reconstitution.

Note: Re-exposure <3 months—no vaccine needed.
>3 months—2 doses, 0 and 3rd day.

The dose of **RIG** (rabies immunoglobulin) **is 20 U/kg for hRIG and 40 U/kg for equine RIG**

RHMAB (rabies monoclonal antibody cocktail) is licensed in India (as Rabisheild, Serum Institute of India; 40 IU/mL). The recommended dose is 3.33 IU/kg body weight, preferably at the time of the first vaccine dose.

Rabies IG should not be used during re-exposure.

CORONAVIRUS VACCINES

- All corona vaccines are safe for pregnant and lactating women.
- All corona vaccines available in India can be transported and stored at normal refrigeration temperatures

COVAXIN

First indigenous vaccine against corona virus produced by Bharat Biotech in collaboration with the National Institute of Virology (NIV) and Indian Council of Medical Research (ICMR) .

- An inactivated vaccine (a vaccine that uses the killed virus)
- 0.5 ml, IM, 2 doses 4–8 weeks apart, booster after 6 months.
- >6 years.
- A nasal covaxin vaccine (iNCOVACC) licensed in India >18 years, 2 doses.

COVISHIELD/COVOVAX

Produced in India by Serum Institute of India (SII).

- Recombinant nanoparticle vaccine
- 0.5 ml, IM, 2 doses 4–8 weeks apart, booster after 6 months.
- >6 years (COVOVAX)

ZYCOV-D

ZYCOV-D is a DNA plasmid-based COVID-19 vaccine developed by Indian pharmaceutical company Cadila Healthcare

- DNA based
- Intradermal injection using a spring-powered jet injector (needle less), 2 doses, 4–8 weeks apart, 0.1 ml
- >12 years

CORBEVAX

A protein subunit COVID-19 vaccine developed by Texas Children's Hospital, Texas. It is licensed to Indian biopharmaceutical firm Biological E Limited (BioE) for development and production

- Subunit (recombinant)
- 0.5 ml, IM, 2 doses 4–8 weeks apart, booster after 6 months.
- >5 years.
- *Note:* Different vaccine could be taken for different dose. Heterologous booster is allowed.
- **Soon vaccine would be available for all ages.**
- It is more likely that Booster may be recommended yearly

NATIONAL IMMUNIZATION SCHEDULE

Age	Vaccines
Birth	BCG, OPV0 (for institutional delivery), HepB
6 weeks	DTwP1/HepB1/Hib1 **(Pentavalent 1), Rota 1,** (BCG if not given at birth), **PCV1, fIPV1**/bOPV1
10 weeks	DTwP2/HepB2/Hib2 **(Pentavalent 2), Rota 2,** (BCG if not given at birth), bOPV2
14 weeks	DTwP3/HepB3/Hib3 **(Pentavalent 3), Rota 3,** (BCG if not given at birth), PCV 2, **fIPV2**/bOPV3
9–12 months	MR1, **JE1,** Vit A (1 Lac IU), **PCV B, fIPVB**
16–24 months	DTwP B1/OPV B, MR2, **JE2**
5–6 years	DTwP B2/OPV B2
10 years	Td
16 years	Td

Contd.

Age	Vaccines
Pregnant women	Td 1 (early in pregnancy) Td 2 (1 month later) Td Booster (if vaccinated in past 3 years)
Vit A	**Total 9 doses** starting at 9 months of age then every 6 months up to 5 years of age

Vit A: <6 months—50,000 IU,
(orally) 6 months–1 year—1 lac IU,
>1 year—2 lac IU.

IAP IMMUNIZATION TIME TABLE

Age	Vaccines
Birth	BCG, OPV0, HepB1
6 weeks	DTwP1/DTaP1, IPV1, HepB2, Hib1, Rota 1, PCV 1
10 weeks	DTwP2/DTaP2, IPV2, HepB3, Hib2, Rota 2, PCV 2
14 weeks	DTwP3/DTaP3, IPV3, HepB4, Hib3, Rota 3, PCV 3
6 months	OPV 1, influenza 1
7 months	Typhoid (TCV), influenza 2
9 months	OPV 2, MMR1
12 months	Hep A1
15 months	MMR-2, PCV booster, varicella-1
16–18 months	DTwP B1/DTaP B1, IPV B1, Hib B
18–19 months	Hep A2, varicella-2
2 years	Influenza
3 years	Influenza
4 years	Influenza
4–6 years	DTwP B2/DTaP B2, IPV B2, MMR-3,
5 years	Influenza
10–12 years	Tdap, HPV 1 and 2
15–18 years	Td, HPV 1, 2 and 3

Note: Newer Recommendation by IAP

1. A booster of the injectable polio vaccine (IPV) is recommended at 4–6 years
2. A uniform dosing of 15 μg (0.5 ml) of inactivated influenza vaccines is recommended for all children older than 6 months.
3. The second dose of varicella vaccine should preferably be administered 3–6 months after the first dose
4. 10-valent pneumococcal conjugate vaccine: Pneumosil. The use of Pneumosil till 2 years of age (not beyond 2 years) in a 3 + 1 schedule, with the booster administered between 12 and 18 months
5. Approves the use of quadrivalent conjugate meningococcal vaccine: Menveo vaccine in the 2–55 years age group. It reiterates the use of this vaccine only in special situations. Menveo is recommended as a single dose schedule after 2 years of age.
6. Use of tetraxim (DTaP/IPV combination vaccine) for the second booster at 4–6 years of age.
7. Use of conjugated typhoid vaccine Typhi BEV for age >6 months and up to 45 years as single dose. There is no recommendation for a booster dose.
8. Recommends the use of rabies monoclonal antibody cocktail for post-exposure prophylaxis of rabies as twinrab over RIGs in the management of category 3 bites. Human monoclonal rabies antibody (rabishield) and murine cocktail monoclonal rabies antibodies (twinrab), both are available in India and approved for the post-exposure management of suspected rabies exposure.

IAP recommended vaccines for High-risk* children (Vaccines under special circumstances):

1. Meningococcal vaccine
2. Japanese encephalitis vaccine
3. Cholera vaccine
4. Rabies vaccine
5. Yellow fever vaccine
6. Pneumococcal polysaccharide vaccine (PPSV 23).

***High-risk category of children:**

- Congenital or acquired immunodeficiency (including HIV infection)
- Chronic cardiac, pulmonary (including asthma if treated with prolonged high-dose oral corticosteroids), hematologic, renal (including nephrotic syndrome), liver disease and diabetes mellitus.
- Children on long-term steroids, salicylates, immunosuppressive or radiation therapy
- Cerebrospinal fluid leak, cochlear implant, malignancies
- Children with functional/anatomic asplenia/hyposplenia
- During disease outbreaks
- Laboratory personnel and healthcare workers
- Travellers

COMBINATION VACCINE

Two or more separate immunogens that have physically combined in a single preparation.

Example: DTwP + Hib, DTwP + Hep B, DTwP + Hib+ Hep B, Hep A + Hep B, MMR, DTwP, DTwP + IPV + Hib + HepB

Electronic Vaccine Intelligence Network (eVIN)

The government of India has rolled out an electronic vaccine Intelligence Network (eVIN) system that digitises the entire vaccine stock management, their logistics and temperature tracking at all levels of vaccine storage—from national to the sub-district.

Intensified Mission Indradhanush (IMI 6.0)—aims at increasing the full immunisation coverage to 90% and covers 12 vaccine preventable diseases.

Future Vaccines

- Dengue virus vaccine (DENGVAXIA/QDENGA)
- HIV vaccine
- HCV vaccine
- Malaria vaccine
- Cancer vaccine

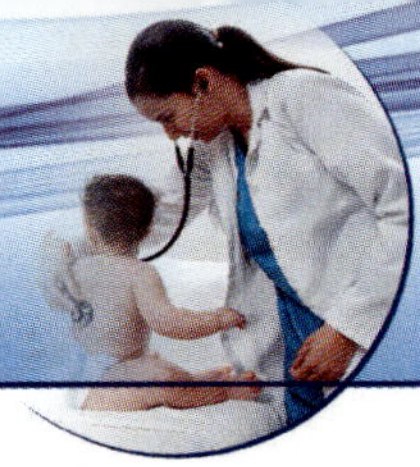

CHAPTER

5

Socioeconomic Status Scale

SOCIOECONOMIC HISTORY

- Kachcha/pukka house
- Number of rooms/family members
- Ventilation—adequate/not adequate
- Water supply—well/tap water/bore well
- Sanitation—toilet/open air defaecation

Modified Kuppuswamy's Socioeconomic Status Scale:

IJCMPH: 2023

Occupation	Score
1. Legislators, senior officials and managers	10
2. Professional	9
3. Technicians and associate professionals	8
4. Clerks	7
5. Skilled workers and shop and market sales workers	6
6. Skilled agricultural and fishery workers	5
7. Craft and related trade workers	4
8. Semi-skilled worker	3
9. Unskilled worker	2
10. Unemployed	1

Education	Score
1. Profession or honours	7
2. Graduate or postgraduate	6
3. Intermediate or post high school diploma	5
4. High school certificate	4
5. Middle school certificate	3
6. Primary school certificate	2
7. Illiterate	1

Family income per month (in Rs)	Score
1. ≥146, 104	12
2. 109, 580–146, 103	11
3. 73, 054–109, 579	10
4. 68, 455–73, 053	9
5. 63, 854–68, 454	8
6. 59, 252–63, 853	7
7. 54, 651–59, 251	6
8. 45, 589–54, 650	5
9. 36, 527–45, 588	4
10. 21, 914–36, 526	3
11. 7, 316–21, 913	2
12. <7315	1

Total score	Socioeconomic class
26–29	Upper (I)
16–25	Upper middle (II)
11–15	Lower middle (III)
5–10	Upper lower (IV)
<5	Lower (V)

FAMILY HISTORY

PEDIGREE

1st degree: Parents/children/siblings (50% shared genes)
2nd degree: Uncle/aunt/niece/nephew/grand-parents (25%)
3rd degree: Cousins (12.5% shared genes)

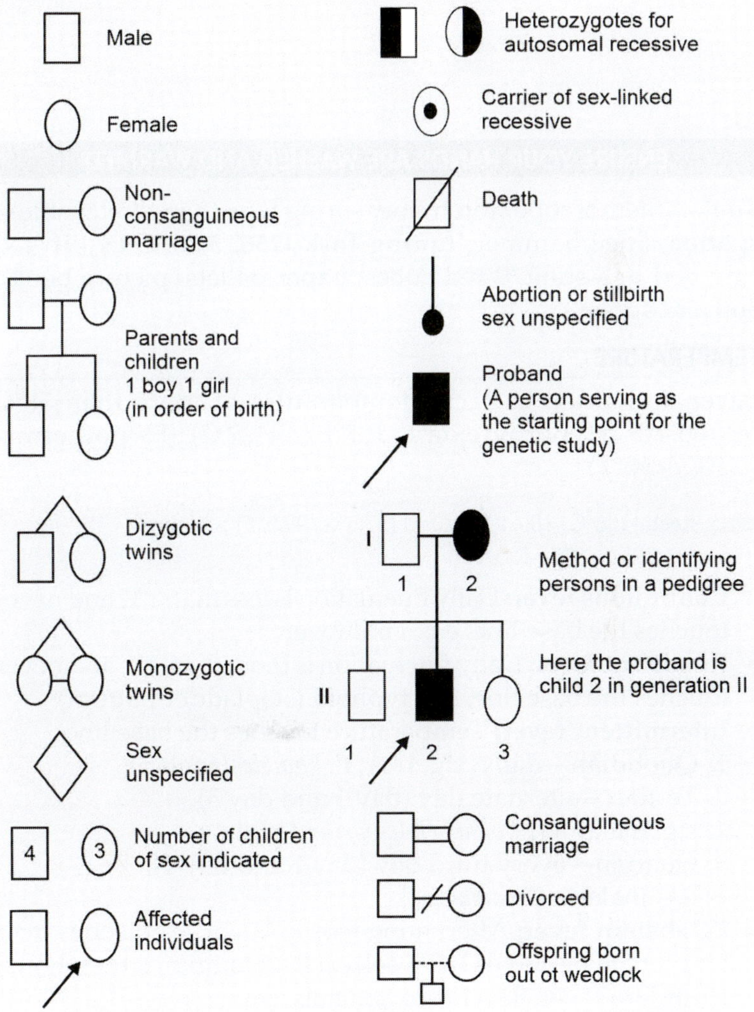

Pedigree chart

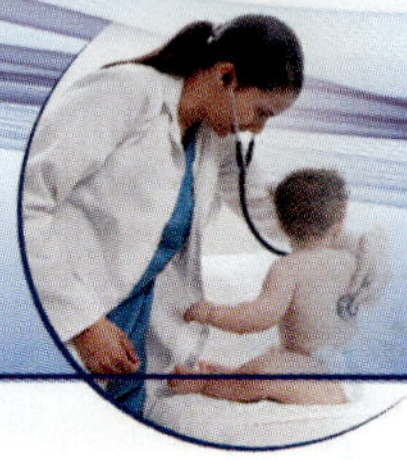

CHAPTER

6

Vitals

ENSURE YOUR HANDS ARE WASHED AND WARMED

Tools—Stethoscope/torch/measuring tape (non-stretchable)/spatula/knee hammer/**tuning fork (256, 512)/CNS kit**/red ring tied to a sting/9 red cubes/paper pallets/picture book/cup and spoon.

TEMPERATURE

Fever is defined as rectal temperature of more than 38°C or 100.4°F. Hyperpyrexia (>107°F/>41.5°C) (Hypothermia <35°C/<95°F)

> Rectal (38°C/100.4°F) >Oral (37.5°C/99.5*F) >Axillary (37.2°C/99°F)—ROA

- **Continuous fever:** Daily fluctuation is less than 1°C and never touches the base line, e.g. viral fever.
- **Remittent fever:** Daily fluctuation is more than 2°C and never touches the base line, e.g. typhoid (stepladder pattern)
- **Intermittent fever:** Temperature touches the base line
  1. Quotidian—daily, e.g. JRA, *P. knowlesi* malaria
  2. Tertian—alternate day (day 1 and day 3) e.g. malaria (*P. vivax/falciparum*/ovale)
  3. Quartan—every third day (day 1 and day 4), e.g. malaria (*P. malariae*)
- **Pelebstein fever:** Alternating febrile/afebrile episodes over an average period of 1–2 week each—Hodgkin's lymphoma
- **Undulant fever:** Fever rises and falls like a wave—Brucellosis
- **Saddle back fever (biphasic fever):** Alternating febrile/afebrile episodes of 1–3 days each—Dengue

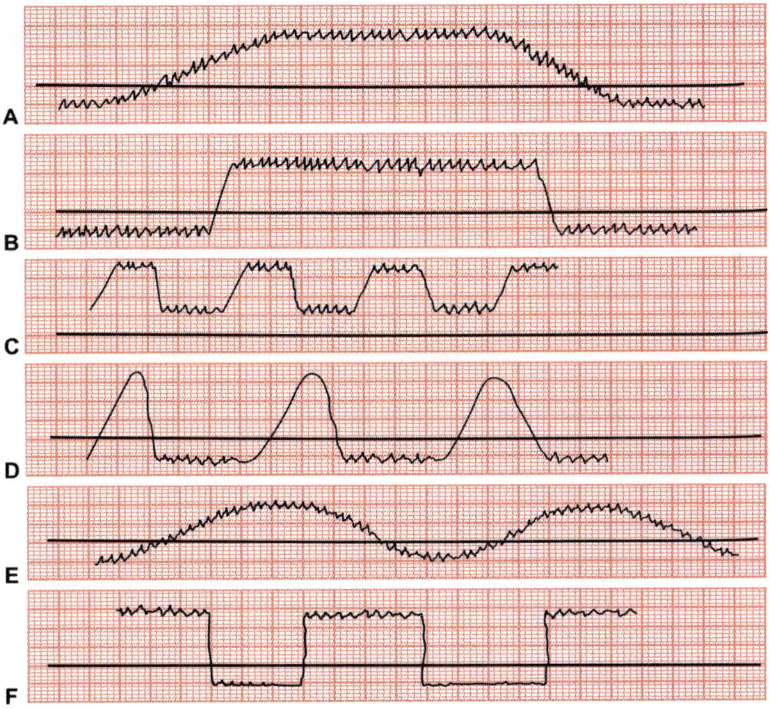

Fever graph

A. Fever continues
B. Fever continues to abrupt onset and remission
C. Remittent fever
D. Intermittent fever
E. Undulant fever
F. Relapsing fever

> With every degree F rise in temperature
> Pulse rate increases by 10 and respiratory rate by 4.
> Normal PR: RR ratio is 4:1

PUO/FUO (pyrexia/fever of unknown origin)—child with documented fever for which no cause could be identified even after 1 week of evaluation in hospital.

Note: Repeated febrile episodes in less than 5 years normal child, 4–6 times a year is common.

PULSE RATE

Rate—count for one min by palpating radial artery by index (rate/rhythm), middle (volume) and ring finger (used to obliterate the artery)

	Tachycardia	Normal HR
NB	>160/minute	120–160
<1 year	>140/minute	110–140
1–5 years	>120/minute	100–120
>5 years	>100/minute	60–100

In infants, heart rate can be counted by auscultation of heart or by assessing the femoral pulse.

- **Rhythm** (by palpating radial artery)—regular/irregular.
- **Volume** (by palpating radial artery)—normal/high (PDA/AR/Anaemia/Fever)/low volume (CCF/shock/COA).
- **Character** (by palpating carotid artery)—normal/pulses alternans (LVF)/collapsing pulse (AR/PDA)/pulsus paradoxus (severe BA).

Note: To palpate carotid A the thumb is pressed backwards at the medial border of SCM muscle at the level of thyroid cartilage (both carotid A should never be palpated simultaneously).

- **Radio-femoral delay**—COA (coarctation of aorta)
  (Normally femoral pulses felt before radial)
- **Radio-radial delay:** Normally both radial pulses felt simultaneously e.g., COA
- **Peripheral pulses**—Palpate bilaterally brachial, radial, posterior tibial, dorsalis pedis pulses.

BLOOD PRESSURE

Width of the bladder of BP cuff should cover at least 2/3rd of the length. Smaller cuff will give higher false reading and bigger cuff will give lower reading.

Plot the recorded systolic and diastolic BP against BP centile chart (based on height, age and sex percentile)—>95 percentile at least 3 different occasions indicate hypertension.

Age	Normal BP	Cuff size
NB	70/50 mm Hg	2.5 cm
<1 year	80/60 mm Hg	5 cm
>1 years	100/70 mm Hg	7.5–12.5 cm

Note: Cuff should be inflated to about 20–30 mm Hg above the level when radial pulse is not felt→ palpatory method.

BP IN CHILDREN >1 YEAR

Upper limit of systolic BP—90 + (age × 2)
Upper limit of diastolic BP—60 + (age × 2)
Lower limit of systolic BP—70 + (age × 2)

Note: For LLBP stethoscope is placed on the popliteal A.

KOROTKOFF SOUNDS

1. Clear and tapping
2. Soft murmur (swishing sound)
3. Murmur becomes louder
4. Muffling of sounds
5. Disappearance of sounds

- Systolic BP corresponds to phase 1 and diastolic to phase 5 but in case of AR phase 4 is taken as diastolic BP because phase 5 may reach zero.
- Its better to take all 4 limb BP in suspected cardiac cases and standing BP to r/o postural drop

RESPIRATORY RATE

Newborn	40–60/minute
<1 year	30–50/minute
1–5 years	20–40/minute
>5 years	20/minute

TACHYPNOEA ACCORDING TO WHO

<2 months	>60/minute
2–12 months	>50/minute
1–5 years	>40/minute

TYPE OF RESPIRATION

Newborn	Abdominal
<5 years and females	Thoraco-abdominal
>5 years	Abdomino-thoracic

DEPTH OF RESPIRATION

Normal	Inspiration-expiration-pause
Shallow	Narcotic poisoning
Deep and rapid (Kussmaul's breathing)	Metabolic acidosis (diabetic ketoacidosis)

RHYTHM OF RESPIRATION: REGULAR/IRREGULAR

Periodic breathing	
Cheyne–Stokes	Cardiac failure (Hyperpnoea/hypopnoea followed by apnoea)
Biot's	Increase ICT (apnoea followed by 4–5 normal breaths)

Note: In neonates periodic breathing is normal (apnoea <20 seconds and not associated with cyanosis/bradycardia)

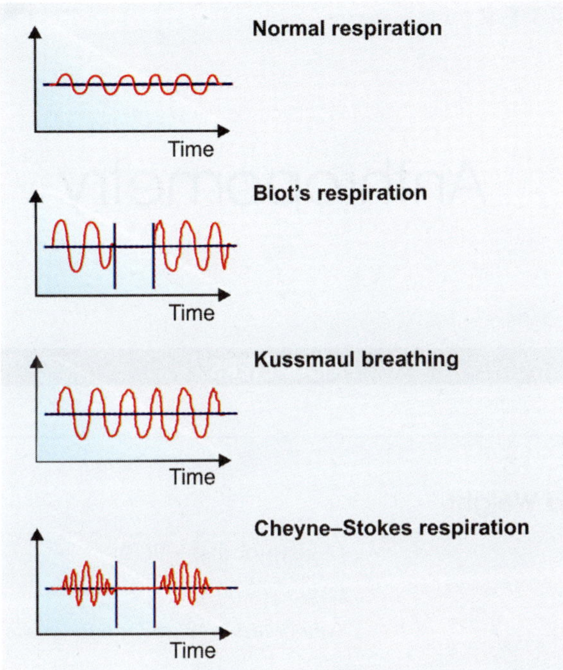

Respiration pattern

Note: Do not forget to mention use of accessory muscles.

- **Paradoxical breathing:** Normally abdomen moves out during inspiration, but in diaphragmatic paralysis opposite happens—sea saw movements.

CHAPTER

7

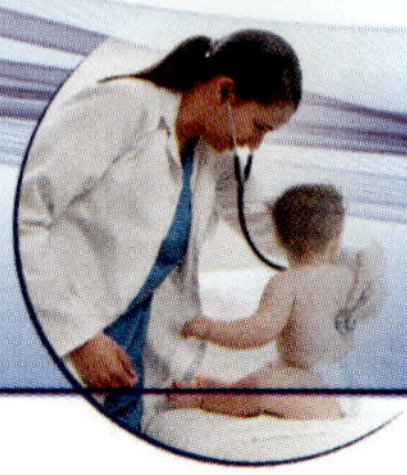

Anthropometry

PARAMETERS

WEIGHT

LBW: <2.5 kg

Expected Weight

<1 year	{Age (months) + 9}/2
1–7 years	{Age (years) + 4} × 2
7–12 years	Age (years) × 3 or 7 × age (years) –5/2

For example, 4 years old child expected weight = (4 + 4) × 2 = 16 kg

> Weight becomes 2X of birth wt by 5 months,
> 3X by 1 year, 4X by 2 years, 5X by 3 years, 6X by 5 years,
> 7X by 7 years and 10X by 10 years

For example, 1 year child with birth weight of 2.5 kg expected weight = 3 × 2.5 = 7.5 kg

IAP Classifiaction of Malnutrition (PEM)

K is postfixed in presence of oedema, e.g. PEM grade II (K)

Grade	% of expected weight
Normal	>80
Grade 1	71–80
Grade 2	61–70
Grade 3	51–60
Grade 4	<50

MODERATE ACUTE MALNUTRITION (MAM)

Wt for Ht between –3SD and –2SD or MUAC of 11.5–12.4 cm and has no B/L pitting oedema.

SEVERE ACUTE MALNUTRITION (SAM)

Among children 6–59 months of age as defined by WHO and UNICEF any of the follow 3:
1. WT for HT below –3SD on the WHO growth standard, or
2. Presence of bipedal oedema, or
3. MUAC (mid upper arm circumference) below 11.5 cm

For **severe acute malnutrition (SAM)** treat in
- 3 phases—(3 Rs: Resuscitation, Restorative, Rehabilitation)
- 10 steps—Mnemonic (3HIDE CMS follow I)
  1. Hypothermia
  2. Hypoglycaemia
  3. Hypokalaemia, hypo/hypernatraemia
  4. Infection
  5. Dehydration
  6. Enteric feeding
  7. Catch up growth/micronutrients
  8. Sensory stimulation
  9. Follow up
  10. Immunization

Note: (1) RUTF: Ready to use therapeutic food (5 times of F100)
(2) F75 (75 kcal + 1 g protein in 100 ml)
(3) F100 (100 kcal + 3 g protein in 100 ml)

HEIGHT

Length till 2 years (infantometer)

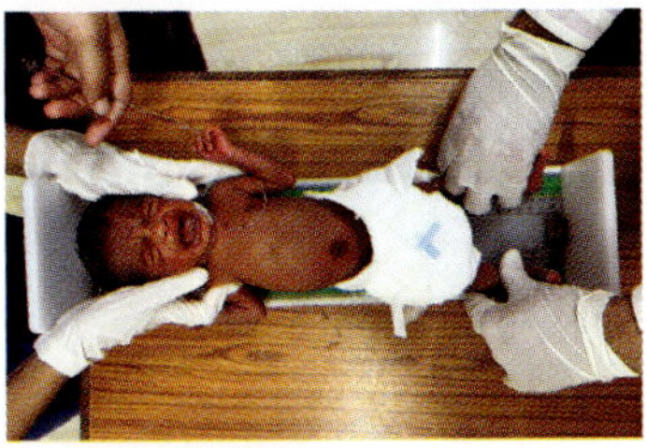

Infantometer

Height >2 years (stadiometer)

• Birth	50 cm
• 6 months	65 cm
• 1 year	75 cm
• 2 years	85 cm
• 3 years	95 cm
• 4 years	100 cm
• 8 years	125 cm
• 12 years	150 cm

OR

2–12 years {Age (years) × 6} + 77 cm

Height doubled by 4 years, tripled by 13 years

2–12 years Ht velocity = 5–6 cm/year

Short Stature

Height <3rd centile or <–2 SD below the median height for that age and sex.

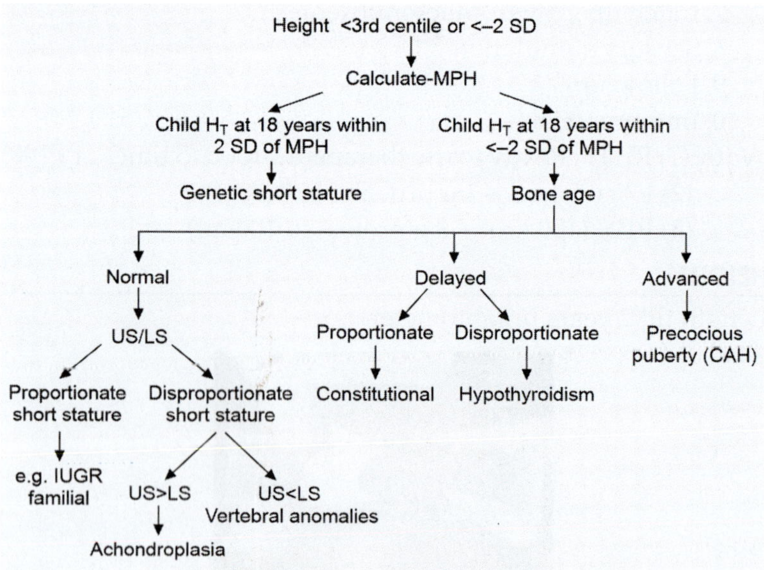

An approach to short stature

Proportionate Short Stature

IUGR, malnutrition, chronic infection (TB), endocrine deficiency (hypothyroidism, GH deficiency, Cushing's syndrome), familial, constitutional

Disproportionate Short Stature

Achondroplasia/vertebral anomalies (Klippel–Feil syndrome).

MPH (mid parental height)

$$\text{Male} = \frac{(\text{Fathers height in cm} + \text{Mothers height in cm}) + 13\text{ cm}}{2}$$

$$\text{Female} = \frac{(\text{Fathers height in cm} + \text{Mothers height in cm}) - 13\text{ cm}}{2}$$

Predicted adult height would be—MPH ± 8.5 cm

OR

2 × (Length at 2 years (in cm) ± 2.5 cm

Ponderal index PI = Weight (g)/Length^3 (cm) × 100

>2.5 = normal, 2–2.5 = symmetrical IUGR,
<2 = asymmetrical IUGR

Normally bone age (BA) = Chronological age (CA), also in familial short stature
CA > BA (delayed bone age): Chronic illness, hypothyroidism, hypopituitarism constitutional growth delay
CA < BA (advanced bone age): CAH, hyperthyroidism
Bone age = height age in constitutional delay, malnutrition
Bone age < height age in growth hormone deficiency, hypothyroidism

Physiological Short Stature/Normal Variant

Feature	Familial	Constitutional
Birth wt	Low	Normal
Family h/o	Short stature but pubertal onset normal	Delayed puberty
Ht velocity	Normal	Normal

Contd.

Feature	Familial	Constitutional
BA relation with CA/HA	CA = BA > HA	CA > BA = HA
Final height	Normal	Short but normal for target Ht

Waterlow Classification of Malnutrition

	Ht for age (stunting)	Wt for Ht (wasting)
Normal	>95% of expected	>90%
1st stunting/wasting	95–90%	80–90%
2nd stunting/wasting	90–85%	70–80%
3rd stunting/wasting	<85%	<70%

$$\text{Ht for age} = \frac{\text{Ht of the child}}{\text{Expected Ht for that age}} \times 100$$

$$\text{Wt for Ht} = \frac{\text{Wt of the child}}{\text{Wt of a normal child at same height}} \times 100$$

WHO Classification of Malnutrition

	Moderate malnutrition (MAM)	Severe malnutrition (SAM)
Symmetrical oedema	No	Yes
Weight-for-height (measure of wasting)	Between –3 SD and –2 SD score (70–79%)	SD-score <–3 (<70%) (severe wasting)
Height-for-age (measure of stunting)	Between –3 SD and –2 SD score (85–89%)	SD-score <–3 (<85%) (severe stunting)
MUAC	11.5–12.4 cm	<11.5 cm

SD score, standard deviation score

Waterlow Classification (Interpretation of Indicators)

Wt for Ht	Ht for age	Inference
>80%	>90%	Normal
>80%	<90%	Stunted (chronic)
<80%	>90%	Wasted (acute)
<80%	<90%	Wasted and stunted (Acute on chronic)

Grade	Kwashiorkor (Wt 60–80% with oedema)	Marasmus (Wt <60% without oedema)
1	Peripheral oedema only	Loose skinfolds in axilla and groin
2	1+ mooning of face	1+ loose skinfolds in thigh and buttocks
3	2+ presacral and abdominal wall oedema	2+ loose skinfolds in chest and spine
4	3+ ascites	3+ loose skinfolds in buccal pad of fat

Under nutrition: (Wt 60–80% without oedema)
Marasmic kwashiorkor: (Wt <60% with oedema)
Failure to thrive (FTT): Child with weight for age below 3rd centile or a downward change in growth that has crossed two major growth percentile in a short time.
Rapid weight loss: >10% Wt loss in 6 months.

HEAD CIRCUMFERENCE (HC)

[From occipital protuberance to supraorbital ridge/glabella]

• Birth	35 cm
• 6 months	43 cm
• 1 year	46 cm
• 2 years	49 cm
• 2–7 years	0.5 cm/year
• 7–12 years	0.3 cm/year

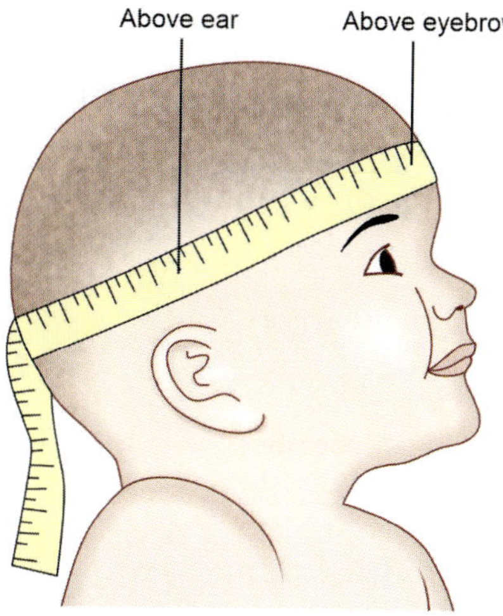

Macrocephaly: >2 SD above the median HC for that age
Example: Hydrocephalus, mucopolysaccharidosis, fragile X syndrome, intracranial tumours
Microcephaly: <–3 SD below the median HC for that age
Primary: Familial (AR/AD), syndromes (5, 18, 21), malformation
Secondary: **M**aternal DM, meningitis
Congenital—TORCH intrauterine infection
HIE
Radiation
Drugs—phenytoin, alcohol
(Mnemonic: **MCH RD**)

One SD is approx 2.5% of the expected HC for that age and sex. For example, if the expected HC is 50 cm, one SD =1.25 cm.

Till 1 year HC for length = (Length in cm/2) ±2.5 cm

Craniotabes: Softened and parchment like skull bones –indented like a ping pong ball—*Rickets, Hypervitaminosis A*
Bossing of skull: *Rickets, thalassemia major*

Note: 90% brain growth occurs within 2 years of age

MID UPPER ARM CIRCUMFERENCE (MUAC)—(ONLY FOR 6 MONTHS TO 5 YEARS)

Midway between tip of acromion process of scapula and olecranon of ulna

Observed	Inference	Shakir tape
>12.5 cm	Normal	Green
11.5–12.4 cm	Moderate	Yellow
<11.5 cm	Severe	Red

BODY MASS INDEX (BMI)

Wt (kg)/Ht^2 (m)

For <12 years

<15	Malnutrition
>22	Overweight
>25	Obesity

WAIST HIP RATIO

A waist hip ratio of >1.0 in male and >0.85 in female in adolescent is associated with metabolic syndromes.

CHEST CIRCUMFERENCE (CC)

Just below the level of nipple in mid inspiration

Newborn	HC > CC
9–12 months	HC = CC
>1 year	HC < CC

UPPER SEGMENT: LOWER SEGMENT RATIO

Birth	1.7:1
2 years	1.5:1
3 years	1.3:1
9 years	1:1
>10 years	0.9:1

Lower segment is measured from ASIS to lower of medial malleolus.

Infantile US/LS, e.g. achondroplasia, hypothyroidism, rickets, sexual prematurity
Advanced US/LS, e.g. Turner, Klinefelter, Pott's spine, kyphoscoliosis, mucopolysaccharidosis

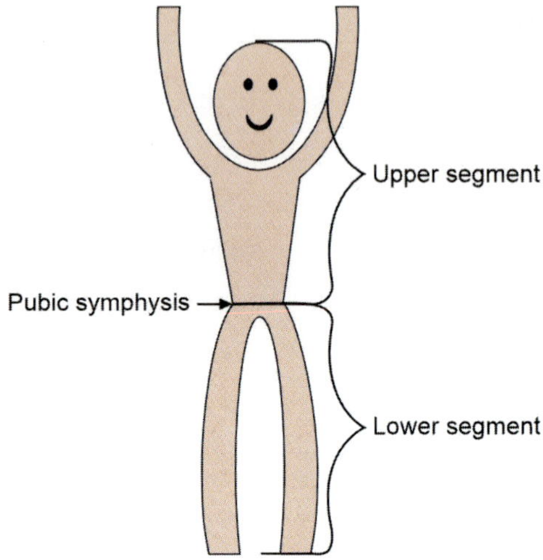

ARM SPAN

- From the tip of the middle finger of one arm to the tip of the middle finger of the other arm with the arms outstretched

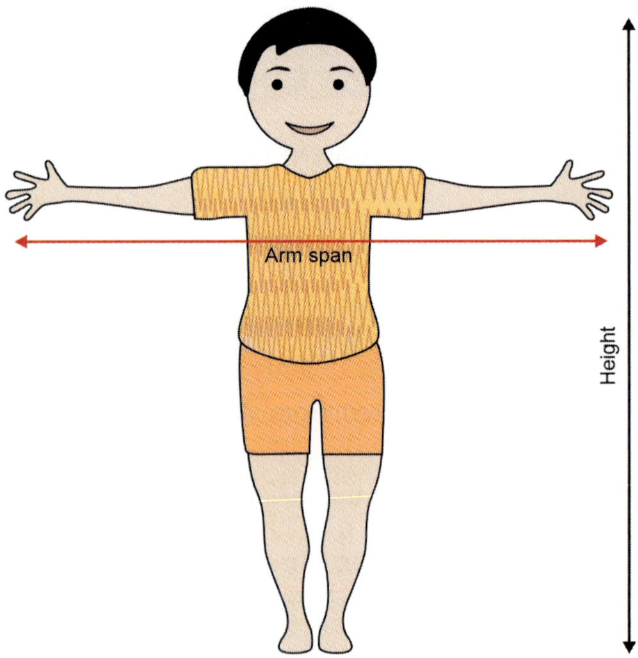

- At birth arm span is shorter than length, it becomes equal to height around 10 years of age.

Arm span remain shorter in Marfan syndrome, COA, Klinefelter, homocystinuria.

Ht > Arm span before 10 years—precocious puberty

BODY SURFACE AREA (BSA)

Weight (kg)	Formula
1–5 kg	$0.05 \times wt + 0.05$
6–10 kg	$0.04 \times wt + 0.1$
11–20 kg	$0.03 \times wt + 0.2$
21–40 kg	$0.02 \times wt + 0.4$

For 15 kg BSA = 0.5, 20 kg = 0.8, 30 kg = 1, and 40 kg = 1.3.

or child weighing (3–30 kg) $BSA\ (m^2) = \dfrac{Wt\ (in\ kg) + 4}{30}$

CHAPTER

8

General Examination

PICCLE

- **Pallor:** Undue paleness of the skin/mucous membrane
  - Seen in lower palpebral conjunctiva, dorsum of tongue, palms, oral mucosa, nails.
  - Can comment on severe pallor if palmar/plantar creases are also pale.

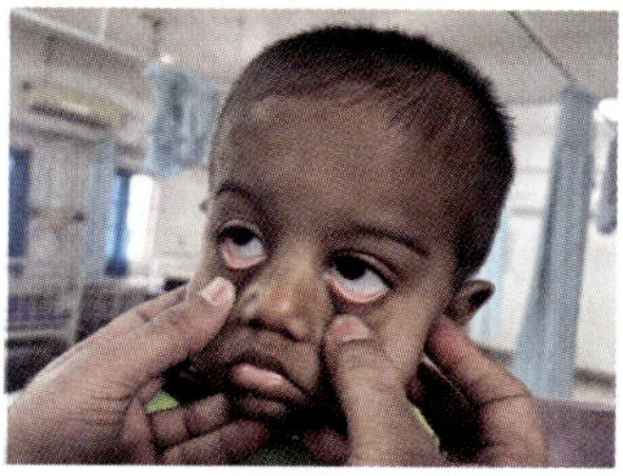

Pallor

- **Icterus:** Yellowish discoloration of the skin/mucous membrane
  - S. bilirubin >2 mg/dl
  - Upper Bulbar conjunctiva, ventral surface of tongue at the junction of soft and hard palate, palms and soles

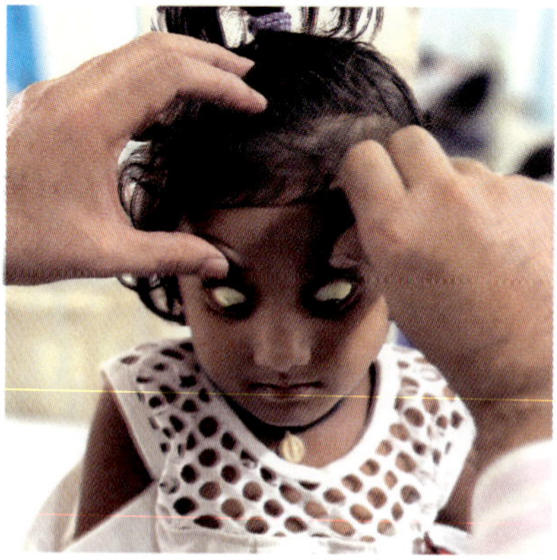

Icterus

- **Cyanosis:** Bluish discoloration of the skin/mucous membrane due to >5 g/dl of reduced Hb seen at lips, nail beds, ear lobes.
- **Mixed cyanosis:** Decreased oxygenation due to sluggish blood flow, e.g. cardiogenic shock/CCF
- Differential cyanosis: Preductal (right UL) SPO_2 > postductal, e.g. PDA, PPHN
- Central: Cyanosis of mucosa and extremities, e.g. high altitude/BA/cyanotic CHD
- Peripheral: Cyanosis of extremities but not of mucosa, e.g. COLD/PVD
- **Clubbing:** Selective bulbous enlargement of the distal portion of the distal phalanx

Grade 1	Softening of the nail bed (increased fluctuation)
Grade 2	Obliteration of the nail bed angle (normal 160°) Lovibond angle (Schamroth's sign)
Grade 3	Parrot beak/drumstick appearance
Grade 4	Hypertrophic pulmonary osteoarthopathy (HPOA)

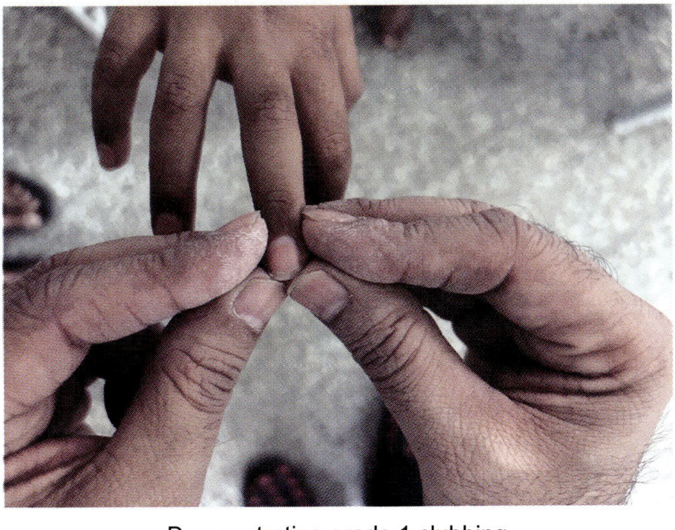

Demonstrating grade 1 clubbing

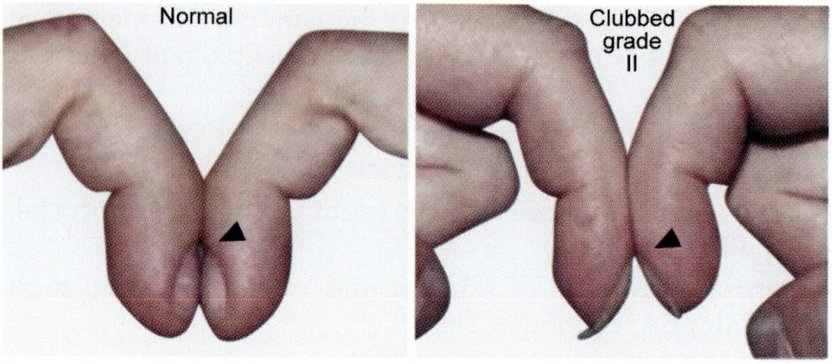

Example: Congenital heart disease, infectious endocarditis, lung abscess, bronchiectasis, Crohn's disease

Pseudoclubbing—*hyperparathyroidism*

- ***Unilateral clubbing*** found in brachial A-V fistula, thoracic outlet syndromes.

- **Lymphadenopathy**
  - Number/site/size/shape/surface/temperature tenderness/consistency/mobility/matted or discrete/discharge/skin over the lymph node/drainage area.
  - *Palpate bilaterally*—Submental/submandibular/cervical (anterior and posterior)/suboccipital/pre- and post-

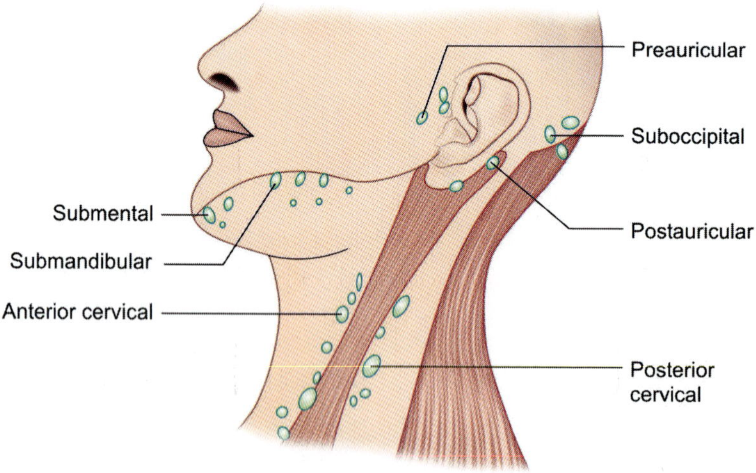

Sites of lymph nodes

auricular/axillary (apical, ant., post, medial, lateral)/ epitrochlear/inguinal.

- ***Cervical Lymph nodes should be examined***
  - **From behind:** Examine the submental/submandibular/ preauricular/tonsillar/supraclavicular and deep cervical glands in the anterior triangle of the neck.
  - **From front:** Examine the post-triangle up to the back of the neck/post-auricular and occipital.

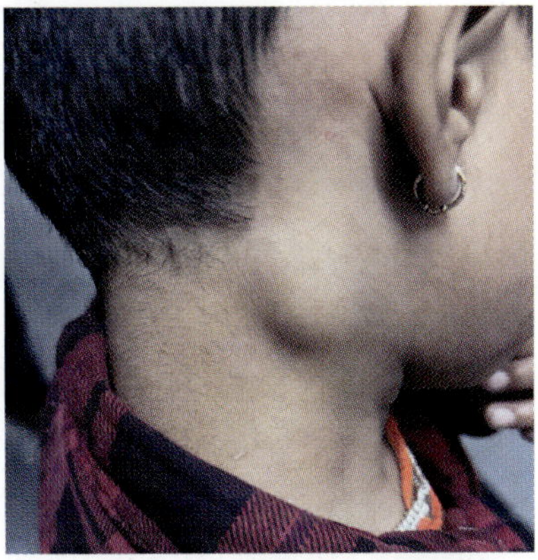

A case of TB cervical lymphadenitis

- **Axillary:** Sit in front of the child, support the arm, palpate the right axilla with the left hand and *vice versa*.

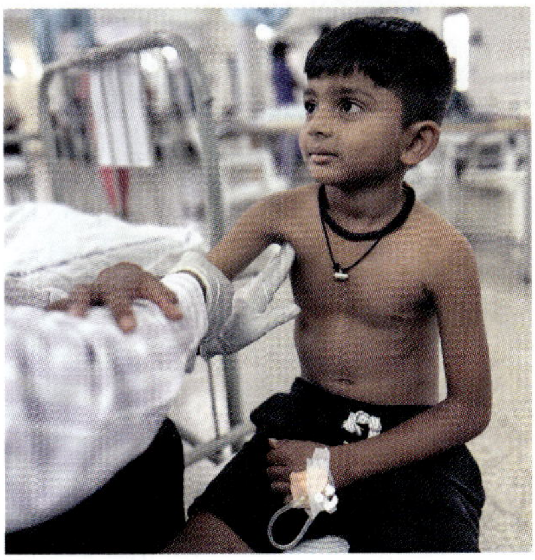

Examination of axillary lymph node

- **Epitrochlear:** Located on the medial side of the arm above the medial epicondyle of the humerus. While supporting the child right wrist with the left hand, grasp the partially flexed elbow with the right hand and use the thumb to feel the epitrochlear.

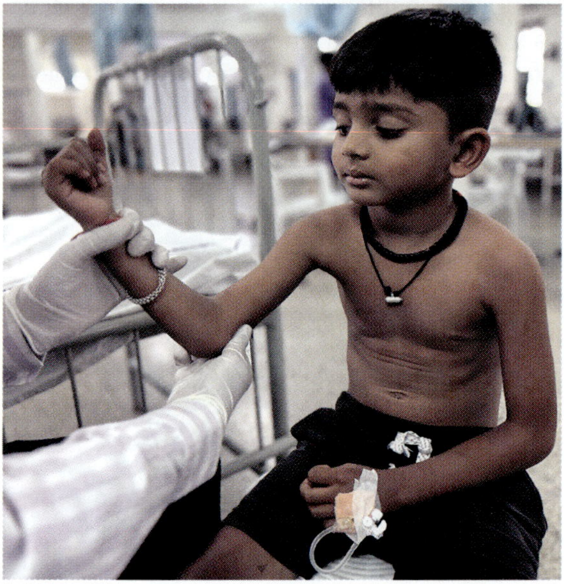

Examination of epitrochlear lymph node

  Examine the left epitrochlear with the left thumb.
  - ***Localized L/N:*** Only one area involved
  - ***Generalized L/N:*** 2 or more noncontiguous area involved
  - ***Persistent L/N:*** >3 months duration
  - ***Significant L/N:*** >1 cm in cervical, axillary and other (inguinal >1.5 cm, **epitrochlear of any size**)
- **Oedema:** Swelling due to excess fluid in body tissue
  - Over medial malleolus/shin/dorsum of feet
  - Apply pressure with thumb/index finger for 5 seconds
  - Pitting/nonpitting
  - Generalised/localised
  - Pedal (cardiac), around eyes (renal),

- Ascites (hepatic), anasarca (nephrotic)
- Note-non pitting oedema is due to lymphatic obstruction *Example:* Milroy syndrome, Turner syndrome

SIGNS OF DEHYDRATION

	No dehydration	Some	Severe
General condition	Alert/active	Restless/ irritable	Lethargic/ drowsy
Weight reduction	<5%	5–10%	>10%
Thirst	Thirsty	Extremely thirsty	Not able to drink
Urine output	Normal	Decreased	Not passed >12 hours
Eyes	Normal	Lustreless	Sunken
Tongue/oral cavity	Moist	Dry	Dry and parched
Tear	Normal	Normal	Dry
Anterior fontanelle	Normal	Slightly depressed	Depressed
Skin turgor/ pinch	Normal	Goes back slowly	Goes back very slowly
Extremities	Warm	Warm	Cold clammy
PR	Normal	Increased	Rapid thready feeble
RR	Normal	Decreased	Deep sighing
BP	Normal	Decreased	Not recordable
Treatment plan	Plan A	Plan B	Plan C

Skin turgor/pinch test is of no value in case of marasmus/ kwashiorkor and in obesity (pinch child abdominal skin)
Plan A: Continue feeding as usual/encourage breastfeeding + give WHO ORS

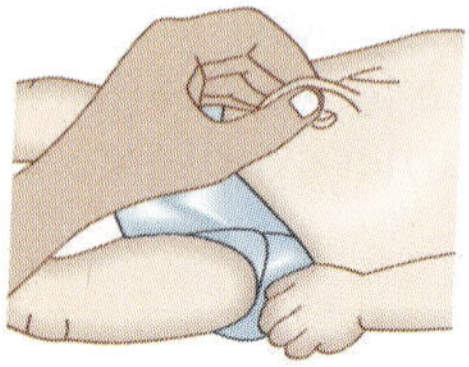

Pinching the child's abdomen to test for decreased skin turgor

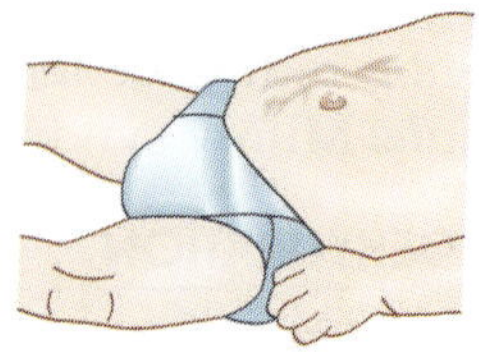

Slow return of skin pinch in severe dehydration

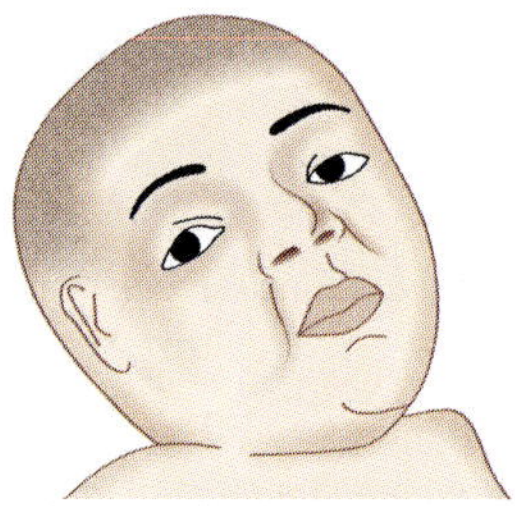

Sunken eye

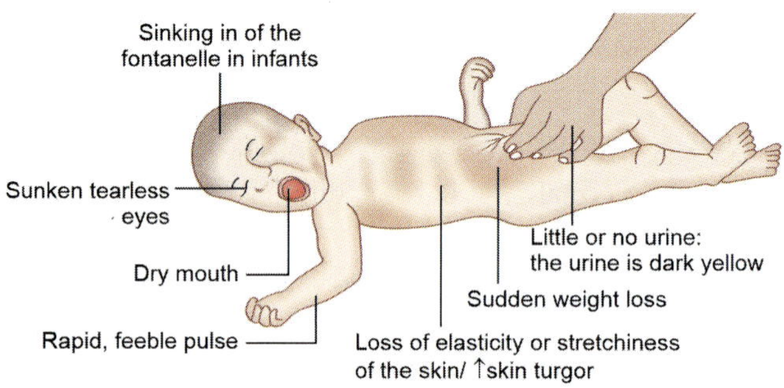

Signs of dehydration

Age	ORS/each stool
<2 years	50–100 ml
2–10 years	100–200 ml
>10 years	As much as one wants

Or if you know the weight: 10 ml/kg of ORS/each stool episode

Note: If not drinking ORS can give rice water/vegetable soups/dal water/lassi/coconut water/plain water with pinch of salt and one teaspoon sugar.

Plan B: Continue feeding as usual/encourage breastfeeding +Give 75 ml/kg of ORS in the first 4 hours.

Reassess after 4 hours:

- If no dehydration—plan A
- If some dehydration—plan B

Plan C: Start IV fluids immediately (RL with 5% dextrose)

Age	1st give	Then give
<1 year	30 ml/kg in 1 hour	70 ml/kg in 5 hours
1–5 years	30 ml/kg in 1/2 hour	70 ml/kg in 2 1/2 hours

WHO ORS

Ingredients	Old (mmol/L)	New low Osmolarity (mmol/L)
Sodium (Na)	90	75
Potassium (K)	20	20
Chloride	80	65
Citrate	10	10
Glucose	111	75
Osmolarity	311	245

Once Made Should be used within 24 hours

2 types of sachet available 1L/sachet or 200 ml/sachet

Give zinc to all: <6 months 10 mg/day, >6 months 20 mg/day OD dose for 14 days. (5 ml syp contain 20 mg Zn)

Zinc decreases both the quantity and frequency of stool and prevent further episodes as given in flowchat on page 62.

Probiotics: Dietary supplement of living microorganism, helps in improving host microorganisms colonisation.

Example: *Lactobacillus, Bifidobacteria S. boulardii*

Prebiotics: Dietary supplement of substrates that selectively stimulate the growth and activity of beneficial gut micro-organisms.

Example: Fructo/galacto/oligosaccharides.

Synbiotics: Probiotics + Prebiotics

Persistent diarrhoea: >14 days

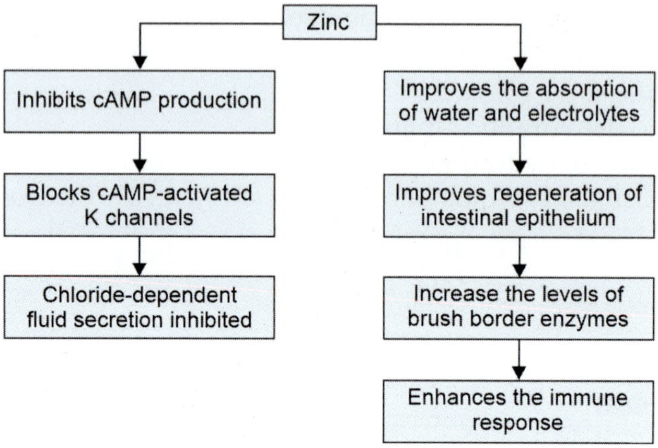

Mechanism of action of zinc in dehydration

Look for Vitamin Deficiency Signs

Vitamin A	**Bitot spots**/xerophthalmia/keratomalacia/toad skin (phrynoderma—also seen in essential fatty acid deficiency)
Vitamin B_1 (Thiamine)	**Dry beriberi** (polyneuritis/ptosis/sluggish DTR) Acute—WE, chronic—KS **Wet-beriberi** (palpitation/dyspnoea/cardiomegaly/oedema)
Vitamin B_2 (Riboflavin)	Glossitis/cheilosis/scaly dermatitis/peripheral neuropathy
Vitamin B_3 (Niacin)	**3D**-diarrhoea/dermatitis/dementia
Vitamin B_6 (Pyridoxine)	Anaemia (microcytic hypochromic)/FTT
Vitamin B_{12} (Cobalamine)	Anaemia (megaloblastic)/thrombocytopenia Subacute combined degeneration (SACD)
Folic acid	**Anaemia (megaloblastic)**/thrombocytopenia/glossitis/decreased immunity
Vitamin C	**Scurvy**—characterized by irritability/pseudo-paralysis/scorbutic rosary/scorbutic beads Poor wound healing, maculosquamous dermatitis

Contd.

Vitamin D	**Rickets** features (bossing of skull/craniotabes/delayed closure of AF/rachitic rosary/Harrison sulcus/knock knees/coxa vara/pot belly/stunting
Vitamin K	Deficiency of clotting factors 2, 7, 9, 10
Vitamin E	Myopathy, neuropathy

Look of Trace Mineral Deficiency (Micro-nutrients)

Iron	H/o **Pica,** easy fatigability, irritability, reduced work capacity, dyspnoea on exertion. O/E impaired growth and development, pallor, koilonychia or spooning of nails
Calcium	**Tetany,** carpopedal spasms, muscle cramps, weakness, rickets and stunting, ECG may show prolonged QT
Iodine	Simple—**Goitre,** stunting, neuromotor retardation, learning disorder, deafness, coarse skin, cold intolerance and constipation
Zinc	Stunting, acrodermatitis enteropathica, mucocutaneous ulcers, poor wound healing, hypogonadism, recurrent infection, decreased immunity
Fluoride	Dental caries, osteoporosis
Phosphorus	Rickets, bone pain, pulp defects in the teeth

Note: X-linked dominant familial hypophosphataemic rickets—most common form of non-nutritional rickets.

Vitamin A Deficiency (WHO Classification)

XN: Night blindness
X1A: Xerosis of conjunctiva
X1B: Bitot's spot
X2: Xerosis of cornea
X3A: Keratomalacia involving <1/3rd of cornea
X3B: Keratomalacia involving >1/3rd of cornea
XS: Corneal scar
XF: Xerophthalmic fundus

Hypervitaminosis A

- Excess intake of vit A
- Acute:
  - In infant—it causes pseudotumor cerebri present with buldging AF, vomiting and irritability
  - In older children—diplopia and headache
- Chronic: Skin desquamation, alopecia, HS, ↑ICT, bone swelling
- Remedy—discontinue taking vit A

FACIES ASSOCIATED WITH DISEASES

Typical facies	Associated with
Potter	B/L Renal agenesis
Gargoylism-coarse facies	Mucopolysaccharidosis
Risus sardonicus	Tetanus
Cretinoid	Hypothyroidism
Adenoid	Adenoid hypertrophy
Haemolytic	Thalassaemia and other haemolytic anaemia
Mongoloid	Down syndrome
Cushingoid	Cushing's syndrome
Expressionless face	B/L Facial nerve palsy

Epicanthal fold: A fold of skin extending downwards from the upper eye lid to cover the inner canthus of eye, e.g. Down syndrome.

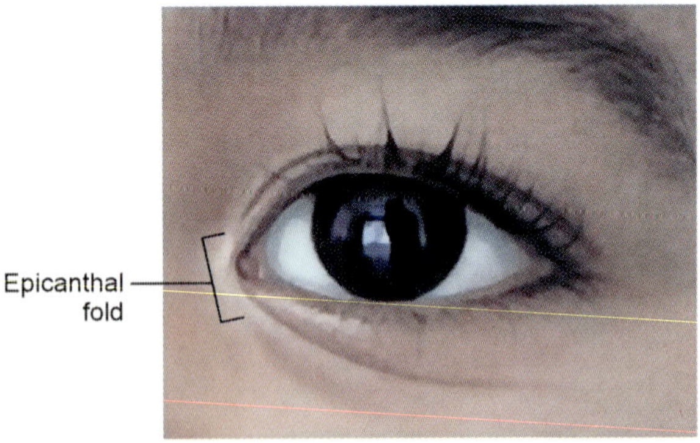

Epicanthal fold

Mongoloid slant: The outer canthi lies above the line joining the inner canthi as in Down syndrome.

Anti-mongoloid slant: The outer canthi lies below the line joining the inner canthi as in Turner syndrome, Noonan's syndrome.

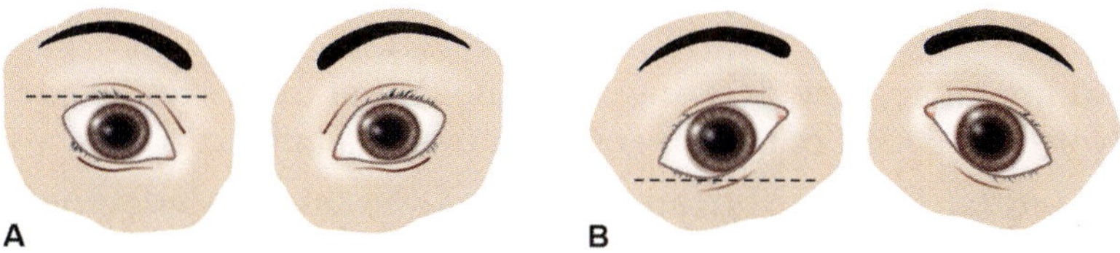

(A) Mongoloid slant; (B) Antimongoloid slant

Hypertelorism

Due to hypertrophy of the lesser wing of sphenoid. Always, suspect hypertelorism if the distance between the medial canthi of the two eyes is more than the width of each eye.

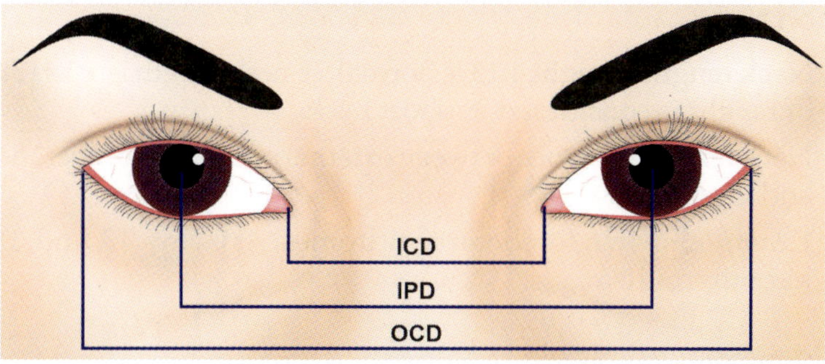

Hypertelorism

Use transparent sheet to measure the distances.

- ICD: Inner canthal distance
- IPD: Inner pupillary distance
- OCD: Outer canthal distance

$$\frac{ICD}{IPD} > 0.6 \quad \text{OR} \quad \frac{ICD}{OCD} > 0.38$$

Example: Down/Turner/Apert/Noonan syndrome/Thalassaemia major/cretinism

Hypotelorism

$\frac{\text{ICD}}{\text{OCD}} < 0.33$ (Normal 0.33–0.38), e.g. craniosynostosis.

Low Set Ears

An imaginary line drawing from the lateral canthi to the ear. Normally 1/3rd of the ear comes above this line.

Example: Down/Marfan/Fragile X/Noonan syndromes, Trisomy 13 (Patau syndrome) and 18 (Edward's syndrome), Cri-du-chat syndrome (5)

Low Hair Line

Hairline in the back extending **below C_4** spine.

Example: Turner syndrome.

Short Neck

- **Neck length: Height 1:13** is normal. If neck length is <1/13th of height is considered as short neck.
- **Neck length:** Distance between external occipital protuberance and C_7 spine.
- *Example:* Down/Noonan syndromes, Trisomy 13 and 18, hypothyroidism.

Widely Spaced Nipple

- Space between nipples >25% of chest circumference.
- *Example:* Turner's syndrome.

  Megalocornea >13 mm (diameter of cornea)

  Microcornea <10 mm

High-arched Palate

If the roof of the palate is not seen when the examiner's eye are at the level of the upper incisor of the child when the mouth is kept open. Seen in—Down/Marfan/Turner syndrome.

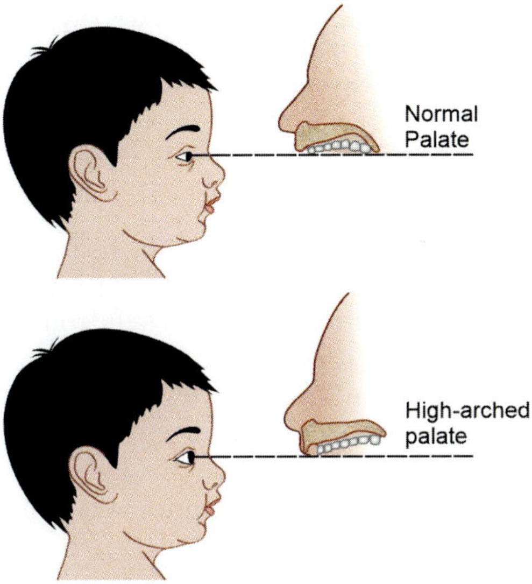

Normal and high-arched palate

Anterior Fontanelle

- The average of anteroposterior diameter (length) and transverse diameter (width) [normal (0.6–3.6 cm) <0.6 small >3.6 large]
- Use transparent sheet on the baby's scalp to mark AF

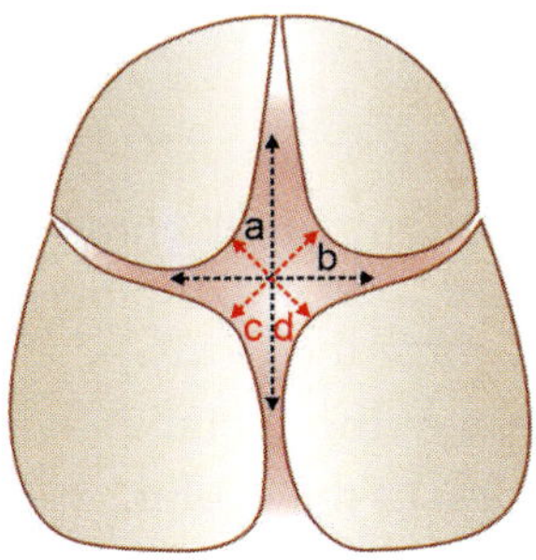

Anteroposterior (a) and transverse (b) diameters

$\frac{a+b}{2}$ =anterior fontanelle size

Diameters dimension of fontanelle

Note: Other method c × d (normal AF = 2.5 cm × 2.5 cm)

Delayed closure of anterior fontanelle—rickets/hypothyroidism/malnutrition/hydrocephalus/trisomy 13, 18 and 21 syndromes
Early closure of anterior fontanelle—craniosynostosis

Polydactyly associated with thumb or big toe are preaxial and those associated with little fingers are post-axial.

- **Thumb sign:** Ask the child to clench the fist with the thumb held inside the palm. The tip of the thumb protrudes past the ulnar border of the palm, e.g. Marfan syndrome.
- **Wrist sign:** The child can encircle his wrist by grasping it with the thumb and the 5th finger, it will overlap each other.
- **Blue sclera:** Osteogenesis imperfecta, glaucoma, marfan syndrome.
- **Proptosis:** (Forward protrusion of the eyeballs) retinoblastoma, thytoxicosis, orbital cellulitis.
- **Ptosis:** Turner/Noonan and Horner syndrome, MG, snake, bite, U/L—III N palsy.

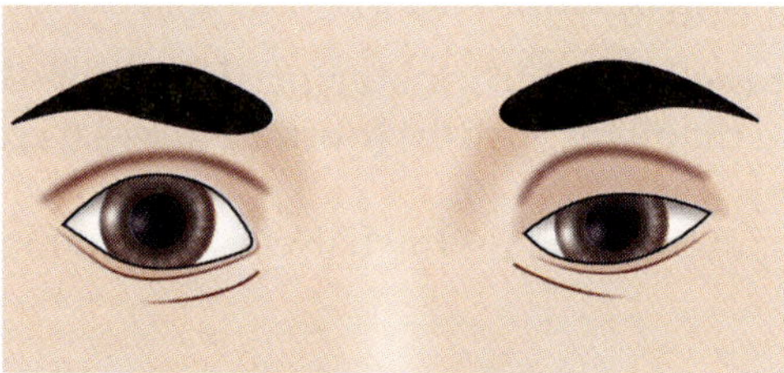

Ptosis in a child

- Normally only about 2 mm of the limbus of cornea is covered by the upper lid when the child looks straight. If more than >2 mm is covered consider ptosis.
- **Ectropion:** Eversion of the eyelid
- **Entropion:** Inversion of the eyelid.

Cystic Hygroma—Lymphangioma

- Appears early in life at lateral side of neck
- Unilocular/multilocular
- Thin, transparent cyst
- Compressible, nontender

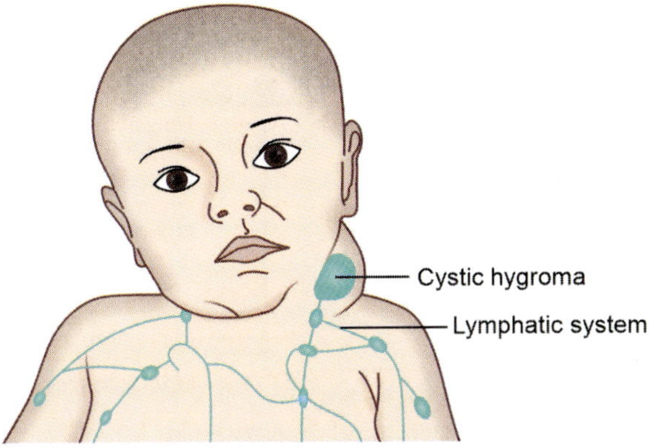

Cystic hygroma

- Donot resolve spontaneously
- Need surgical correction

Thyroglossal Cysts

- Midline of the neck
- On moving tongue out swelling moves upward
- On deglutition swelling moves upward as in thyroid gland swelling

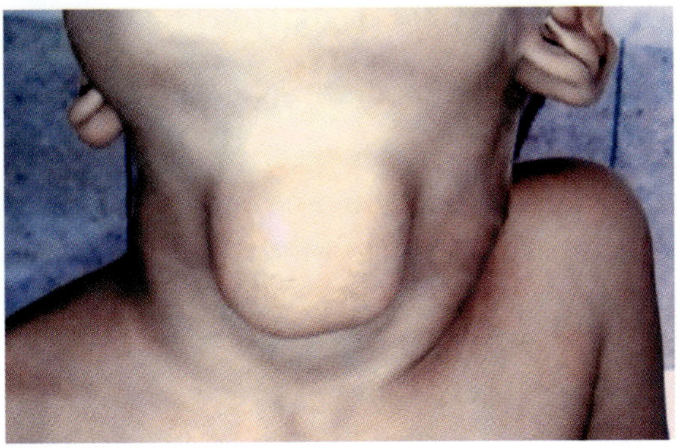

Thyroglossal cysts

- **Anotia:** Absence of ears
- **Microtia:** Incompletely formed external ear canal
- **Aural atresia:** Absence of ear canal
- **Aniridia:** Absence of IRIS, e.g. Wilms' tumour

- Microstomia and macrostomia

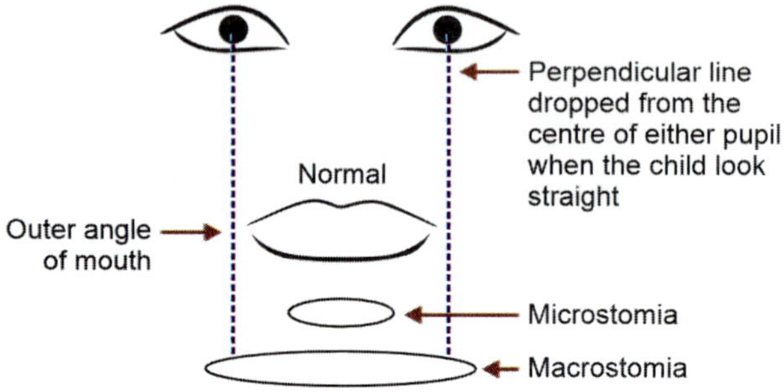

Micro- and macrostomia

- IRIS coloboma: Abscence of part of IRIS, e.g. charge syndrome
- LISCH nodules: Pigmented/non-pigmented elevated, dome shaped nodules in the IRIS, e.g. NF-I
- Brush field: Whitish speckling of IRIS (salt and peper speckling), e.g. Down syndrome
- Miosis: Seen in OP/barbiturate/opium poisoning, Horner's syndrome
- Mydriasis: Atropine, B/L III N palsy, ↑ICT
- Anophthalamia: Abscence of U/L or B/L eyeballs
- Lagophthalamus: Child unable to close eyes completely-hyperthyroidism.
- Enophthalamos: Recession of the eye balls, e.g. Horner's syndrome.

Doll's Eye Phenomenon (Oculo-cephalic Reflex)

- Turn the head suddenly to Rt, Lt, up, down—observe the movements of the eye ball—abscence of Doll's eye movement suggestive of increase ICT

KF RING Kayser-Fleischer Ring

- Greyish brown or golden ring
- Located at the limbus of cornea, e.g. Wilson disease

Strabismus (Squint)

- Nonparallelism of the visual axis in different field of gaze
- Convergent (ESOTROPIA)

- Divergent (EXOTROPIA)
- Seen in refractory errors/hereditary
- Physiological strabismus is common till 2 years of age
- Test to do:
  - Light reflex test
  - Red reflex test
  - Cover/uncover test

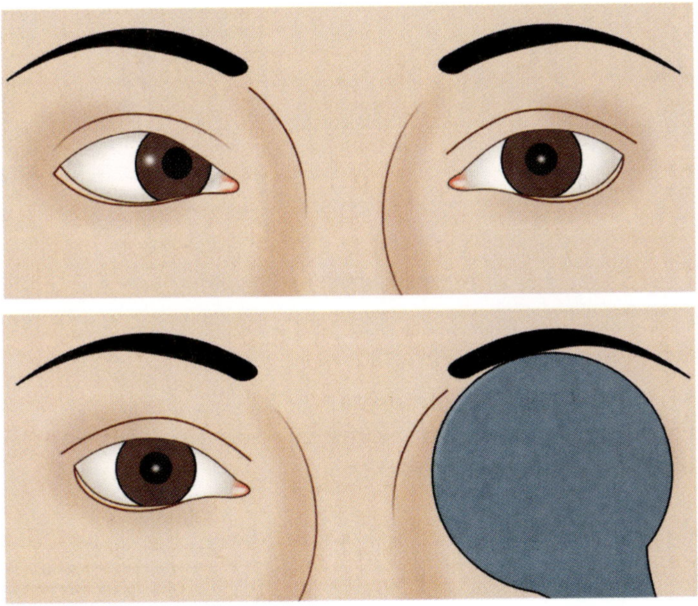

Strabismus—cover/uncover text

Nystagmus

- Rhythmic rapid movements of the eye balls
- Observe the eye balls at straight gaze for 5 sec then lateral gaze for 5 sec, e.g. cerebellar lesion

Normal Human Karyotype

- Consists of 22 pairs of autosomes and two sex chromosomes (total 46 chromosomes)
- Male 46, XY
- Female 46, XX

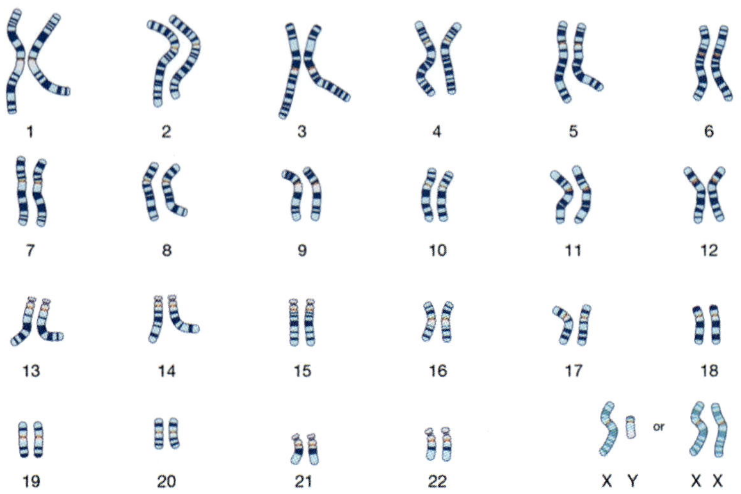

Normal human karyotype

Down Syndrome—Trisomy 21

- M/C chromosomal abnormal
- Extra-copy of chromosome 21 due to nondisjunction, translocation/mosaicism

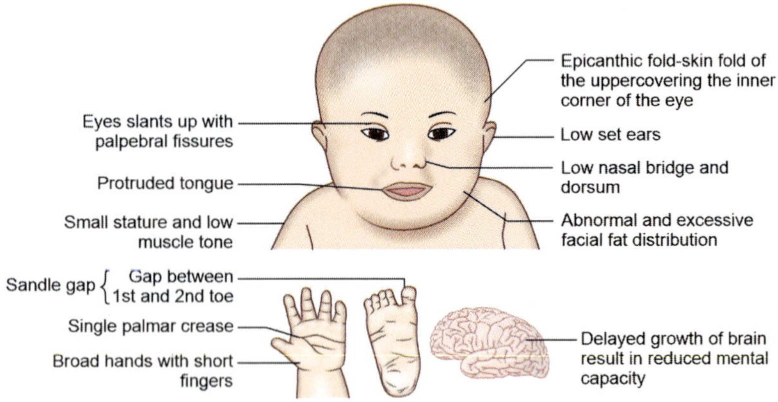

Down syndrome

Klinefelter Syndrome—47XXY

- Male born with an extra-copy of the X chromosome
- Meiotic nondisjunction of chromosome

Turner Syndrome—45X

- A female born with only one X chromosome (monosomy)

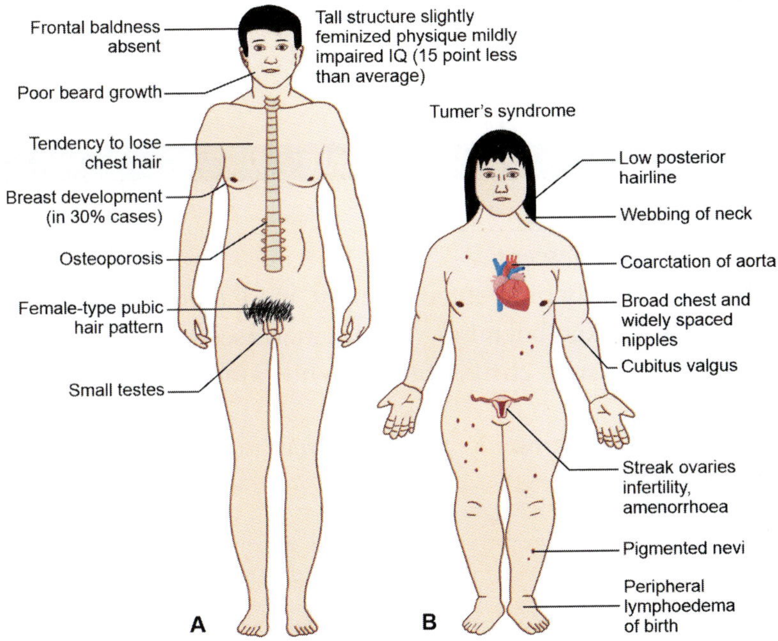

(A) Klinefelter syndrome; (B) Turner syndrome

CHAPTER

9

Sexual Maturity Rating: (SMR): Tanner Staging

SMR—FEMALE

PUBIC HAIR

Stage I: Preadolescent

Stage II: Lightly pigmented, straight, medial border of labia

Stage III: Darker, beginning to curl, increased amount

Stage IV: Coarse, curly, abundant but amount less than in adult

Stage V: Adult feminine triangle, spread to medial surface of thighs

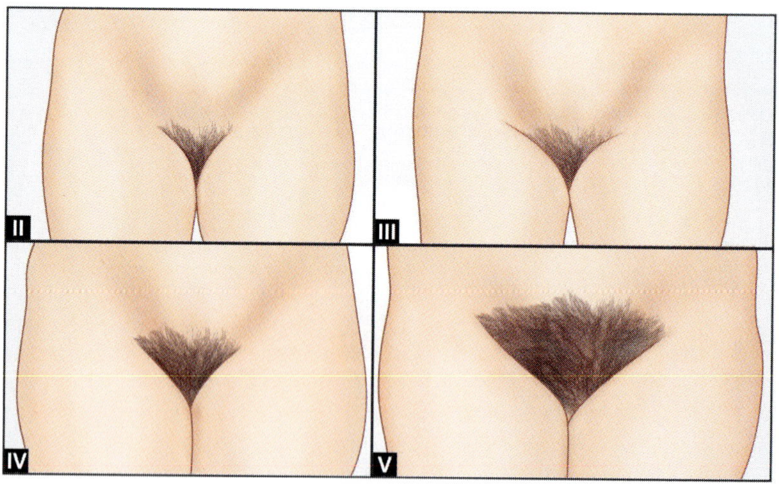

Female sex maturity—pubic hair

BREAST DEVELOPMENT

Stage I: Preadolescent

Stage II: Breast and papilla elevated as small mound; areolar diameter increased

Stage III: Breast and areola enlarged, no contour separation

Stage IV: Areola and papilla form secondary mound

Stage V: Mature, nipple projects, areola part of general breast contour

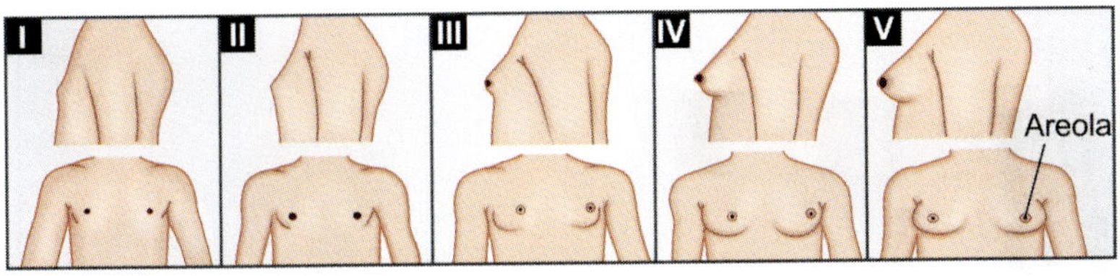

Female sex maturity—breast

SMR—MALE

Stage	Pubic hair	Scrotum/testicular volume	Penis
Stage I	Preadolescent	Preadolescent (<4 ml)	Preadolescent
Stage II	Scanty, straight, slightly pigmented	Scrotum, pink, texture altered (4–10 ml)	Enlarged
Stage III	Darker, starts to curl, small amount	Larger (10–15 ml)	Longer
Stage IV	Resembles adult type but less in quantity; coarse, curly	Larger, scrotum dark (15–20 ml)	Larger glans and breadth increase in size
Stage V	Adult distribution, spread to medial surface of thighs	Adult size (>20 ml)	Adult size

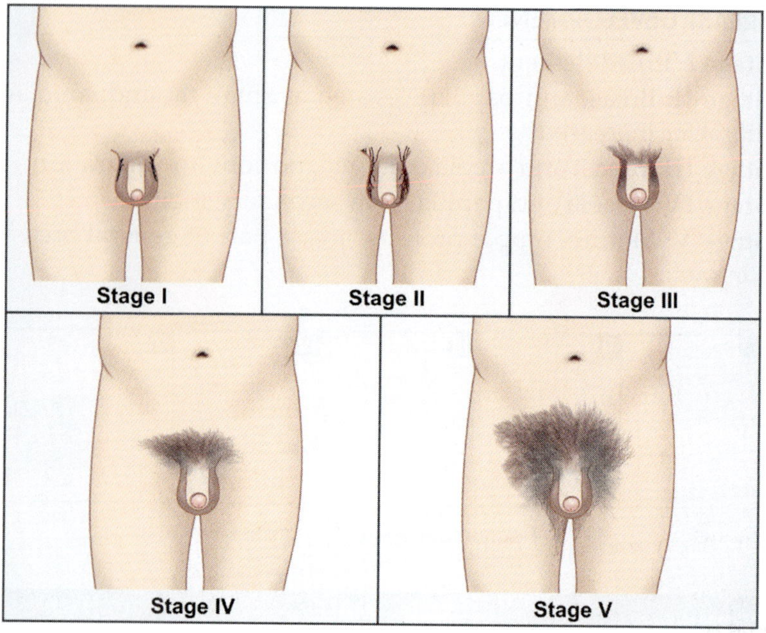

Male sex maturity—pubic hair, scrotum and penis

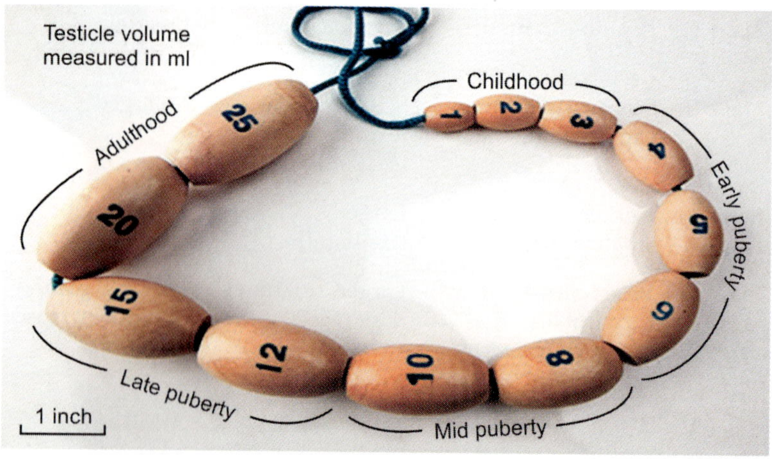

Orchidometer

In male growth spurt—stages III and IV
In female growth spurt—stages II and III

Female 2nd sexual character sequence is:
Thelarche–Pubarche–Menarche (TPM)
Male 2nd sexual character sequence is: **Testicular enlargement—pubic hairs–axillary hairs–facial hairs, Penile enlargement—spermarche**

Delayed puberty: No 2nd sexual character in female by 13 years (or no menarche by 16 years) and in male by 14 years.

Precocious puberty: In girls, thelarche before 8 years and menarche before 10 years of age. **In boys**, pubertal onset before 9.5 years.

For **bone age estimation (<8 years)** take left wrist X-ray
Age (year) = Number of ossification centres in wrist-1
She looks too pretty, try to catch her
Medial to lateral (ossification at **age in year**)
Scaphoid(**5**)/lunate(**4**)/triquetral (**3**)/pisiform (**12**)
trapezium (**5**)/trapezoid (**5**)/capitate (**1**)/hamate (**1**)

Gynecomastia

- Presence of glandular breast tissue >1 cm in males
- Physiological in the adolescents and elderly

Disorders of Sex Development (DSD)

Group of conditions where the genetic sex of the baby does not match with clinical phenotype, e.g. congenital adrenal hyperplasia (most common) 46, XX.

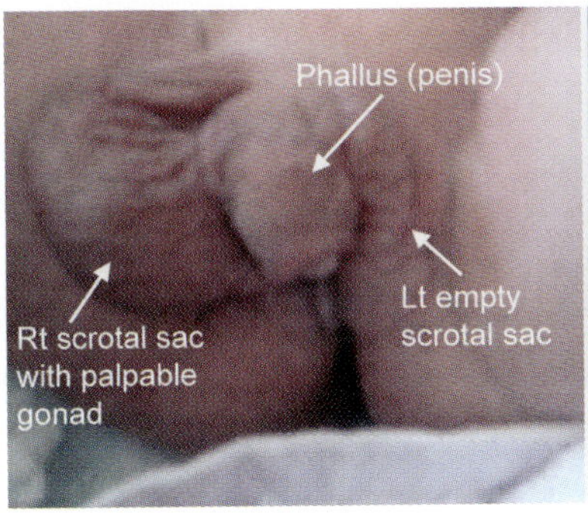

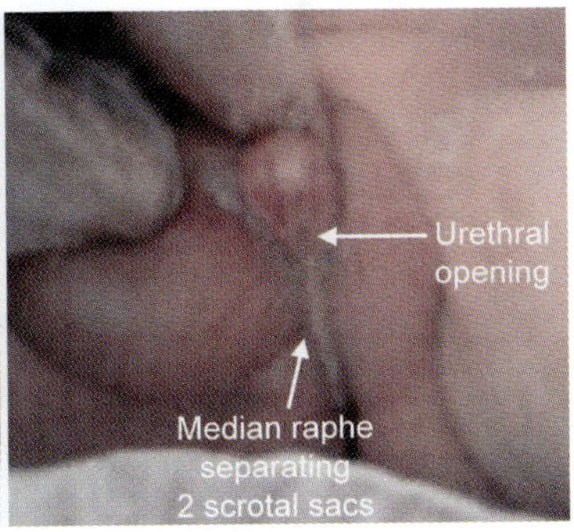

Micropenis

Length of phallus <2.5 SD (<2 cm at birth).

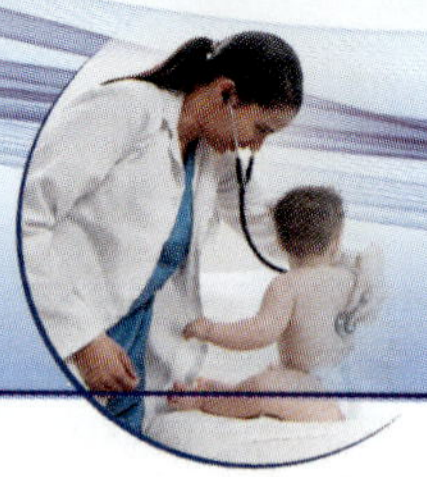

CHAPTER

10

Skin Diseases

DEFINITIONS OF SKIN LESIONS

- **Exanthem:** Eruption of the skin
- **Enanthem:** Eruption of mucosa
- **Macule:** Flat nonpalpable area of altered colour or texture.
- **Papule:** Small palpable lesion <0.5 cm in diameter
- **Nodule:** Large palpable lesion >0.5 cm in diameter
- **Vesicle:** Small fluid filled lesion <0.5 cm in diameter
- **Bullae:** Large fluid filled lesions >0.5 cm in diameter
- **Pustule:** A visible accumulation of pus in the skin
- **Petechiae:** Skin bleed <2 mm
- **Purpura:** Skin bleed 2–10 mm
- **Ecchymosis:** Skin bleed >10 mm
- **Telangiectasia:** Dilatation of superficial blood vessels.
- **Wheal:** Elevation of the skin caused by acute oedema of the dermis.
- **Erosion:** Partial loss of epidermis which heals without scarring.
- **Ulcer:** Discontinuity in the full thickness of the epidermis.
- **Sinus:** A small opening in a cavity through which it drains out.
- **Fissure:** Linear slit in the skin due to loss of epidermis and dermis as found in eczema.

- **Burrows:** Short, linear, elevation of the epidermis, characteristic of scabies disease.

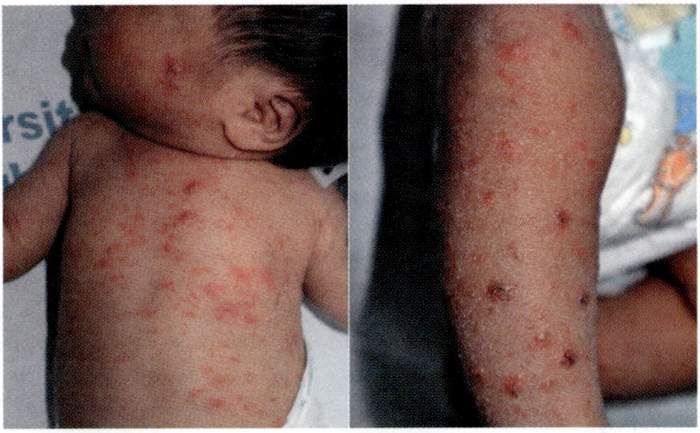

Scabies

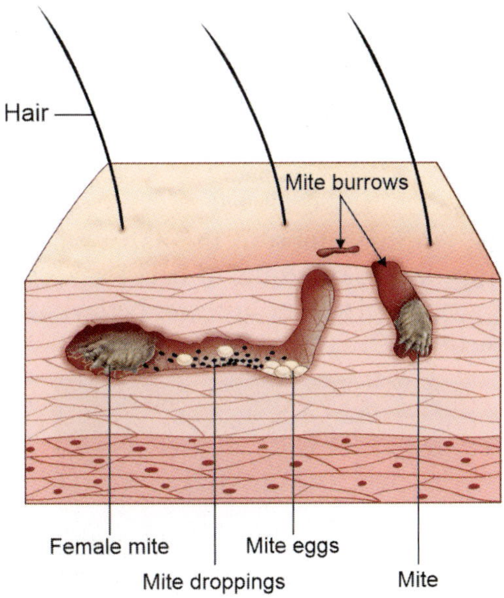

Burrows

- **Erythema nodosum:** Painful, tender, red nodules, mostly seen over the skin. Fade over few weeks leaving bruises seen in—TB, IBD, lymphogranuloma venereum, Behçet's disease.

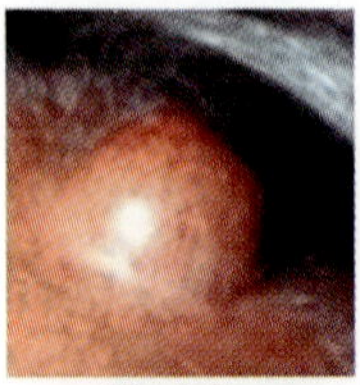
Nodule

Cyst

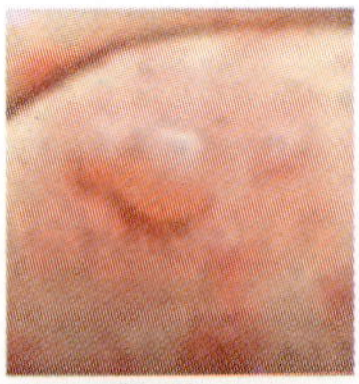
Bullae

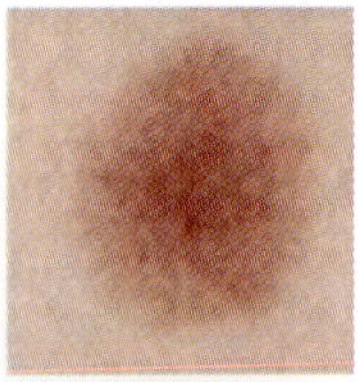
Macule

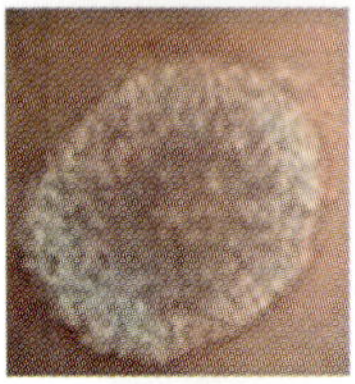
Plaque

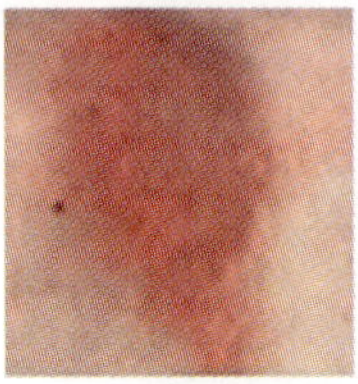
Wheal

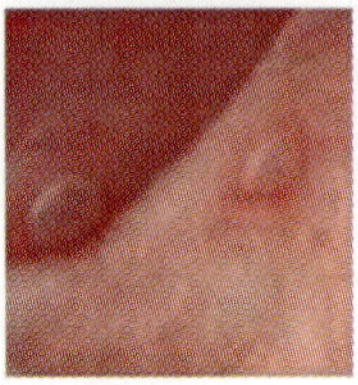
Vesicle

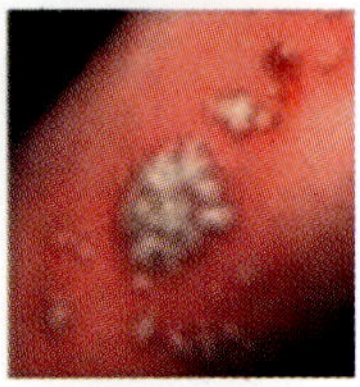
Pustule

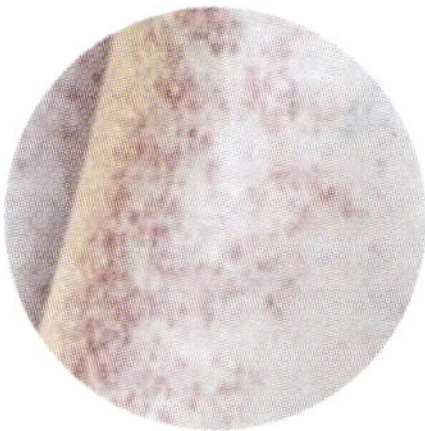
Petechiae (<2 mm)

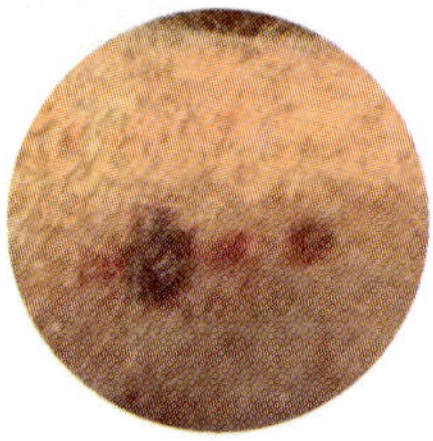
Purpura (2–10 mm)

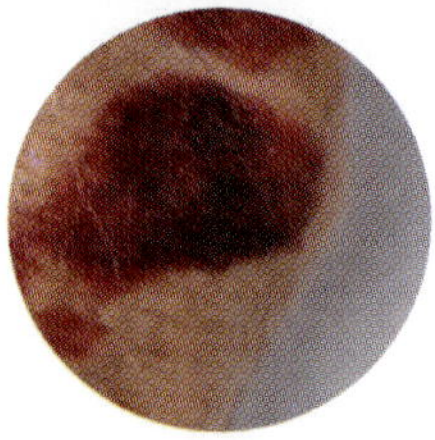
Ecchymosis (>1 cm)

- **Pediculosis:** An infestation of the hairy part of the body with the eggs, larvae or adults of lice. Rx—1% permethrin medicated soap, malathion, linoane, benzyl alcohol rarely oral ivermectin.

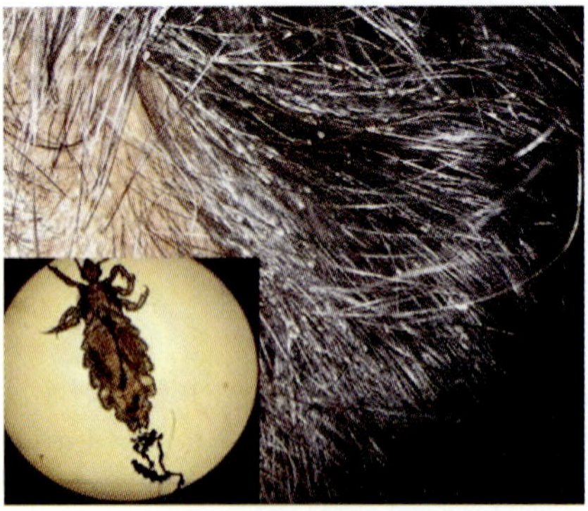
Pediculosis with lice

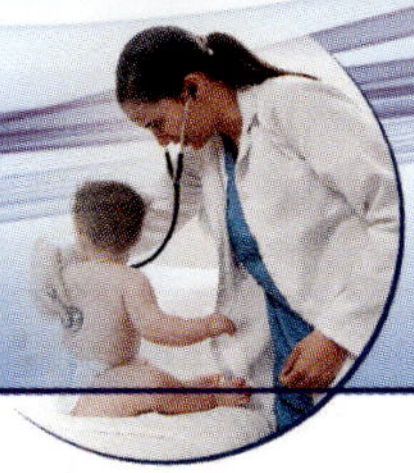

CHAPTER

11

Respiratory System

HISTORY AND GENERAL EXAMINATION

UPPER RESPIRATORY TRACT EXAMINATION

- Nose-discharge/bleed/DNS/turbinates
- Cottle test:
  - To check nasal obstruction due to abnormality of nasal valve
  - Check is drawn laterally while child breathes quietly, if child's breathing improves—the test is positive
- Paranasal sinuses—tenderness (maxillary/frontal/ethmoid)
  - Frontal sinus: Palpate below the lower border of eyebrow (floor of frontal sinus)

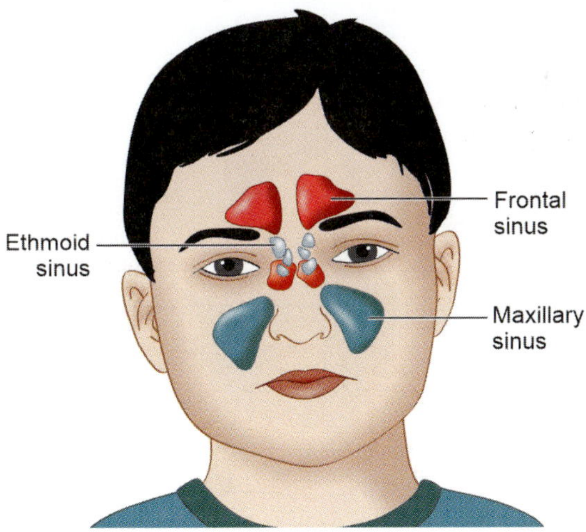

Paranasal sinuses

- Ethmoid sinus: Palpate between root of nose and medial canthus
- Maxillary sinus: Palpate canine fossa/maxillary area

- Throat-tonsils/pharynx (peritonsillar abscess, quinsy, PND)
- Ear: Look for any discharge, examine tympanic membrane with otoscope

For Ear Examination
Newborn and infants: Pull the pinna of the ear with thumb and index finger towards downward and laterally
Older children: Upward and backward.

LOWER RESPIRATORY TRACT

Trachea can be surface marked anteriorly from the cricoid cartilage to the sternal angle and posteriorly from the C6 to T4 vertebrae; thereafter; trachea is divided into two principal bronchi (carina).

Inspection

- Respiratory rate/rhythm (regular/irregular)/character
- Type—abdominal/thoraco-abdominal/abdominothoracic
- Audible sounds—grunt/stridor/wheeze

1. Shape of the chest:
   Normal: Circular/cylindrical
   Barrel: Emphysema
   Funnel: Rickets

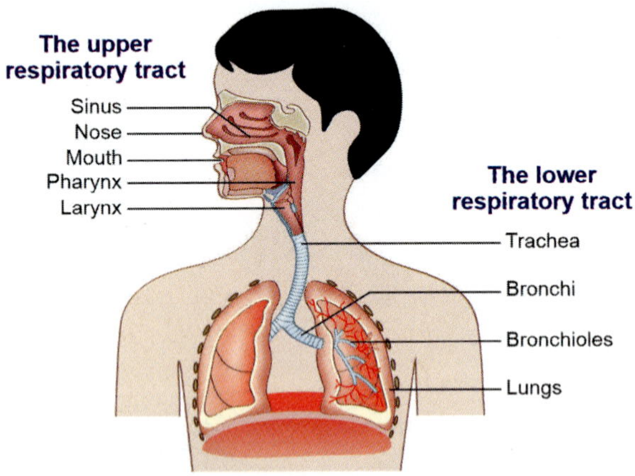

Schematic diagram of respiratory tract

2. Symmetry of the chest—B/L symmetrical/asymmetrical.
3. Trachea—appears to be central/deviated to side (trail sign).
4. Use of accessory muscle/flaring of alar nasi/intercostals indrawing/subcostal retraction/suprasternal retraction
5. Apex beat appears to be in 4th (<3 years)/5th ICS medial to mid clavicular line.
6. Drooping of shoulder/supraclavicular hollowing/infraclavicular flattening/infrascapular wasting/crowding of ribs
7. Spine appears to be central/scoliosis or kyphosis
8. Visible scars/sinuses/dilated veins/pulsations
9. Movement appears to be equal B/L or diminished in:

Areas of lung
Supraclavicular
Infraclavicular (up to level of 2nd rib)
Mammary (up to level of 5th rib)
Inframammary
Axillary (up to level of 4th rib)
Infra-axillary
Suprascapular
Interscapular
Infrascapular areas.

Palpation

1. Trachea confirmed to be central/deviated to__ side (trail sign).
2. Apex beat confirmed to be in 4th/5th ICS medial to mid clavicular line.
3. Movement are equal B/L or diminished in ______________ area.
4. Vocal fremitus—tell child to repeat 99-99-99—are equal B/L or diminished in____________area.
5. Bony/intercostal tenderness
6. Palpable—rub/rhonchi/crepitation

7. Measurement

AP diameter ______ cm
T diameter ______ cm
Chest circumference ______cm
Chest expansion ______cm (normal 2–5 cm)
Hemithorax ______cm
Hemithorax expansion ______cm

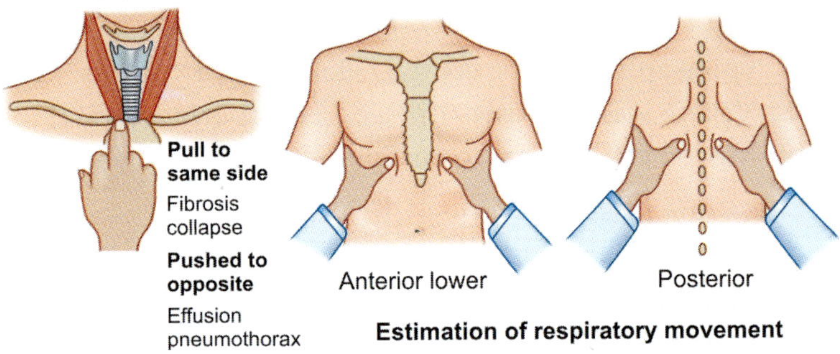

Estimation of respiratory movement

Percussion

1. Resonant/impaired/hyperresonant note/dull/stony dull in supraclavicular/infraclavicular/mammary/inframammary/axillary/infra-axillary/suprascapular/interscapular/infrascapular areas
2. Upper border of liver corresponds to right 5th ICS
3. Liver span ___ cm
4. Left heart border corresponds to apex beat
5. Right heart border corresponds to right lateral border of sternum
6. Specific test if indicated—shifting dullness/tidal percussion (liver dullness varies with respiration)/Traube's space (crescent shape)
   - Upper border: Left 6th Rib
   - Lateral: Left anterior axillary line
   - Inferior Left costal margin
   - It overlies the fundus of the stomach, hence normally tympanic on percussion. If dull suspect, PE, splenomegaly

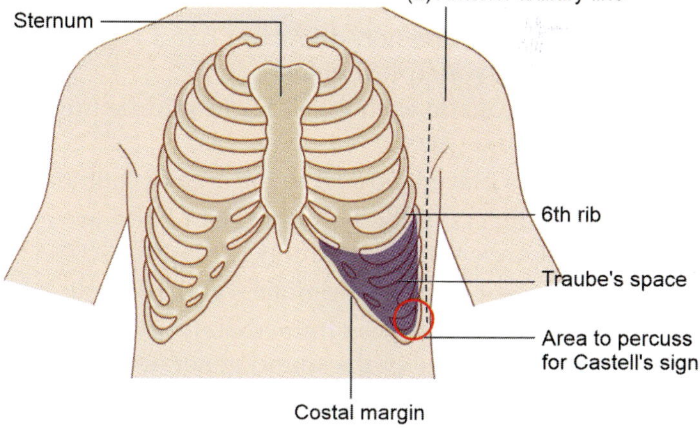

Auscultation

Auscultate anteriorly from above the clavicle down to the 6th rib, laterally from the axilla to the 8th Rib, posteriorly down to the level of the 11th rib.

1. Character of breath sounds-—vesicular/bronchial
2. Intensity of breath sounds—normal/diminished/high in ___ area
3. Adventitious sounds—crepitation (during inspiration)/ rhonchi (during exp)/pleural rub (both during Ins/Exp) heard in ______area.
4. Vocal resonance—are normal/increased/diminished in _______________area. Bronchophony (increase in the intensing and clarity of spoken words heard when auscultating the lungs, e.g. consolidation pneumonia)/whispering pectoriloquy (whispered words are heard clearly when auscultating the lungs, e.g. consolidation, pneumonia, lung tumors, bronchopulmonary fistula)/aegophony (E to A change, e.g. area above PE, consolidation).
5. Specific test—coin test (friction test—pneumothorax)/ succussion splash (hydro-pneumothorax)

Rules of Percussion

1. Middle finger of the non-dominant hand is placed firmly over the chest wall (pleximeter)
2. Percussion is made with the index or middle finger of the dominant hand (plexor)
3. Pleximeter is placed parallel to the area of dullness.
4. The other fingers of the non-dominant hand are lifted off to avoid dampening of vibration.
5. The movement of stroke originates at the wrist joint.
6. Plexor should be removed immediately after the stroke off to avoid dampening of the sound generated.
7. Clavicle is percussed directly.
8. Percussion must proceed from a resonant area to a dull area.
9. Corresponding areas of both sides are to be percussed and compared.
10. For percussing axillary area, tell child to keep his hands above the head and for scapular area over his opposite shoulders, crossing the arms in front of the chest.

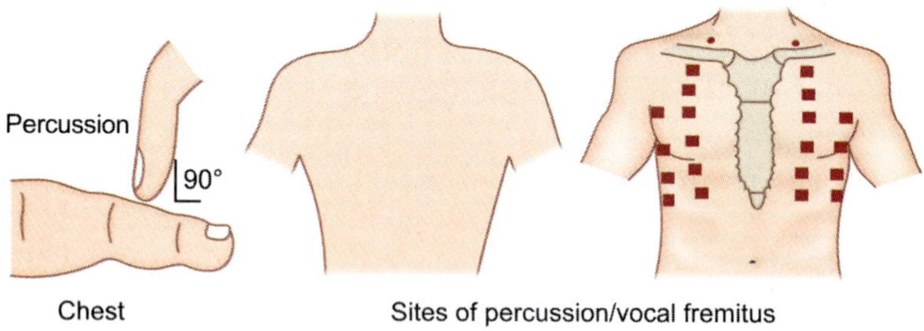

Sites of percussion/vocal fremitus

Grunt	Expiration through partially closed glottis to raise end expiratory pressure (PEEP)
Hyperpnoea	Abnormally deep respiration
Hypopnoea	Abnormally shallow respiration

Contd.

Dyspnoea	Difficulty in breathing
Orthopnoea	Difficulty in breathing in recumbent position
Platypnoea	Difficulty in breathing in upright position
Paroxysmal nocturnal dyspnoea (PND)	Sudden onset of severe dyspnoea with cough and wheezing at midnight in deep sleep relieved by standing upright near good ventilation suggestive of acute left ventricular failure
Stridor	Due to extrathoracic obstruction
Wheeze	Due to intrathoracic obstruction

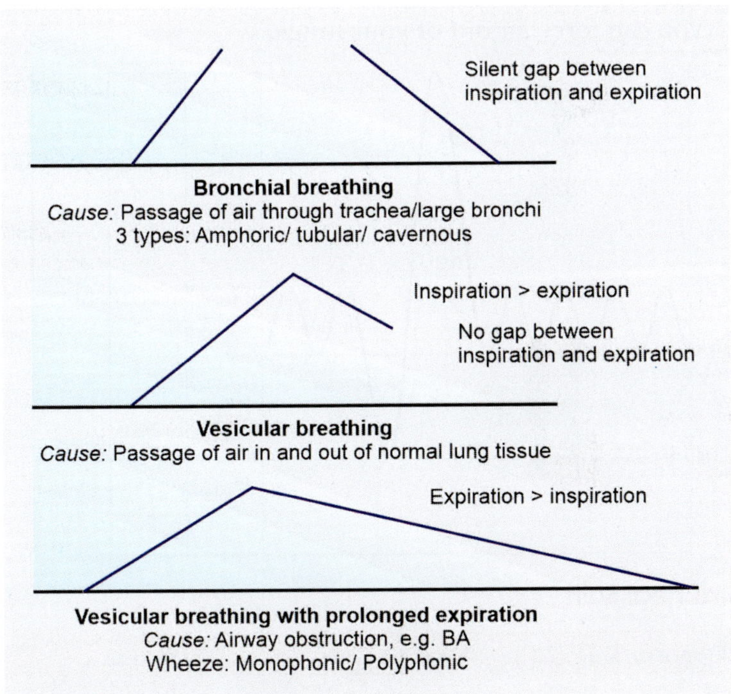

LUNG/PULMONARY FUNCTION TEST

- **Tidal volume (VT):** Volume of air inhaled or exhaled during normal breathing.
- **Vital capacity (VC):** Total volume of air that can be exhaled after inhaling as much as you can.

- **Functional residual capacity (FRC):** Volume of air left in lungs after exhaling normally.
- **Residual volume (RV):** Volume of air left in the lungs after exhaling as much as you can.
- **Total lung capacity:** Total volume of air in the lungs after a maximum inspiration.
- **Forced vital capacity (FVC):** This is the amount of air exhaled forcefully and quickly after inhaling as much as you can.
- **Forced expiratory volume (FEV_1):** This is the amount of air expired during the first second.
- **Peak expiratory flow rate (PEFR):** This is the fastest rate that you can force air out of your lungs.

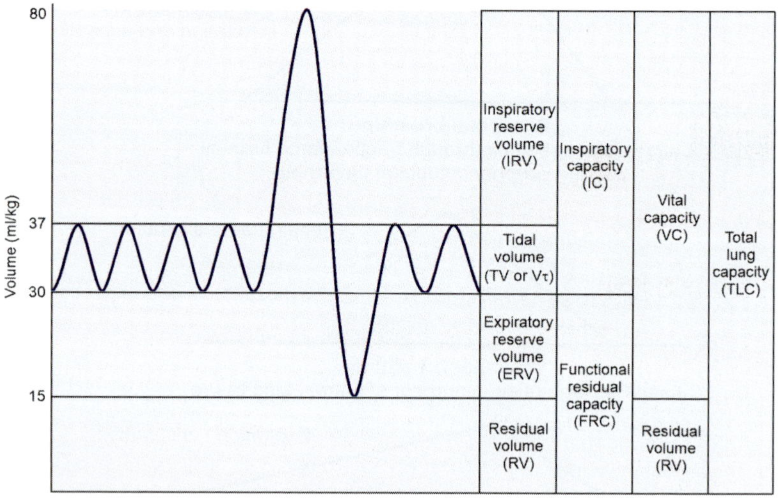

Tracheal Shift

Opposite side	No shift	Same side
Pleural effusion	Consolidation	Collapse
Empyema	Emphysema	Fibrosis
Pneumothorax	Bronchiectasis	
Hydropneumothorax	Bronchial asthma	

Vocal Fremitus

Increased	Absent	Decreased
Consolidation	Pleural effusion	Bronchial asthma
	Pneumothorax	
	Collapse	
	Fibrosis	

Percussion Note

Hyper-resonant	Pneumothorax, bronchial asthma
Resonant	Normal
Impaired/dull	Consolidation Collapse Fibrosis
Stony dull	Pleural effusion Massive collapse/consolidation Solid tumours

Auscultation

Vesicular	Normal
Bronchial	Consolidation Collapse
Bronchovesicular	Bronchial asthma Emphysema

Vocal Resonance

Increased	Absent	Decreased
Consolidation	Collapse Fibrosis	Pleural effusion Empyema, BA Pneumothorax Hydropneumothorax

ACUTE RESPIRATORY INFECTION (ARI) CONTROL PROGRAMME

Classification	Clinical features	Treatment	Place of treatment
No pneumonia	• Cough • No fast breathing • No chest in drawing • Feeding well	Treat like URI. No anti-biotics	Home
Pneumonia	• Cough • Fast breathing • Lower chest indrawing • Drinking well	Oral antibiotics	Home/health care centre Reassess after two days and manage accordingly
Severe pneumonia	• Cyanosis • Fast breathing • Chest indrawing • Not able to drink	Oxygen IV antibiotics	Admit in hospital Assess once daily
Very severe pneumonia	• Cyanosis • Severe respiratory distress • Lethargy/excessive drowsiness/ convulsions	Oxygen IV antibiotics IV fluids	Admit in hospital Assess twice daily

WHO CLASSIFICATION OF PNEUMONIA

There are now just 2 categories of pneumonia:

1. Pneumonia which is treated at home with oral amoxicillin/ cotrimoxazole
2. Severe pneumonia (increase RR , chest indrawing, presence of danger signs) which requires injectable antibiotics.

ASSESSMENT OF ASTHMA SEVERITY

Asthma is a chronic inflammatory disorder characterized by narrowing of airways.

Component of severity	Intermittent	Mild persistent	Moderate persistent	Severe persistent
Day time symptoms	<2 days/ week	>2 days/ week but not daily	Daily	Throughout the day

Contd.

Component of severity	Intermittent	Mild persistent	Moderate persistent	Severe persistent
Nighttime symptoms	<2 times/ month	>2 times/ month	>1 time/ week	Frequent 7 times a week
PEFR%/FEV1	>80%	>80%	60–80%	<60%
PEFR%/FEV1 variability	<20% diurnal variation	20–30% diurnal variation	>30% diurnal variation	>30% diurnal variation
SABA use	<2 days/ week	>2 days/ week but not daily	Daily	>Twice daily
Exacerbations requiring systemic corticosteroids	<1/year	>4 episodes in a <5-year-old child >2 episodes in a >5-year- old child		

Note: PEFR could be done for child >5 years.

CBC in BA

ANC (absolute eosinophil count)

Chest X-ray in BA

- Hyperinflation
- Atelectasis
- Bronchial cuffing

Step up and step down approach in the management of bronchial asthma

Classification	Rx (step)	Medications
Intermittent	1	No ICS , SABA as needed
Mild persistent	2	Low dose ICS, SABA as needed
Moderate persistent	3	Medium dose ICS, + LABA
Severe persistent	4	High dose ICS/oral corticosteroid + LABA

- ICS: Inhaled corticosteroids (budesonide/fluticasone)
- SABA: Short-acting beta agonists (salbutamol/terbutaline)
- LABA: Long-acting beta agonists (salmeterol/formoterol)

DIFFERENCES BETWEEN TRANSUDATES AND EXUDATES PLEURAL EFFUSION

Features	Transudates	Exudates
Appearance	Clear/straw color	Cloudy/opalescent
Protein	<30 g/L	>30 g/L
Specific gravity	<1.015	>1.015
Glucose	>40 mg/dl	<40 mg/dl
LDH	<200 IU/L	>200 IU/L
WBC	<1000/mm^3	>1000/mm^3
Pathogenesis	Increased hydrostatic or decreased oncotic pressure	Inflammation or infiltration
Causes	CCF, NS, cirrhosis of liver	Pneumonia Tuberculosis Empyema

Note: Light's criteria for pleural effusion:

	Transudates	Exudates
Protein Pleural/serum	≤0.5	>0.5
LDH Pleural/serum	≤0.6 Pleural LDH ≤2/3rd upper limit of normal serum LDH	>0.6 Pleural LDH >2/3rd upper limit of normal serum LDH

Bobbling of Head

Movement of head synchronous with breathing as seen in severe respiratory distress.

Pediatric Respiratory Severity Score (PRESS)

Score component	Operational definition	Scoring
RR	RR at rest, on room air according to age	0–1
Wheezing	Presence or absence	0–1
Accessory muscle use	Any visible use of accessory muscle	0–1

Contd.

Score component	Operational definition	Scoring
SPO_2	>95% or <95%	0–1
Feeding prob	Yes/No	0–1
Press score	Mild Moderate Severe	0–1 2–3 4–5

History of Contact with Tuberculosis

- Is difined as any household with sputum positive or taking ATT or have taken ATT in the past 2 years

Test to Diagnose Tuberculosis

- CBC (↑TLC, ↑L), ↑ESR
- Sputum—AFB/culture (L–J medium)/fluorescence microscopy
- CBNAAT (cartridge based nucleic acid amplification test)
- Mantoux test
- Chest X-ray/CT scan

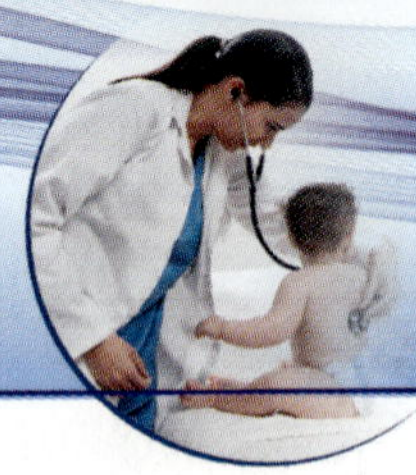

CHAPTER

12

Coronavirus Disease

Coronavirus disease-19 (COVID-19) is the infectious disease caused by the coronavirus, SARS-CoV-2 (RNA), which is a respiratory pathogen.

Most children infected with the virus will experience mild-to-moderate respiratory illness and recover without requiring special treatment. However, some will become seriously ill and require medical attention. Children with underlying medical conditions like cardiovascular disease, diabetes, chronic respiratory disease, or cancer are more likely to develop serious illness. Anyone can get sick with COVID-19 and become seriously ill or die at any age.

MODES OF SPREAD

Coronavirus mainly spread through respiratory droplets or aerosols even though some suggest air pollution particles could help coronavirus travel further in the air.

The virus can spread from an infected person's mouth or nose in small liquid particles when they cough, sneeze, speak, sing or breathe. These particles range from larger respiratory droplets to smaller aerosols.

Hands touch many surfaces and can pick up viruses. Once contaminated, hands can transfer the virus to eyes, nose or mouth. From there, the virus can enter and infect.

Incubation period: 2–14 days

Infective period: 2 days before the onset of symptoms to 14 days after.

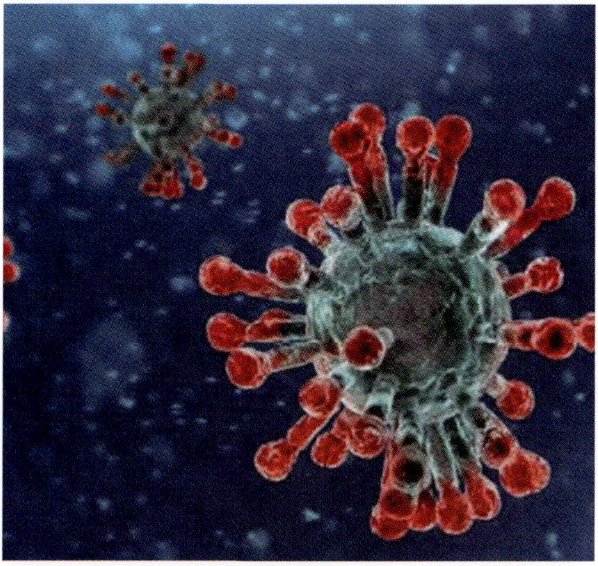

Coronavirus

Entry through: Eyes, nose and mouth.

Pathogenesis: The moment corona virus enters into the body, its spike protein connect with ACE2 receptors found on the surface of our cells. ACE2 receptors are found in many organs of the body. Once the virus enters the cell, it turns the cells into a factory, making millions of copies of coronavirus. Hyperactive immune response results in cytokine storm.

Coronavirus typically attacks respiratory system but can damage any organ.

Clinical Features

- Asymptomatic/presymptomatic and mild-to-moderate illness constitute >80% of cases.
- Most of the children present with URTI.

Most Common Symptoms

- Fever
- Dry cough
- Fatigue

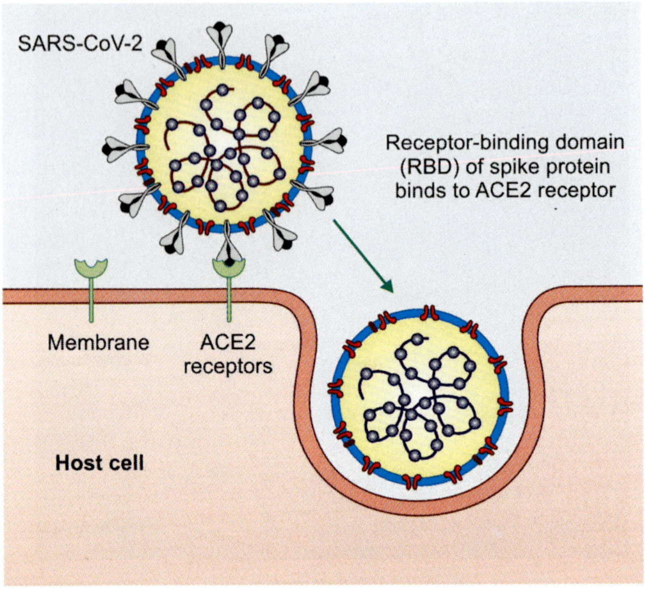

COVID-19: Pathogenesis

Less Common Symptoms

- Decreased appetite
- irritability
- Loss of taste or smell
- Nasal congestion
- Conjunctivitis (also known as red eyes)
- Sore throat
- Headache
- Muscle or joint pain
- Different types of skin rash
- Nausea or vomiting
- Diarrhoea
- Chills or dizziness

Severe Symptoms

- Shortness of breath
- Loss of appetite
- Confusion

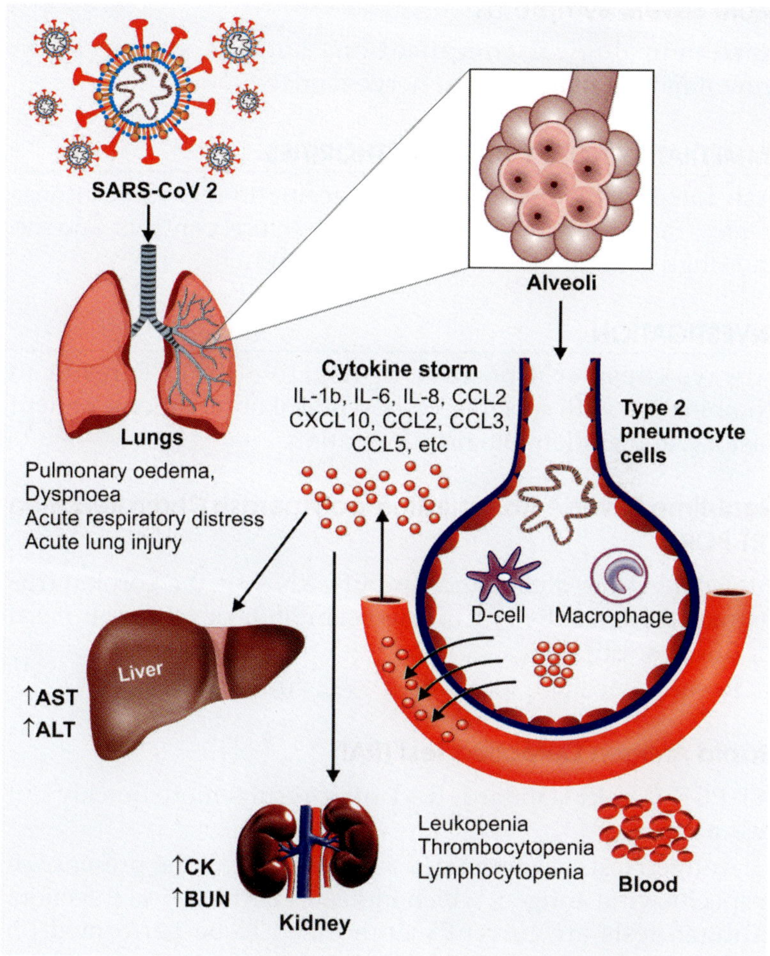

Coronavirus attacks on various systems of our body

- Persistent pain or pressure in the chest
- High temperature (>38°C)
- Irritability
- Reduced consciousness (sometimes associated with seizures)
- Anxiety
- Depression
- Sleep disorders

More Severe Symptoms

Rare neurological complications such as stroke, brain inflammation, delirium and nerve damage.

IMMEDIATELY NOTIFY TO THE AUTHORITIES

Ask for past history of illness/vaccination/chronic illness if any/family history/travel history/close contacts and do thorough general /systemic examination.

INVESTIGATION

Always consider a positive or negative RT-PCR result in combination with specimen type, clinical observations, patient history, and epidemiologic information.

Real-time Reverse Transcription-polymerase Chain Reaction (RT-PCR)

Molecular tests detect and amplify RNA of the coronavirus extracted from saliva or mucus (sample taken through nasal or throat swab).

Results—positive for SARS-CoV-2 viral RNA

Rapid Antigen Detection Test (RAT)

RT-PCR is gold standard, RAT offer results more quickly but less accurate.

Antigen tests are immunoassays that detect the presence of a specific viral antigen, which indicates current viral infection. Antigen tests are currently authorized to be performed on nasopharyngeal, nasal swab, or saliva. Specimens placed directly into the assay's extraction buffer or reagent.

Results—positive for SARS-CoV-2 virus antigen.

Antibody Tests

Also known as a serology test, can detect IgG/IgM antibodies to SARS-CoV-2 in blood, can be taken at home or anywhere, are easy to use, and produce rapid results.

Interpretation—positive for SARS-CoV-2 virus antibodies

Antibody test not recommended

- If you have a current infection.
- If you have immunity to SARS-CoV-2 following COVID-19 vaccination.
- Whether you need to get a booster following COVID-19 vaccination.
- Whether you need to quarantine after a known or suspected exposure to COVID-19.

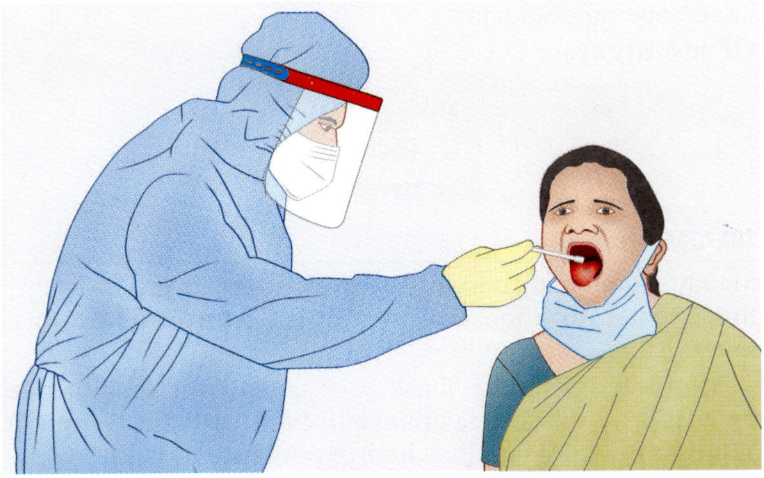

RT-PCR test

Other Investigations

CBC: Lymphopenia, leukocytosis, leukopenia, thrombocytopenia, decreased eosinophils, decreased haemoglobin.

Pulse oximeter: Decreased SpO_2

ABG: May show low partial oxygen pressure

LFT/KFT/electrolytes: Elevated liver enzymes, elevated total bilirubin, renal impairment, hypoalbuminemia, electrolyte derangements.

Thyroid function test: Elevated TSH, low free T_3/T_4

Blood glucose level: Hypo/hyperglycaemia

Serum LDH/ESR/CRP/ferritin/procalcitonin: Elevated in severe illness

Serum- IL-6/amyloid A level/ CK/myoglobin: Elevated in severe illness

Coagulation profile: Elevated D-dimer, prolonged prothrombin time, elevated fibrinogen, prolonged INR

Blood and sputum cultures: Negative for bacterial infection

Chest X-ray: Ground-glass opacity, consolidation

CT scan: B/L peripheral patchy ground glass opacities with lower lobe predominant.

CT severity score

<8	Mild
9–15	Moderate
>15	Severe

TREATMENT

Mainly symptomatic and supportive. Rest, isolation, paracetamol, fluids, good nutrition, oxygen that is all you need except in severe cases.

Most of the drugs previously used are now not recommended by WHO as remdesivir, favipiravir (Fabi-flu), tamiflu, ivermectin, azithromycin, doxycycline, hydroxychloroquine, chloroquine, convalescent plasma, lopinavir-ritonavir combination, long-term use of vit C, zinc.

Recommended drugs are:

- Corticosteroids
- Low-molecular-weight heparin
- 2-Deoxy glucose (2-dG)
- Immunomodulators
- Cytokine-based therapies

PREVENTION

1. Maintain at least a 1–2 metres distance
   The farther away, the better.
2. Make wearing a mask a routine.
   N95 mask is the best but can use any triple layer mask.

3. Avoid the 3Cs: Spaces that are closed, crowded or involve close contact.
4. Do not forget the basics of good hygiene.

   Regularly and thoroughly clean your hands with an alcohol-based hand rub or wash them with soap and water for minimum of 20 seconds.
5. Avoid touching your eyes, nose and mouth.
6. Clean and disinfect surfaces frequently especially those which are regularly touched, such as door handles, faucets and phone screens.
7. Stay home and self-isolate even if you have minor symptoms such as cough, headache, mild fever, until you recover.
8. Both isolation and quarantine are methods of preventing the spread of the disease.
9. Reject infodemics/fake news.
10. Get vaccinated. (Vaccine against coronavirus is discussed in Chapter 4: Immunization; pages 30–31)

COMPLICATIONS

1. Mental trauma—COVID-19 and its negative impact on mental health-shadow pandemic
2. Increased blood viscosity
3. Persistent hypoxia
4. Post-COVID syndrome
7. MODS
8. Multisystem inflammatory diseases (MIS-C)

MULTISYSTEM INFLAMMATORY SYNDROME IN CHILDREN (MIS-C)

Also known as paediatric post-COVID-19 inflammatory syndrome is a condition where different body parts can become inflamed, including the heart, lungs, kidneys, brain, skin, eyes, or gastrointestinal organs in a child with h/o COVID-19 and no other plausible diagnosis.

Diagnostic Criteria

Diagnostic criteria MIS-C

- Children and adolescents 0–19 years of age with fever ≥3 days

AND two of three

- Rash or bilateral, non-purulent conjunctivitis or mucocutaneous inflammation signs (oral, hands or feet)
- Hypotension or shock
- Features of myocardial dysfunction pancarditis, valvulae, or coronary abnormalities (including ECHO findings or elevated troponin/NT-pro BNP)
- Evidence of coagulopathy (by PT, PTT, elevated D-dimers)
- Acute gastrointestinal problems (diarrhoea vomiting, or abdominal pain)

AND

- Elevated markers of inflammation such as ESR, C-reactive protein or procalcitonin

AND

- No other obvious microbial cause of inflammation, including bacterial sepsis/staphylococcal or streptococcal shock syndromes

AND

- Evidence of COVID-19 (RT-PCR antigen test or serology positive), or likely contact with patients with COVID-19

Danger Signs

- Severe stomach pain
- Difficulty breathing
- Pale, blue-coloured skin, lips or nail beds
- New confusion/seizures
- Inability to wake up or stay awake

Investigation and Treatment as Discussed Above

Actually prevention is the best weapon against COVID-19- *"Do gaj ki duri, hath dhona, vaccine, mask hai zaruri"*.

A FEW IMPORTANT DEFINITIONS

- **Quarantine:** Separates and restricts the movement of people who were exposed to a contagious disease to see if they become sick.

- **Isolation:** Separates sick people with contagious disease from people who are not sick.
- **Endemic:** A disease outbreak is endemic when it is consistently present but limited to a particular geographical region.
- **Epidemic:** An unexpected increase in the number of disease cases in a particular geographical region.
- **Pandemic:** An epidemic that spreads over multiple countries or continents.
- **Telemedicine:** The delivery of healthcare services, where distance is a critical factor, by healthcare professionals using information and communication technologies for the exchange of valid information for the diagnosis, treatment, and prevention of disease and injuries, research and evaluation, and the continuing education of healthcare workers, with the aim of advancing the health of individuals and communities.

CHAPTER

13

Cardiovascular System

HISTORY AND GENERAL EXAMINATION

Again mention PR/RR/BP/JVP/CFT/SpO_2

Its better to take all 4 limbs BP/SpO_2 in suspected cardiac cases and standing BP to rule out postural drop.

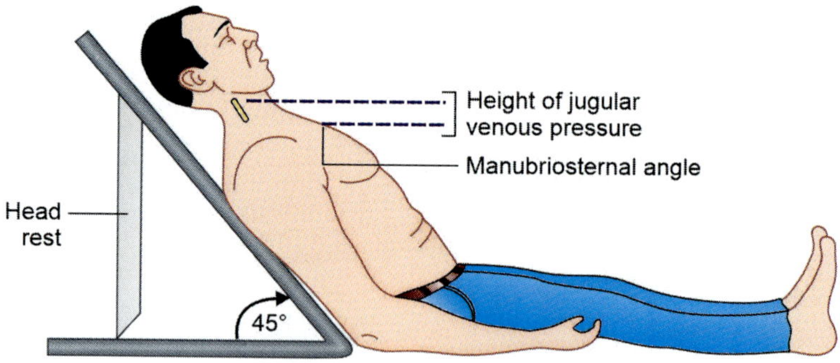

Patient position for examination

JVP measurement: Raised in RVF, TS/TR, fluid overload

PP (Pulse pressure) = systolic BP–diastolic BP

- Wide PP in AR, PDA and narrow PP in AS, MS

Mean arterial pressure (MAP) =
Diastolic pressure + (Pulse pressure/3)

For newborn its GA in weeks +10

New York Heart Association Grading (NYHA) of Dyspnoea

Class I	No symptoms with ordinary activity
Class II	With ordinary physical activity, e.g. walking to school
Class III	With activities of daily living, e.g. bathing/going to toilet
Class IV	Symptoms at rest

Nada's criteria: Presence of one major or two minor criteria indicates heart disease.

Major	**Minor**
Systolic murmur grade III or more	Systolic murmur less than grade III
Diastolic murmur	Abnormal 2nd heart sound
Cyanosis	Abnormal ECG
CCF	Abnormal X-ray Abnormal BP

Acyanotic CHD (Left to **R**ight Shunt): PDA, ASD, VSD, COA

Cyanotic CHD (**R**ight to Left Shunt): **5T PE** -TA, TOF, TGA, TAPVC, Truncus Arteriosus, PA, Ebstein's anomaly

Eisenmenger syndrome: Untreated left to right shunt lesions develop features of bidirectional or right to left shunt due to development of pulmonary-veno-occlusive disease (PVOD).

Inspection

Note any abnormal facies:

1. Shape of the precordium/visible precordial bulge.
2. Symmetry of the chest
3. Position of trachea
4. Apex beat appears to be in—4th (<3 years)/5th ICS medial to midclavicular line.
5. left parasternal lift
6. Visible pulsation (suprasternal, 2nd left space, epigastric)/ scars/sinuses/dilated veins.
7. Spine appears to be central/scoliosis or kyphosis

Palpation

Angle of Louis corresponds to 2nd rib at manubrio-sternal joint.

1. Apex beat confirmed to be in—4th/5th ICS medial to mid clavicular line (Finger tips)
   - Localised/not localized
   - Character—Normal/Absent/Tapping/Heaving/Hyperdynamic

   Character of apex beat
   - **Normal:** Confined to 1 ICS, <1/3 of systole, not forceful
   - **Absent: (Mnemonic—PRODE)**

     P—Pericardial effusion

     R—Behind the Rib

     O—Obesity

     D—Dextrocardia

     E—Emphysema
   - **Tapping:** Confined to 1 ICS, <1/3 of systole, not forceful + palpable S_1 as felt in MS
   - **Heaving apex beat:** Confined to 1 ICS, >2/3 of systole, forceful, sustained, felt in LVH—AS, COA
   - **Diffuse or hyperdynamic apex beat:** >1 ICS, forceful ill-sustained, felt in volume over load condition as AR/MR/VSD/PDA/anaemia/thyrotoxicosis
2. Epigastric pulsation [(RV dilatation (tip of finger), aortic aneurysm (pulp of finger)]

   2nd left ICS pulsation—Pulmonary A (artery) dilatation

   Suprasternal pulsation—AS/AR/PDA
3. Thrill—Base of fingers/hypothenar aspect of palm

   If felt in mitral area—MS/MR

   Tricuspid area—VSD

   Aortic area—AS

   Pulmonary area—PS/PDA
4. Palpable left parasternal heave—(wrist/ulnar border of palm)—due to hypertrophy of RV/LA
5. Venous hum at the base of the neck (turbulent flow of blood in IJV)—felt in high cardiac output state
6. Carotid-pulsation/thrill

7. Palpate B/L brachial/radial/femoral/dorsalis pedis/ posterior tibial and popliteal artery pulsation.
8. Palpable sound—S_1(MS) at apex, S_2 (PAH) at pulmonary area
9. Pericardial rub—pericarditis

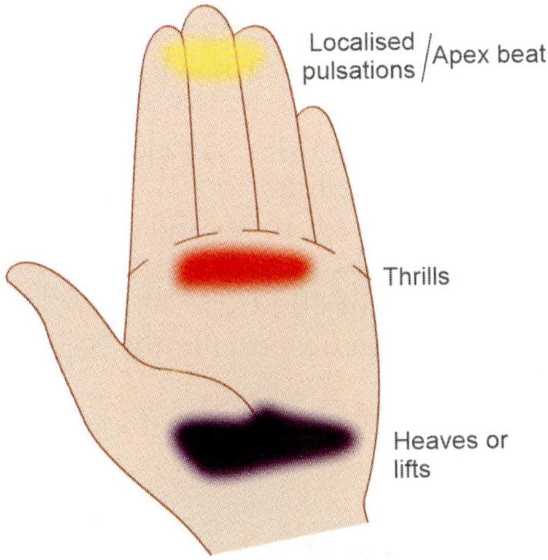

Percussion

1. Left heart border corresponds to apex beat (percuss from left mid axillary line)—dullness before apex beat s/o pericardial effusion
2. Right heart border corresponds to right lateral border of sternum (percuss from right middle of clavicle)—dullness before RSB s/o RAH/pericardial effusion
3. Upper border of liver-corresponds to right 5th ICS.
4. Liver span ______ cm
5. Dullness of left 2nd intercostal space (if >2.5 cm beyond LSB suspect PAH/PDA/LAH)

Auscultation

1. **Mitral area** (corresponds to the apex beat) S_1 and S_2 heard, S_1 loud/S_2 normal split
   Any murmur
2. **Tricuspid area** (lower end of the sternum to its left), i.e. 4th/5th left parasternal area/ICS

S_1 and S_2 heard, S_1 normal/S_2 normal split
Any murmur
3. **Aortic area** (right of the sternum in the 2nd ICS)
S_1 and S_2 heard, S_1 loud/S_2 normal split
Any murmur
4. **Pulmonary area** (left of the sternum in the 2nd ICS)
S_1 and S_2 heard, S_1 loud/A_2 normal, P_2 loud

Any murmur

- Look for opening snap (MS/TS)/ejection click (AS/PS)/ precordial rub (pericarditis)
- Also auscultate over the carotids and wherever appropriate into the axilla and back.
- Look for signs of ARhF/IE/CCF
- Examine the **abdomen** especially for hepatomegaly and ascites.
- Examine **chest** especially for basal crepitation.
- Examine **fundus.**

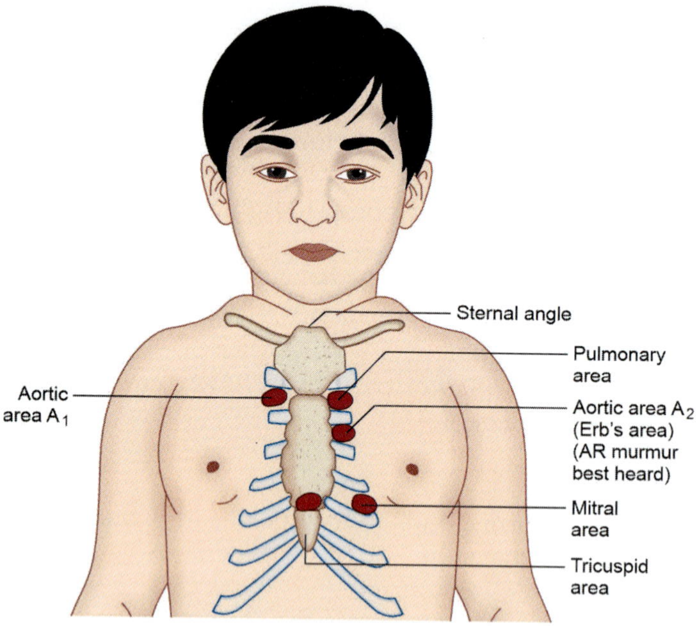

Areas where murmur can be best heard

Apical Impulse/Apex Beat

Lower most, outermost, definitive cardiac impulse

Apical Impulse Displaced to

- In case of LVH: Lateral and inferior displacement
- In case of RVH: Lateral displacement

Heart Sounds

S_1—due to closure of AV valve, i.e. mitral and tricuspid valve (low pitched, prolonged—LUB)
S_2—due to closure of semilunar valve, i.e. aortic and pulmonary valve (high pitched, short—DUB)
S_3—due to rapid ventricular filling: heard in CCF, myocarditis
S_4—due to rapid atrial emptying (always pathological—HTN/HCM)

Heart Sounds Variation

- Loud S_1—MS/TS/PAH
- Soft S_1—MR/TR
- Loud A_2—HTN/AR
- Soft A_2—aortic atresia
- Delayed closure of A_2—AS/LBBB/PDA/AR
- Early Closure of A_2—VSD/MR
- Loud S_2—PAH/VSD/ASD
- Soft S_2—PS/TS
- Delayed closure of S_2—PS/RBBB/ASD

S_2 heart sound normally split into A_2 and P_2 during inspiration

- Single S_2—TOF/TGA/PAH
- Wide and fixed S_2 splitting—ASD
- Wide and variable S_2 splitting—VSD
- Wide and reverse (paradoxical) S_2 splitting—PDA

Heart Murmurs

Caused by normal flow through a abnormal valve or abnormal flow through a normal valve.

Points to note in a Murmurs

Mnemonic—PQRST VBG

1. **P**itch/frequency
2. **Q**uality/character

3. **R**adiation
4. **S**ite
5. **T**iming
6. **V**ariation with respiration/posture/exercise
7. **B**ell or diaphragm
8. **G**rading

1. Pitch/Frequency

- High pitch—AR
- Low pitch—MS

2. Quality/Charactor of Murmurs

- Diamond shape—AS
- Crescendo—MS
- Decrescendo—AR
- Pansystolic/holosystolic—MR/TR/VSD
- Machinary/continuous—PDA/venous hum/AV fistula

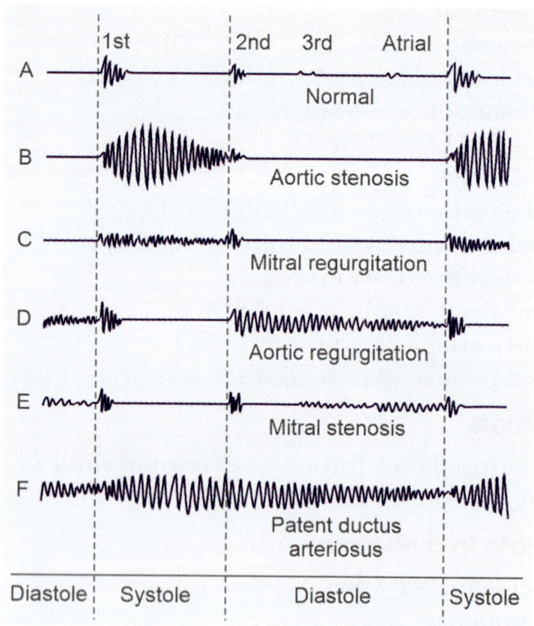

3. Radiation of Murmur

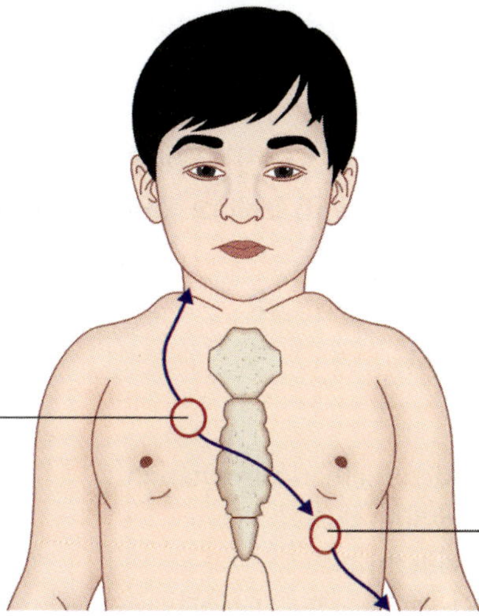

Radiation of murmur

4. Site of Murmurs

Location of maximum intensity of murmurs

- Mitral area: MR/MS/MVP
- Tricuspid area: VSD/TR/TOF
- Pulmonary area: ASD/PDA/PS
- Aortic area: AS/AR

5. Murmur Based on Timing

- Ejection systolic murmur—AS/PS
- Pansystolic murmur—VSD/MR/TR
- Late systolic murmur—MVP
- Early diastolic murmur—AR/PR
- Mid diastolic murmur—TS/MS

Note: Murmur audible with carotid pulse are systolic murmur/ S_1.

6A. Variation of Murmur with Respiration

- All left-sided murmurs best heard in expiration
- All right-sided murmurs best heard in inspiration

6B. Variation of Murmurs with Posture

- MDM of MS best heard in left lateral position at apex by bell
- EDM of AR best heard in sitting and learning forward position at aortic area by diaphragm

7. Murmur Best Heard with Bell or Diaphragm

- Low pitch—Bell-MS
- High pitch—Diaphragm-AR

8. Grading of Murmur

1. Very faint
2. Faint but easily identified on auscultation
3. Loud murmur without thrill
4. Loud murmur with thrill
5. Audible even when one edge of stethoscope is off the chest
6. Audible even when stethoscope is fully taken off the chest

Innocent Murmers

- Short
- Systolic grade <3
- Normal S_1 and S_2
- No radiation
- No haemodynamic instability

Example: Low pitched, rumbling, MDM grade 2 murmur, best heard during expiration, in mitral area, in left lateral position with bell, no radiation, presystolic accentuation present.

Grading of Parasternal Heave

1. Lift visible not palpable
2. Visible and palpable, lift can be obliterated
3. Visible and palpable, lift cannot be obliterated

Diagnosis

1. Type of heart disease (acyanotic or cyanotic congenital heart disease/rheumatic heart disease)
2. Valve involvement—MR/MS/AS/AR

3. Evidence of pulmonary HTN
4. Evidence of IE
5. Evidence of CCF
6. Sinus rhythm

Example: Rheumatic heart disease with mitral stenosis with pulmonary hypertension with no evidence of IE. Not in CCF in sinus rhythm.

MODIFIED DUKE CRITERIA FOR INFECTIVE ENDOCARDITIS*

Major	1. 2 or >2 separate positive blood culture 2. Echo evidence of endocarditis—vegetation, abscess, valvular regurgitation
Minor	1. Predisposing heart condition 2. IV drug abusers, presence of nonfeeding central or peripheral lines 3. Fever 4. Vascular phenomena—emboli, mycotic aneurysm, Janeway lesions, neurological deficit 5. Immunological phenomena—AGN, Osler nodes/Roth spots 6. Pallor/clubbing/splenomegaly/splinter haemorrhages 7. High ESR/CRP 8. Positive blood culture but does not meet the major criteria 9. Echo evidence of endocarditis but does not meet the major criteria 10. Microscopic haematuria

***2 major or 1 major + 3 minor or 5 minor criteria is diagnostic.**

DIFFERENCES BETWEEN CENTRAL AND PERIPHERAL CYANOSIS

	Central cyanosis	Peripheral cyanosis
Site	Lips, tip of tongue, palatal and conjunctival mucosa, nails	Tip of nose, ear pinna, tips of fingers and toes

Contd.

	Central cyanosis	Peripheral cyanosis
Touch of limbs	Warm	Cold
Mechanism	Reduced Hb >5%	Sluggish blood flow
CFT	<3 seconds	>3 seconds
Clubbing	Present	Absent
On warming	No change	Disappear
On giving 100% O_2	No change except Pulmonary causes	Decreases

DIFFERENCES BETWEEN RHEUMATIC CARDITIS AND INFECTIVE ENDOCARDITIS

Features	Rheumatic carditis	Infective endocarditis
Onset	Acute	Chronic
Fever	High grade	Low grade
Vegetation	Large Sessile Along the valves Not friable	Small Pedunculated Along the wall Friable, easily dislodged
Blood culture	Positive for streptococci	Positive for causative agents (HACEK)
Sequela	Valvular stenosis	Wall defects, aneurysms

Alfred DE Musset's Sign

Due to sudden filling and emptying of the corotid artery—causing up and down movements of the head with each beats as in AR.

Hess Test/Fragility Test/Tourniquet Test

Sphygmomanometer cuff is tied and pressure is elevated to a point between systolic and diastolic BP for 5 minutes if >20 petechiae/purpurae appear in 2.5 cm^2 area—test is positive for dengue haemorrhagic fever.

CHAPTER 14

Gastrointestinal System

HISTORY AND GENERAL EXAMINATION

UPPER GIT

- **Lips:** Cheilitis/angular stomatitis/fissuring/vesicles (herpes)/pigmentation
- **Gum:** Gingivitis/bleeding/hypertrophy
- Oral hygiene
- **Teeth:** No of permanent/milk teeth/discolouration/caries
- **Tongue:** Moist/dry/pallor (dorsal surface)/icterus (ventral or under surface)/cyanosis/thrush/papillae
- **Oral mucosa:** Ulcers/bleed/pigmentation (Peutz–Jeghers syndrome/Addison's disease)
- Tonsils—normal/hypertrophied
- Pharynx—normal/inflamed

LOWER GIT

Divided into: Epigastrium/right and left hypochondriac region/umbilical area/right and left lumbar region/hypogastrium/right and left iliac region.

Epigastrium	Left lobe of the liver, stomach, part of pancreas and kidney
Right hypochondrium	Liver, gallbladder, right kidney
Left hypochondrium	Stomach, spleen, left kidney
Umbilical area	Stomach, pancreas, small intestine, transverse colon

Contd.

Right lumbar region	Right kidney, small intestine, ascending colon
Left lumbar region	Left kidney, small intestine, descending colon
Hypogastrium	Bladder, small intestine and sigmoid colon
Right iliac region	Small intestine, caecum, ascending colon, appendix
Left iliac region	Small intestine, descending and sigmoid colon

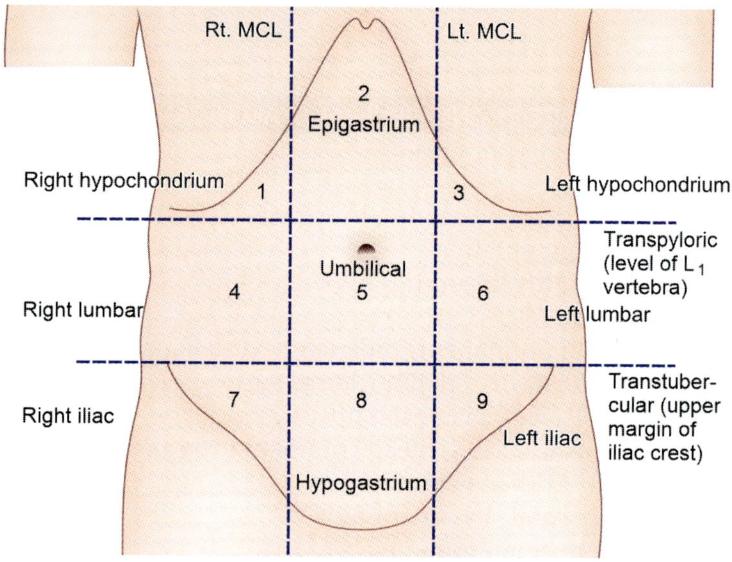

Lower GIT region

INSPECTION

i. **Shape:** Normal (scaphoid shape)/distended
ii. **Flanks:** Full/not
iii. **Movement with respiration:** All quadrants move equally with respiration
iv. **Umbilicus:** Central inverted/shifted everted
v. **Skin:** Normal/stretched/shiny
vi. Visible pulsation/scars/sinuses/dilated veins/mass/peristalsis

vii. **Hernial orifices:** Protrusion of viscus or part of viscus through a normal or abnormal opening—inguinal/femoral/umbilical/incisional

vii. **Genitalia**

viii. **Signs of liver failure:** Alopecia/altered sensorium/ascites/bleeding tendency/caput medusa/distension of abdomen/oedema/flapping tremors/gynecomastia/haematemesis/icterus/pruritus/palmar erythema/spider angioma/parotid swelling/testicular atrophy/xanthoma

PALPATION

Flex patients knee and hip joint/ask child to take deep breath. The examiner should stand on the right side while the head of the child should be turned to the left side

1. Local rise of temperature
2. Tenderness
3. Soft/guarding/rigidity
4. Rebound tenderness
5. **Palpate liver**—Palpate for the liver with radial border of palm from right iliac fossa moving upward with each inspiration towards the lower costal margin—cm below costal margin in right midclavicular line/towards rt iliac fossa
   Edge—round/sharp, **surface**—smooth/nodule,
   Consistency—soft/firm/hard
   Tender/nontender, moves with respiration, cannot insinuate finger between mass and costal margins.
   Grading of hepatomegaly (below the RCM)

Mild	<4 cm	Infective hepatitis
Moderate	5–7 cm	Wilson's disease
Massive	>7 cm	CML/hepatoma

6. **Palpate spleen:** Palpate from right iliac fossa towards left hypochondriac along spino-umbilical line with each inspiration
   - For small spleen: Hooking method
   - Presence of ascites: Dipping method
   - ____ cm below costal margin in left midclavicular line
     Towards-downwards/spino-umbilical line.

Edge—notched, **Surface**—smooth/nodule
Consistency—soft/firm/ hard
Tender/nontender, moves with respiration,
Cannot insinuate fingers between mass and costal margins,
Notch palpable/not palpable
Grading of splenomegaly (below the LCM)

Mild	<2 cm	Typhoid
Moderate	2–7 cm	Portal HTN
Massive	>7 cm	CML/kala azar

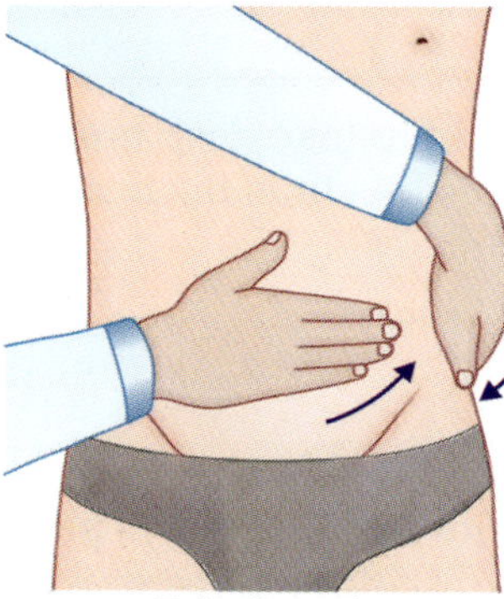

Palpating spleen

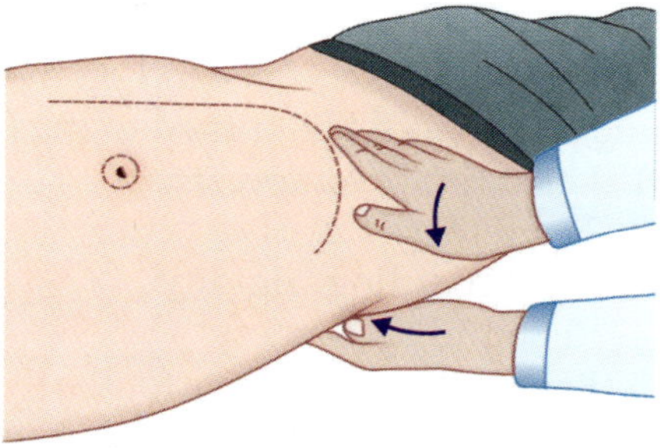

Bimanually palpation of the kidney

Hepatosplenomegaly found in typhoid/GSD/ALL/thalassemia/HODGKIN'S lymphoma

7. No other mass palpable (kidney/UB/para-aortic lymph nodes)

   Any abdominal mass look for—site, size, shape, surface, border/margin, skin over the mass, consistency, tenderness, mobility, pulsation, fluctuation test, reducibility, compressibility, transillumination, pitting.
8. Rectal examination________
9. B/L testes palpable/not palpable

PERCUSSION

1. Upper border of liver—corresponds to right 5th ICS
2. Liver span ___ cm

Normal liver span

<1 year	4–5 cm
1–5 years	6–7 cm
5–12 years	8–9 cm
>12 years	9–11 cm

3. Shifting dullness (500 ml)
   - Percuss from the midline out to left flank until tympanic note change to dullness
   - Mark the point (keep pleximeter at the point of dullness) and ask child to roll towards you
   - Wait for 30 sec then percuss—if dull note becomes tympanic s/o ascites.

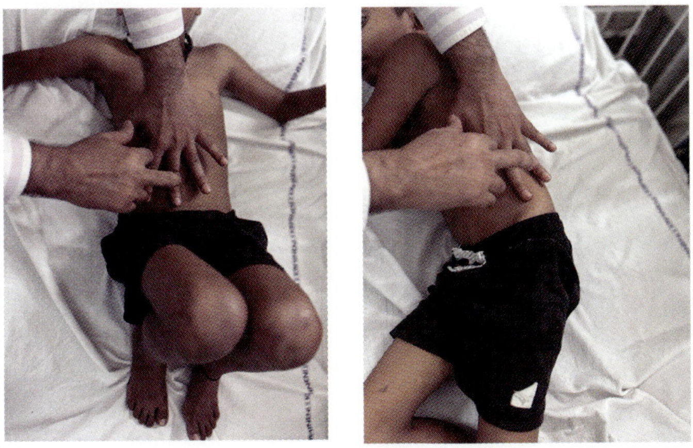

Demonstrating shifting dullness

4. Fluid thrill (1500 ml)
   - Ask the child or attender to place the ulnar border of hand firmly on the centre of abdomen with fingers directed downwards
   - Flick the flank of one side and feel the thrill by the other hand palm on the opposite flank
5. Puddle sign (for minimal fluids <150 ml) (knee-elbow position)
6. Dullness of renal angle

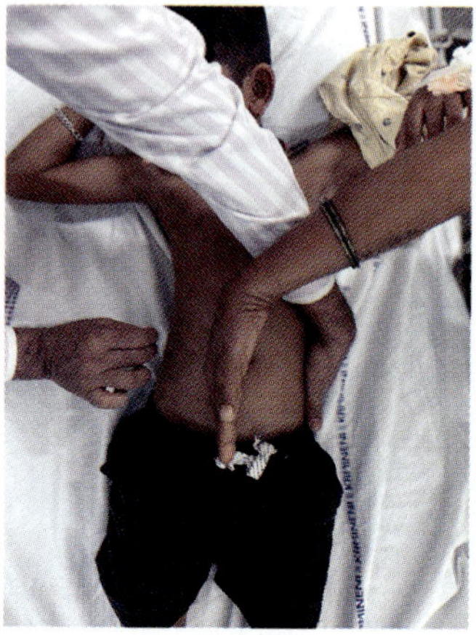

Demonstrating fluid thrill

GRADING OF ASCITES

I. Mild	**Puddle sign + Ascites detected by USG**
II. Moderate	Shifting dullness + No fluid thrill
III. Massive	Fluid thrill + Tense ascites

AUSCULTATION

1. Bowel sounds heard (normal 2–3/min)
   (Try to hear for full 3 min, Rt/Lt side of umbilicus)
2. Bruit
   - Hepatic—hepatoma
   - Spleen—haemangioma
   - Arterial—aneurysm
   - Renal—renal artery stenosis
3. Venous hum-portal vein obstruction

Haematochezia—fresh blood in stool, s/o of lower GI bleeding. (below ligament of Treitz)

Melaena is altered blood in stool, s/o of upper GI bleeding (above duodenojejunal flexure/ligament of Treitz)

Persistent diarrhoea—>14 days

Tenesmus—frequent urge to defaecate but with little evacuation

Bilious **vomiting**	Upper GI obstruction (due to obstruction distal to ampulla of Vater)
Projectile **vomiting** (without nausea)	Raised ICT, pyloric stenosis
Haemoptysis (blood mixed with sputum)	Respiratory system illness
Haematemesis (fresh blood)	Upper GI bleed

Differences between Transudates and Exudates Ascites Fluid

Features	Transudates	Exudates
Appearance	Clear and colourless	Cloudy , white
Protein g/dl	<2.5	>2.5
Specific gravity	<1.018	>1.018
WBC	<1000/mm^3	5000–50000/mm^3

Visible Pulsation/Peristalsis over the Abdomen

Visible gastric peristalsis moving LT → RT	Pyloric stenosis
RT to LT	Transverse colon obstruction
Transmitted pulse (fingers are not separated)	Abdominal mass lies in front of Abdominal aorta
Expansile pulsation (fingers are separated)	Abdominal aortic aneurysm

Comparison between Splenomegaly and Renal Lump

Splenomegaly	Renal lump
Not palpable bimanually	Palpable bimanually
Cannot insinuate fingers between mass and costal margins	**Can** insinuate the finger between enlarged kidney and costal margins
Can cross the umbilicus/midline	Cannot cross the umbilicus/midline
Splenic notch palpable	Not palpable

Chronic Abdominal Pain (CAP)

Continuous or occurring at least once a week for >3 months.

Constipation

2 or more of the following for >1 month

1. <2 defaecation/week in >4 years child
2. Painful defecation
3. Palpable fecal mass in the rectum
4. Fecal incontinence
5. H/o passage of large diameter stool

Complication of Undescended/Ectopic Testes

T Torsion
E Epididymo-orchitis
S Sterility
T Trauma
I Inguinal hernia
S Seminoma

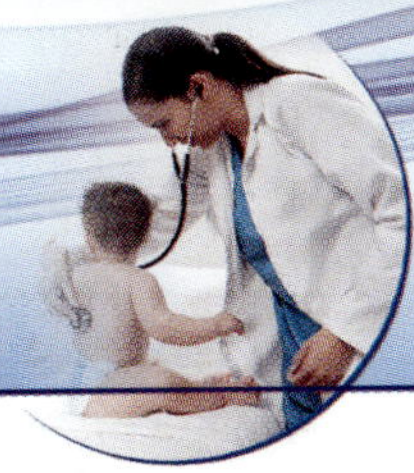

CHAPTER

15

Central Nervous System

HISTORY

1. Developmental history—GM/FM/PS/Language/Vision/ Hearing
2. Weakness/tightness
   a. Duration/onset/progress
   b. Distal weakness—difficulty in buttoning/writing/ feeding with spoon/cannot grip the slippers.
   c. Proximal weakness—difficulty in combing hair/taking bath/getting up from squatting position/climbing stairs
   d. Associated symptoms
3. Sensory disturbance—superficial/deep, B/B disturbance
4. Cranial nerve involvement
   - I—h/o smell disturbances
   - II—h/o visual disturbances
   - III, IV, VI—h/o diplopia/squint/ptosis
   - V—h/o difficulty in feeding
   - VII—h/o dribbling of saliva/deviation of angle of mouth/ inability to close eyes/loss of taste sensation
   - VIII—h/o hearing disturbances
   - XI, X—h/o nasal twang to speech/nasal regurgitation
   - XI—h/o difficulty in shrugging of shoulders
   - XII—h/o dysphagia/dysarthria
5. Higher mental function

6. Seizures—type/onset/duration/progress/B/B disturbance/post-ictal period/episodes.
7. Cerebellar symptoms—h/o swaying/difficulty in taking food to mouth (coordination), ataxia.
8. Headache/vomiting/blurring of vision (raised ICT), fever, altered sensorium (meningoencephalitis).

EXAMINATION

CNS EXAMINATION

1. HMF
2. Cranial nerves
3. Motor system examination
4. Sensory system examination
5. Cerebellar signs
6. ANS examination
7. Skull and spine

HIGHER MENTAL FUNCTION

MNEMONIC (ABCDE MIS OS): Appearance/Behavior/Consciousness Level/Delusion/Emotional Liability/Memory/Intelligence/Speech/Orientation/Sleep

i. Appearance—dressing/hygiene/self neglect
ii. Behaviour—normal/hyperactive/docile
iii. Level of consciousness drowsy/delirium/obtundation/stupor/coma-light/deep/flaccid [DDO SC]
iv. Delusion—(false and firm believe)
    Illusion—(false believe with external stimuli, e.g. snake instead of rope)
    Hallucination—(false believe without external stimuli, e.g. visual/olfactory/tactile)
v. Emotional lability
vi. Memory—immediate/recent/remote
vii. Intelligence
viii. Speech—normal/dysphasia/aphasia/dysarthria
    - BROCA speech—inferior frontal gyrus (understand but cannot write)

- WERNICKE speech—superior temporal gyrus (do not understand but can write)
- Bulbar palsy—9, 10, 12 CN—nasal twang
- Pseudobulbar palsy—craniospinal—slurred
- Cerebellar lesion—scanning
- U/L vocal cord palsy—hoarseness of voice
- B/L vocal cord palsy—aphasia

ix. Orientation to time/place/person

x. Sleep pattern

CRANIAL NERVES

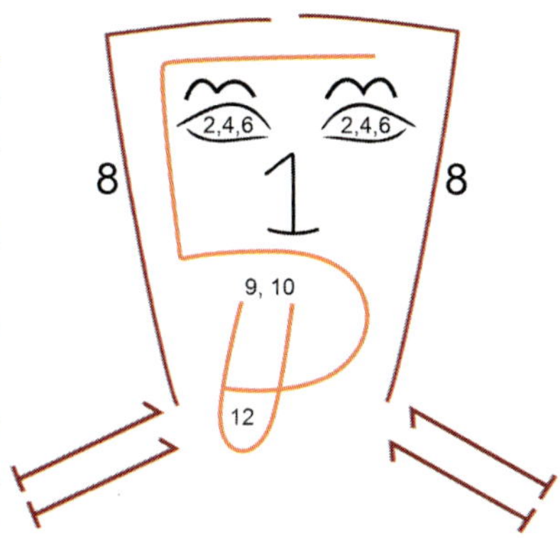

MNEMONIC: OOO to take a family vacation go valley such heaven

All the cranial nerve except I and II originate from brainstem.

1, 2, 8 sensory, 5, 7, 9 and 10 mixed rest all are pure motor

1. **Olfactory (I):** Check that nasal passage is clear/ask child to close eyes/occlude the other nostril, test each nostril separately, use coffee powder (never use pungent substances like ammonia)
2. **Optic (II)**

Gross vision	
Acuity of vision	Snellen's chart (distant vision) Jaeger's chart (near vision) (keep at 30–40 cm) Finger movement/hand movement/perception (stand at 100 cm)
Field of vision Colour vision	Perimetry (>7 years) or confrontation method (>3 years) (sit 3 feet away) (Ishihara test) (>3 years)
Fundus	Look for optic disc, retina, maculae
Reflexes	Pupillary/accommodation (Afferent: CN II; Efferent: CN III)

- Tell child to fix the gaze to examiner eye

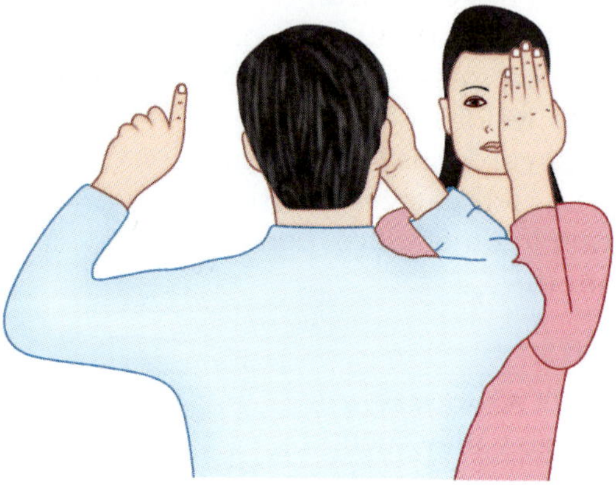

Confrontation test

Snellen's test: The lines can be read at 60, 36, 24, 18, 12, 9, 6 and 5 ms respectively. Visual acuity = d/D. Where d is the distance at which the letters are read (distance between child and examiner) and D is the distance at which they should be read. Normal visual acuity is 6/6.

3. and 4. **Oculomotor (III), trochlear (IV):** (3, 4, 6 cranial nerves are examined together)
5. **Trigeminal (V):** Inspect the muscle of mastication for wasting.
   - **Sensory:** Sensation over face dermatome-mandibular/maxillary/ophthalmic
   - **Motor:** Clenching of the teeth (palpate masseters and temporalis muscle)
     - Lateral movement of jaw (pterygoid muscles)
     - Opening the jaw against resistance (pterygoid/mylohyoid/anterior belly of digastric)
   - **Reflexes:** Corneal reflex/Jaw jerk

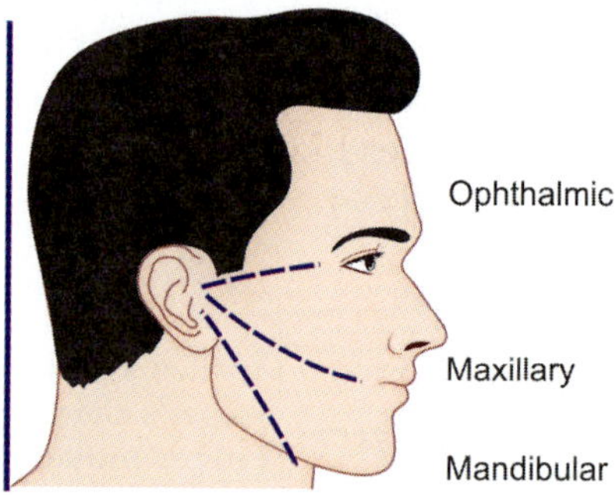

6. **Abducens (VI)**—SO4, LR6. Superior oblique muscle is supplied by IV CN. Lateral rectus muscle is supplied by VI CN. Rest supplied by CN III.

Head should be in neutral position

Ptosis/nystagmus/strabismus **(cover uncover test)**/ movements of eye—follow my finger test (sit 1 foot apart) ________/pupils (size/shape/reflexes-direct/consensual, accommodation)

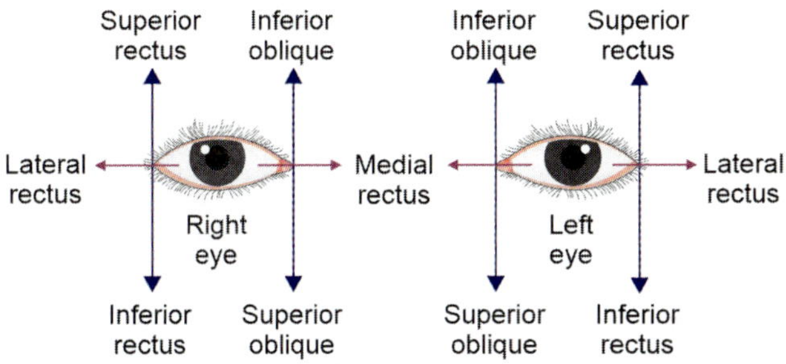

Principal directions of action of extraocular muscles (double H)

Ptosis + mydriasis s/o CN III lesion
Ptosis + miosis s/o sympathetic NS lesion
Note: Levator palpebrae superioris muscle supplied by—CN III. Sup. tarsal muscle supplied by sympathetic NS

7. **Facial (VII):** Ask in history about deviation of angle of mouth/hyperacusis/leaking of food and saliva. Look for any facial asymmetry
   - **Sensory:** Taste sensation over anterior 2/3rd of tongue (ask the child to identify the substance by pointing to the words **written on the card**).
   - **Motor:** Forehead furrowing/eyebrow raising *(frontalis)* *(Keep a hand over the scalp to block occipital head)*
     - *Eyes closure:* Orbicularis oculi, Bell's phenomenon
     - *Teeth showing:* Depressor anguli oris
     - *Blowing the cheek:* Buccinator
     - *Nasolabial fold* (Obliterated on the paralysed side) and eversion of lower lip): Platysma
   - **Secretomotor:** Salivation/lacrimation (**Schirmer's test:** Put a piece of blotting paper under the lower eyelids and remove it after 5 min. Normally after 5 min blotting paper should be marked with 10 mm of tear secretion)

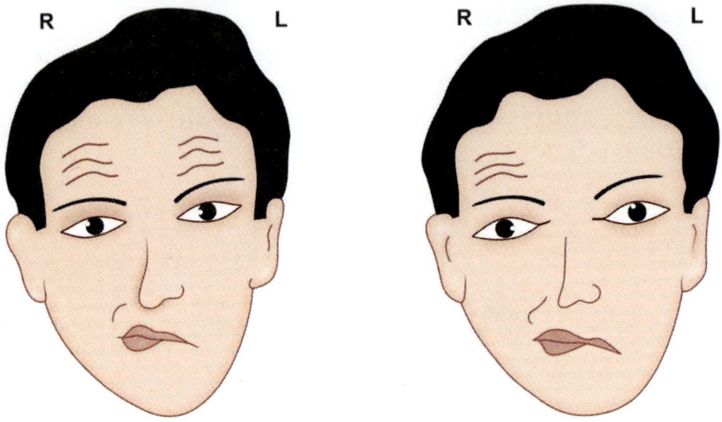

Left upper motor neurone/facial palsy

Left lower motor neurone/facial palsy

Note: In UMN lesion upper part of face is spared

8. **Vestibulo-cochlear (VIII)**
   - Vestibular (h/o vertigo), nystagmus, Romberg's sign, doll's eye (occulo-cephalic reflex), Fukuda step test
   - Vestibulo-ocular Reflex—Afferent: CN VIII; Efferent: CN 3, 4, 6
   - Cochlear (Watch test/Rinne's test/Weber's test) (256 or **512 Hz**)

Test	Normal response	Conductive hearing loss	Sensori-neural hearing loss
Rinne	AC > BC	BC > AC	Cannot be tested
Weber	No lateralisation	Lateralised to defective ear	Lateralised to normal ear

AC: Air conduction; BC: Bone conduction

9. and 10. **Glosso-pharyngeal (IX), Vagus (X) (Longest CN)**
   - **Sensory:** Taste sensation of the posterior 1/3rd (IX) of tongue
   - **Motor:** H/o dysphagia/dysarthria/nasal regurgitation/ nasal twang of voice.
   - Movement of palate/position of uvula (X)/gag reflex—Afferent: CN IX; Efferent: CN X

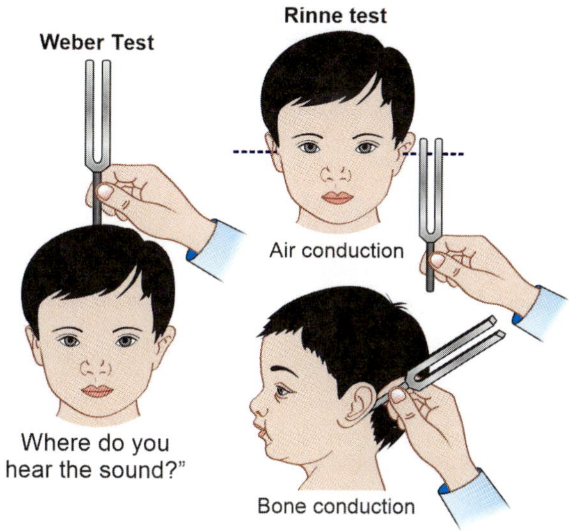

11. **Spinal accessory (XI):** Shrugging of shoulder (trapezius)—check from behind

    Turning the neck against resistance (sterno-cleidomastoid) check from front.

12. **Hypoglossal (XII):**
    - H/o dysarthria
    - Position of tongue/wasting/deviation/fasciculation/movements on protruding out

Remember Rule of 17

10 + 7 =17 (10th and 7th nerve palsy results in deviation to the opposite side)
As in 7th nerve palsy, mouth deviate to the opposite side,
10th nerve palsy uvula deviate to the opposite side
12 + 5 = 17 (12th and 5th nerve palsy results in deviation to the same side)
As in 5th nerve palsy, jaw deviate to the same side (healthy lateral pterygoid push it towards paralysed side), 12th nerve palsy tongue deviate to the same side
(Tongue always tells the truth)

Note: Nerves in the shadows (research going on)
(i) Cranial N XIII: Nervus terminalis/zero nerve/nerve N
(ii) Cranial N XIV: Nervus intermedius

MOTOR SYSTEM

MNEMONIC: ABCD MP GST—Attitude/bulk/coordination/ DTR/ movement (invol)/power/GAIT/sup reflex/tone.

1. **Attitude of limb:** UL

   LL

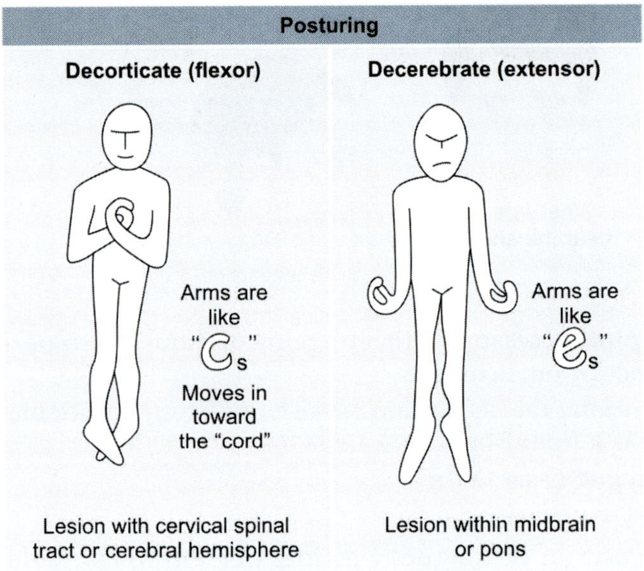

Decorticate/decerebrate rigidity

2. **Nutrition (bulk):** Comment on size/shape and symmetry
   Measurement in cm

	Right	Left
Mid arm		
Mid forearm		
Mid thigh		
Mid calf		

3. **Coordination of movements:** Finger nose test/heel knee test

4. Deep reflexes

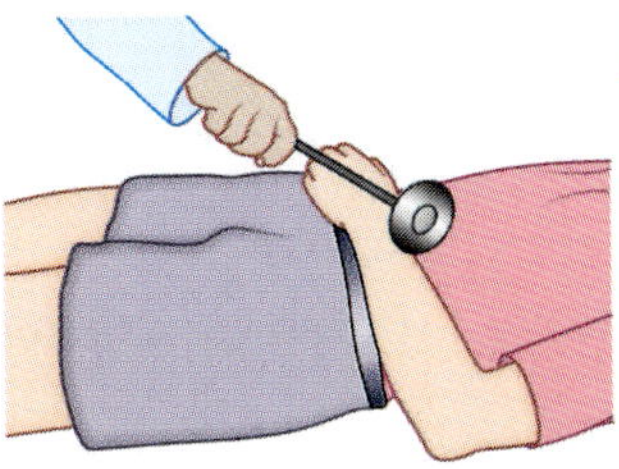

Eliciting the supinator jerk

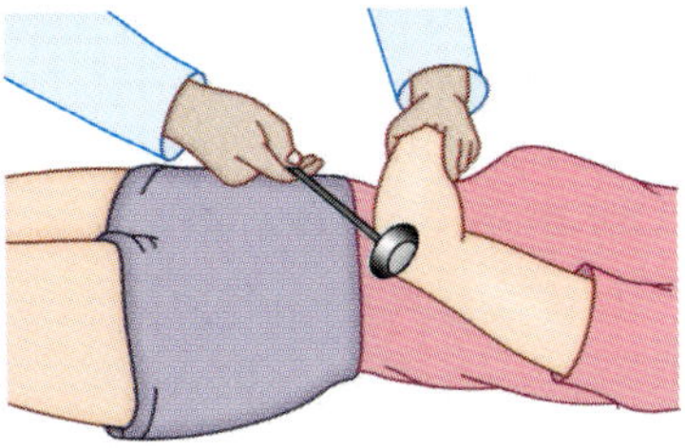

Eliciting the triceps jerk

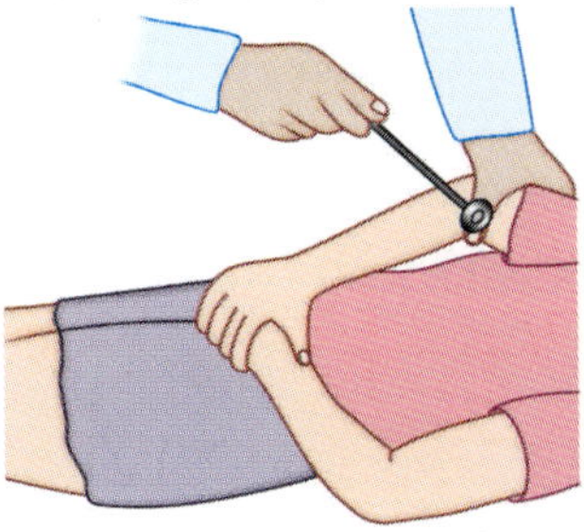

Eliciting the biceps jerk

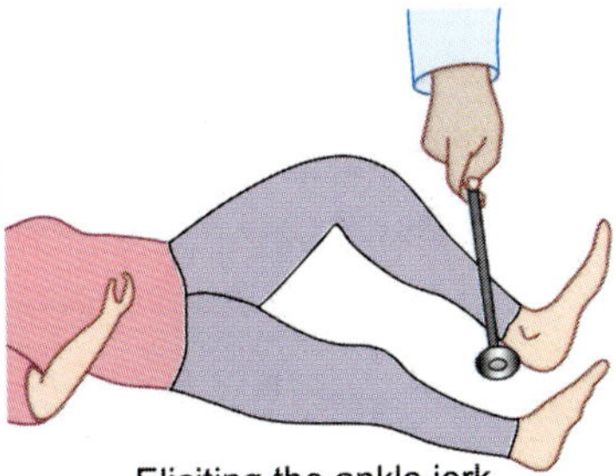

Eliciting the ankle jerk

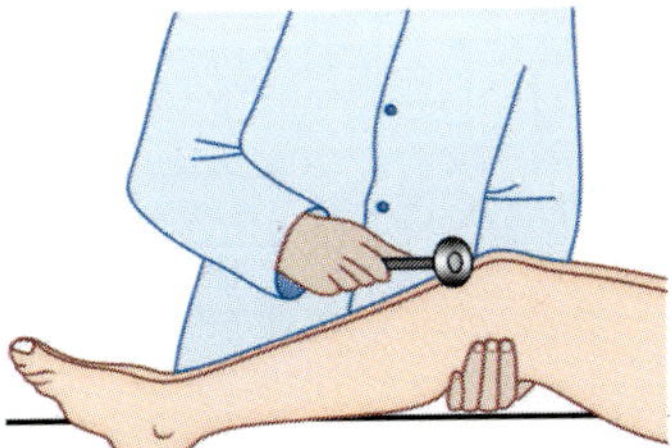

Eliciting the knee jerk

DTR	Root value	Reaction noticed	Rt	Lt
Bicep	$C_5 C_6$	Contraction of the biceps and flexions of the forearm		
Supinator	$C_5 C_6$	Flexion of the elbow		
Tricep	$C_6 C_7, C_8$	Contraction of triceps and extension of forearm		
Knee	$L_3 L_4$	Contraction of quadriceps and extension of the knee		
Ankle	S_1, S_2	Contraction of calf muscles		

Mnemonic

1, 2: Buckle my shoes (Ankle/Achilles reflex)
3, 4: Kick the door (Knee/patellar)
5, 6: Pick up the sticks (Biceps and supinator/brachioradialis)
7, 8: Lay them straight (Triceps)

Note: Jaw jerk—trigeminal (V) nerve (afferent and efferent both)

Grading of DTR

0	Absent
+	Sluggish or present only with reinforcement
++	Readily elicited (like normal ankle jerk)
+++	Brisk (like normal knee jerk)
++++	With clonus

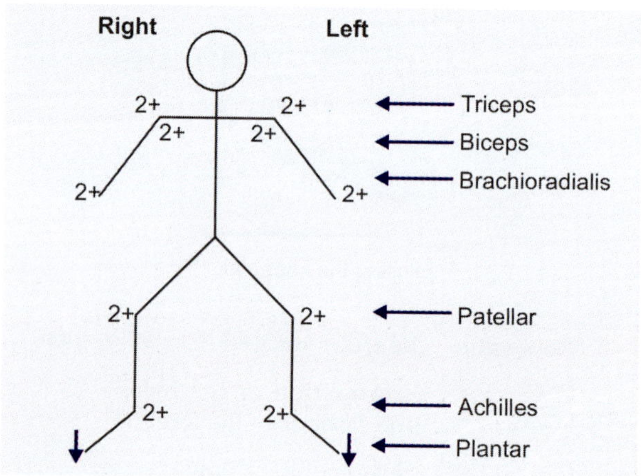

- Clonus—patellar/knee, sustained/ill sustained
- Plantar is extensor till 2 years of age.
  - Reinforcement of reflexes by—Jendrassik manoeuvre

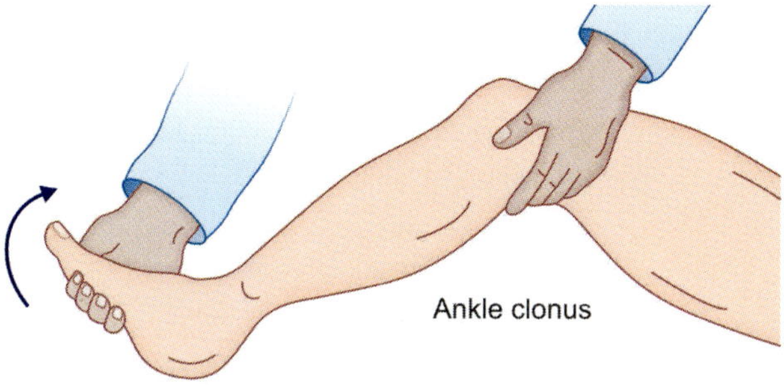

Ankle clonus

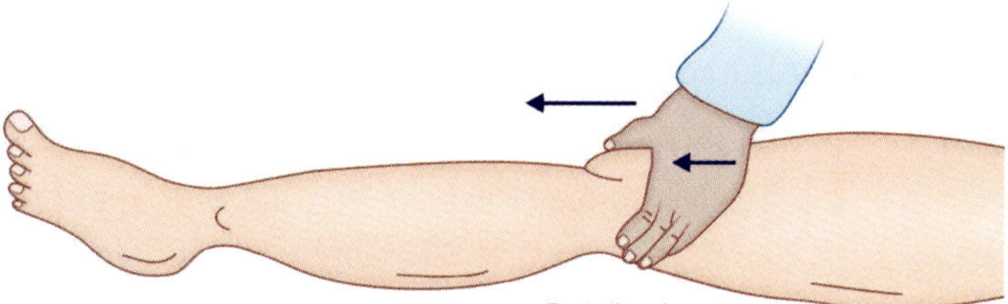

Patella clonus

5. **Involuntary movements:** Mention if any seen fasciculation/tremors/chorea/athetosis/hemiballism
6. **Power**

   Grade the power (Medical Research Council Scale)

0	Absent voluntary contraction
1	Feeble contraction on manoeuvre
2	Movement with gravity eliminated
3	Movement against gravity
4	Movement against partial resistance
5	Normal

Check for movement bilaterally and grade the power

Neck	Extension/flexion
Shoulder	Abduction/adduction/extension/flexion/elevation
Elbow	Extension/flexion/supination/pronation
Wrist	Extension/flexion

Contd.

Grip	
Intercostal muscle	Splinting of diaphragm
Diaphragm	Splinting of chest (intercostal muscle)
Abdomen	Beevor sign
HIP	Abduction/adduction/extension/flexion/internal rotation/external rotation
Knee	Extension/flexion
Ankle	Dorsi flexion/plantar flexion/inversion/eversion

Or you can test the muscle power individually

Muscle	Instruction to the child	Examiner action
Latissimus dorsi	Clasp your hands behind your back	Resist downward backward movement
Serratus anterior	Push forwards against the wall	Observe winging of scapula
Pectoralis major	Stretch your arms in front and clap your hands	Try to hold the hands apart
Deltoid supraspinatus	Lift the arm away from the chest	Resist abduction
Triceps	Flex the forearm first. Now try to straighten out the forearm against the resistance offered by the examiner.	Try to keep the forearm flexed while the child tries to straighten it.
Biceps	Holding your forearm against your side, bend it	Grasp the wrist and offer resistance to flexion.
Brachioradialis	Place the arm between the prone and supine position, now bend the forearm	Grasp the wrist and offer resistance to flexion.
Extensors of wrist	Extension of the hand at the wrist	Grasp the wrist and offer resistance to dorsiflexion/extension of the hand at the wrist
Flexors of wrist	Flexion of the hand at the wrist	Resist flexion of the hand.

Contd.

Muscle	Instruction to the child	Examiner action
Flexors of the fingers	Squeeze my fingers	Present index and middle fingers to the child to squeeze
Adductors of the thigh	Keep leg straight and abduct it fully now bring the leg back to the midline against resistance	Offer resistance to adduction
Abductors of the thigh	Move the leg out against resistance	Offer resistance to abduction
Flexors of the thigh (Psoas)	Keep knee extended lift leg off the bed	Offer resistance to flexion of the thigh
Extensors of the thigh	Keep knee extended lift leg off the bed now push the leg down against resistance	Offer resistance to extension of the thigh
Internal rotation at hip joint	Put child in prone, Keep knee flexed now try to abduct the legs fully	Offer resistance to internal rotation of the thigh
External rotation at hip joint	Put child in prone, Keep knee flexed, now try to cross the legs fully	Offer resistance to external rotation of the thigh

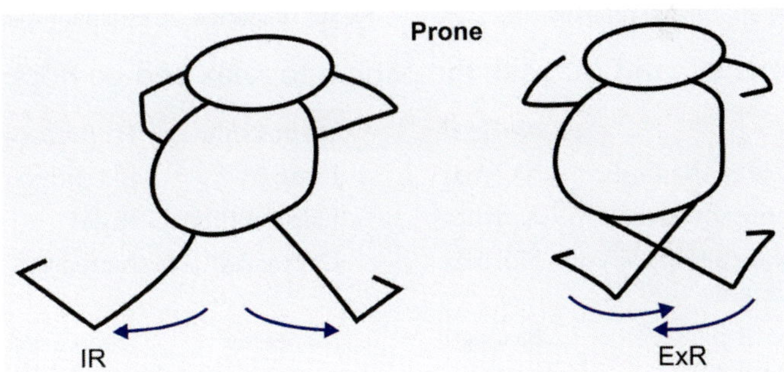

Internal rotation External rotation

7. **Gait:** Hemiparetic/ataxic/shuffling/high stepping/ waddling/spastic.

8. **Superficial reflexes**: Glabellar: Afferent V, efferent VII

	Root value	Right	Left
Corneal	Afferent V/efferent (VII) CN		
Abdominal (stroke towards umbilicus)	T_6 to T_{12} Epigastric - T_6 to T_9 (Absent in UMN lesion)		
Cremasteric (stroke towards upper inner aspect of thigh)	L_1 (Absent in UMN lesion)		
Plantar	S_1 (Babinski/extensor response in UMN lesion)		
Anal	S_3 and S_4		

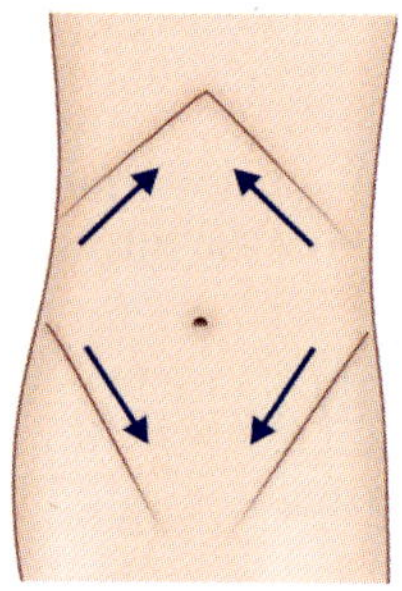
Eliciting abdominal reflexes

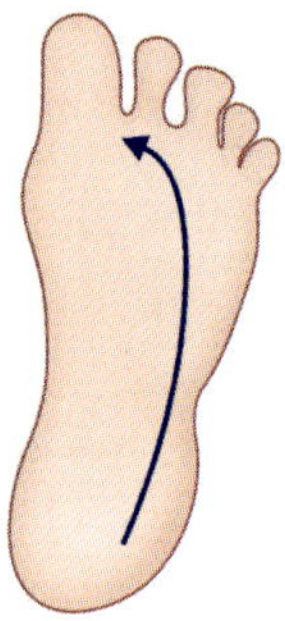

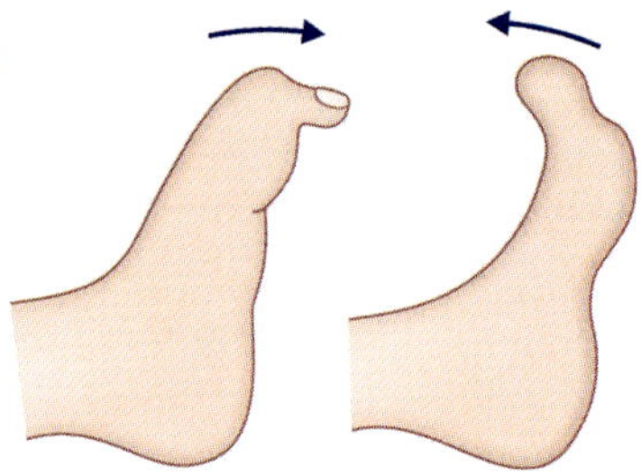
Flexor response Extensor response

9. **Tone:** UL and LL (Ask the patient to relax and go floppy)

Tests	Normal	Hypotonia	Hypertonia
Posture of the limb	Normal	Limp	Extended/stiff
Palpation of muscle	Normal	Flappability	Rigid
Resistance to passive movements	Normal	Decreased	Increased
Range of passive movements	Normal	Increased	Decreased

Hypertonia (spasticity/rigidity)

- Clasp knife, spasticity—pyramidal
- Cog-wheel, lead pipe—rigidity—extrapyramidal

In newborn tone is assessed by scarf sign/heel to ear manoeuvre/adductor angle.

SENSORY SYSTEM

Check for each dermatomes bilaterally, distal to proximal. Tell child to close the eyes and tell him to respond verbally to appreciation of sensation. [Required tools—tuning fork 128 Hz, 2 test tube, safety pin, coin, cotton, wooden tongue depressor, blocks, compass)

Antero Lateral Spinothalamic Tract Column Sensation

- Crude touch (ANT STT)
- Temperature (use two test tubes of worm and cold water)
- Pain (use pin head)

Posterior or Dorsal Column Tract Sensation (PCT)

- Light touch (use cotton wisp)
- Vibration (128 Hz) (check on bony points B/L–medial malleoli/tibial tuberosity/iliac spine/head of ulna/elbow /mastoid)
- Joint sense—upper limb/lower limb
- Position sense (proprioception): Ability to determine the direction of movement of the great toe or fingers of hand—upward and downward with closed eye.
- Romberg's sign (inability to stand with feel together and eyes closed) two senses:
  - Proprioception (PCT) (The ability to know one's body position in space) and
  - Vestibular function (VIII CN) (The ability to know one's head position in space

Note: Romberg test is not a sign of cerebellar lesion it is positive in disturbance of PCT and vestibular lesion

- Pressure sense (use wooden tongue depressor)

Note: **PCT does not carry PCT (pain, crude touch, temp)**

Cortical Sensation

- Tactile localisation
- Tactile discrimination
- Two-point discrimination (use compass)
- Sensory inattention/dissociation (pain and temp lost, crude touch present)
- Stereognosis (give familiar objects, e.g. coin/keys)

- Graphaesthesia (write numbers by your finger on child's palm)
- Extinction (double simultaneous stimulation)
- Construction and dressing apraxia (give him blocks to make, clothes to wear)

Dermatomes

Remember

- Thumb—C_6
- Big toe—L_4
- Nipple—T_4
- Umbilicus—T_{10}
- Anus—S_3, S_4

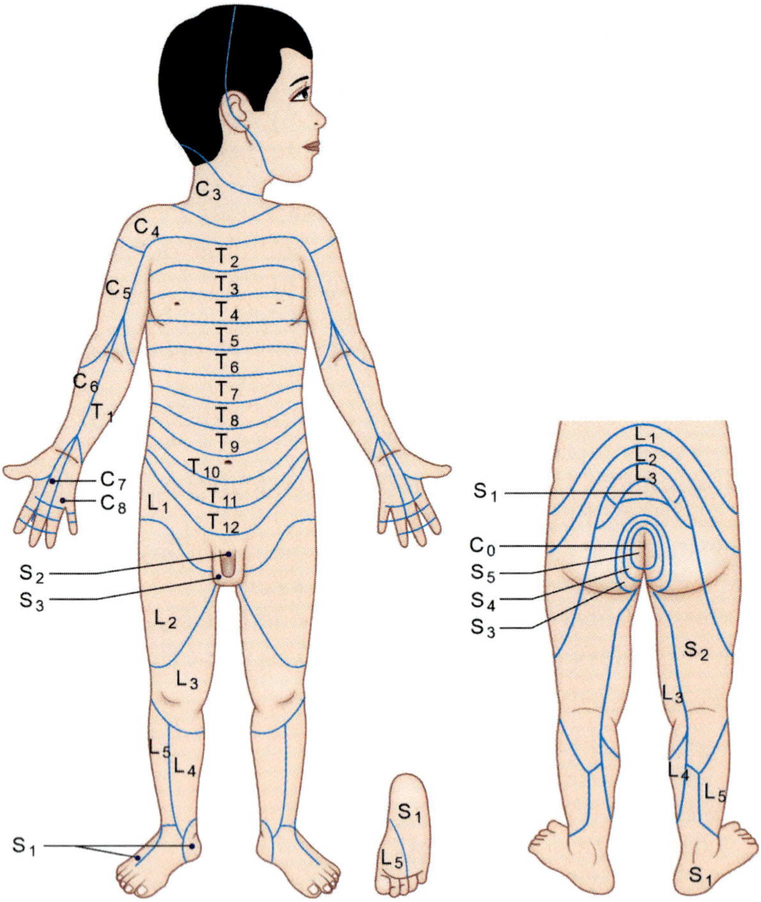

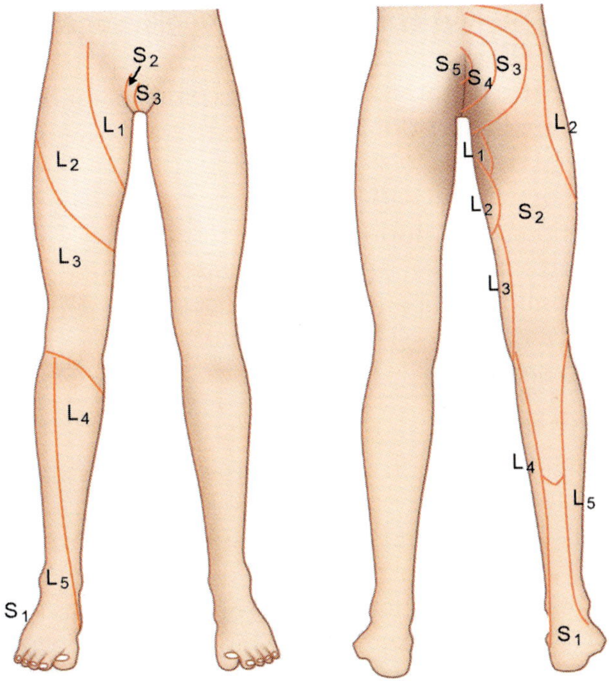

CEREBELLAR SIGNS (MNEUMONIC: ANS DTR)

- Ataxia
- Atonia (hypotonia)
- Ataxic gait
- Nystagmus
- Scanning speech
- Dysmetria/past pointing (finger–finger-nose test)
- Dyssynergia (knee heel test)
- Dysdiadochokinesia (rapid alternating movements)
- Dysarthria
- DTR—(pendular knee jerk)
- Tandem walking
- Tremors intention (essential tremors—senile)
- Rebound phenomenon

Autonomic Nervous System (Head Ganglion of ANS Hypothalamus)

- **Sympathetic:** (Fight and flight) thoracolumbar outflow (T_1–L_2)
- **Parasympathetic:** (Rest and digest) craniosacral outflow (3, 7, 9, 10 cranial nerve and S_2–S_4)
  1. Look for sweating after hot bath
  2. Variation in HR during Valsalva maneuver
  3. Fall in BP >20 mm Hg from supine to standing indicates autonomic neuropathy (normal variation is <10 mm Hg)

SKULL AND SPINE

Meningeal Signs

- **Neck rigidity:** Flexion of head causes spasm in the extensor muscles of neck
- **Kernig's sign:** Painful restriction of extension of leg when the hip is flexed (due to spasm of the hamstring muscles)
- **Brudzinski's:** Neck sign—flexion of knee and hip following flexion of the neck (better elicited in the sitting posture)

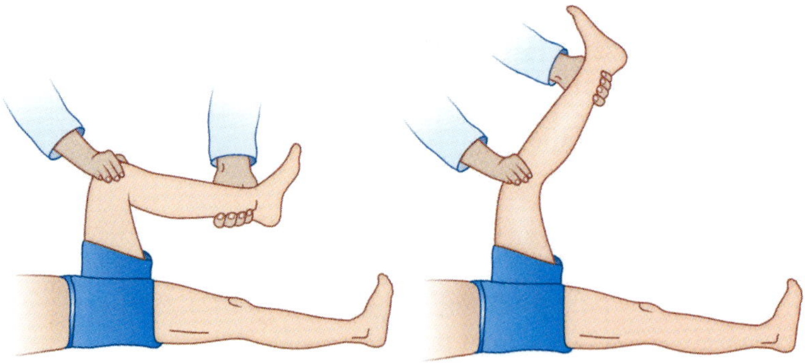

Eliciting Kerning's sign

- **Brudzinski's leg sign:** Flexion of knee and hip of opposite side following flexion of other limb
- **Straight leg raising test**

Note: Meningeal signs in-meningeal irritation are due to stretching of spinal nerve roots causing reflex muscle spasm

*Example:*______ years old male/female child suspected to have TB meningitis with right hemiplegic/convulsion ±/cranial nerve palsies of __________

Features s/o increased ICT with grade III PEM with normal/abnormal development, immunised for age.

Differences between UMN and LMN Lesion

Features	Upper motor neuron lesion	Lower motor neuron lesion
Power	Reduced	Markedly reduced
Distribution of muscle weakness	Diffuse and symmetrical	Patchy and asymmetrical
Muscle tone	Spasticity	Hypotonia/atonia
Muscle wasting	Minimal/absent	Significant
DTR	Brisk ± clonus	Sluggish/absent
Plantar	Extensor	Flexor/absent
Fasciculation/fibrillation	Absent	Seen
Reaction of degeneration	Absent	Seen

In UMN facial nerve palsy forehead is spared.

Differences between Cerebellar and Extrapyramidal Dysfunction

Features	Cerebellar dysfunction	Extrapyramidal dysfunction
Power	Normal	Normal
Muscle tone	Hypotonia	Cog-wheel/dystonia
Muscle wasting	Absent	Absent
Speech	Scanning	Slurred
Gait	Reeling/ataxic	Shuffling
Tremors	Intention	Pill rolling/resting tremors

GLASSGOW COMA SCALE (GCS)

Eye opening	Verbal response	Motor response
4 Spontaneous 3 To voice 2 To pain 1 None	5 Oriented 4 Confused 3 Inappropriate words 2 Incomprehensible sounds 1 No response to pain	6 Obeys commands 5 Localizes to pain 4 Withdraws 3 Flexion response to pain (decorticate) 2 Extension response to pain (decerebrate) 1 No response to pain

Score <7 indicates coma, max score = 15, min score = 3

CRITERIA FOR SIMPLE FEBRILE SEIZURE

1	6 months to 5 years
2	Neurologically normal child
3	Absence of CNS infection
4	Family history
5	Within 24 hours of fever
6	Single episode
7	Generalised tonic clonic seizure (GTCS)
8	<10 minutes
9	No post neurological deficit
10	EEG normal, CT normal

Cerebral Palsy

Nonprogressive, nondegenerative neuromuscular disorder often associated with epilepsy, abnormalities of speech, vision and intellect due to defect or lesion in the developing brain. Types—spastic/ataxic/dyskinetic/atonic/dystonic/mixed.

Acute Flaccid Paralysis

Onset of paralysis (<4 weeks) in a child <15 years of age for which no obvious cause has been found.
Common causes are—polio/GBS/transverse myelitis and traumatic neuritis

Acute Encephalitis Syndrome (AES)

A person of any age, at any time of year with the acute onset of fever and a change in mental status (including symptoms such as confusion, disorientation, coma, or inability to talk) and/or new onset of seizures (excluding simple febrile seizures).

Involuntary Movements

1. **Ballismus:** Throwing movement, rapid, forceful, flingy (disappear in sleep, spare face and trunk)
2. **TICS:** Throat clearing, shrugging of shoulders, eye blinking, increase during stress, can suppress voluntarily
3. **Tremors:** Purposeless rhythmic movement
4. **Athetoid movement:** Stiffening and loosening of the body (rhythmic, irregular, disappear in sleep, increase with activity)
5. Chorea = nonrhythmic, fast abrupt, brief jerky, milk maid grip, darting tongue, piano playing, disappear in sleep, [Sydenham's chorea (St Vitus' dance) seen in Rh fever]

GAIT

- Circumduction gait → Hemiplegia
- High stepping gait → Polio, peripheral neuropathy
- Ataxic/drunken gait → Cerebellar lesion
- Waddling gait → Myopathic gait
  - U/L → Trendelenburg
  - B/L → Hip girdle muscle weakness
- Diplegic/spastic gait → Cerebral palsy
- Parkinsonian gait → Walk of little steps

Specific Investigation to Diagnose CNS Diseases

- **Lumbar puncture**—CSF analysis (pages 223–225)
- **Cranial ultrasonography or neurosonogram (NSG)**—useful in—newborn and infants with open AF
- **Computed tomography scan (CT scan)**
  - Quick and inexpensive than MRI
  - Contrast/Noncontrast → to see structural defects—cerebral palsy/SOL/bleeding
    ↓
    meningitis
- **Magnetic resonance imaging (MRI)**
  - Better anatomic details than CT, espessially for myelination and migration disorders, vascular
  - Better visualisation or posterior fossa/temporal lobes
- **Electroencephalogram (EEG)**—to diagnose and followup of seizures.

CHAPTER

16

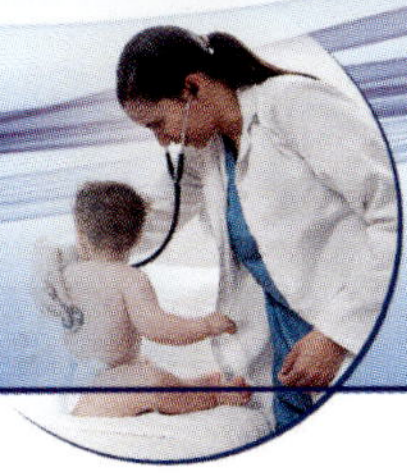

Muscle, Bones, Joints and Rheumatic Disorders*

History and thorough general examination are to be done.

AUTO-ANTIBODIES ASSOCIATED WITH RHEUMATOLOGIC DISEASE

Systemic lupus erythematosus (SLE)	Juvenile rheumatoid arthritis or JIA	Vasculitis
• ANA • Anti-double stranded DNA • Anti-Smith • Anti-RNP • Anti-microsomal Anti-phospholipids	• Rheumatoid factor • Anti-cyclic citrullinated peptide (ACCP) • Anti-citrullinated protein Ab (ACPA) • Anti-perinuclear factor (APF)	• ANCA cyto-plasmic/PR3 • ANCA Perinuclear/MPO

DUCHENNE MUSCULAR DYSTROPHY

Most common hereditary neuromuscular disorder. X-linked recessive, dystrophin deficiency predisposes to destruction of muscle fibres.

(Lyon hypothesis—One X chromosome becomes inactive. Why some Genetic disorders as DMD, colour blindness, haemophilia mostly found in males? explained by Lyon hypothesis)

Males are Commonly Affected

- **Age:** 3–10 years.

*Written by Dr Fazeel Ahmed Khan (MBBS, D Ortho, DNB orthopaedics), Senior Clinical Fellow, University Hospital Birmingham, Birmingham, UK

- **C/F:** Gradual proximal muscle weakness
  - Pseudohypertrophy of calf muscle
  - Valley sign
  - Positive Grower sign
  - Intellectual impairment
  - DTR absent except ankle
  - Waddling gait, lordosis/scoliosis
  - Cardiomyopathy
  - Acute respiratory failure

Investigation

- Increase serum creatinine kinase (CK)
- Normal CK is 160 U/L in DMD >10000 U/L
- Muscle biopsy/molecular genetics
- EMG/NCV/MRI/ECG

Treatment

Supportive/steroids/treatment of complication/myostatin inactivation/myoblast transfer/genetic counselling.

Prognosis

With advance cardio-respiratory treatment, patient can survive till early 30s.

JUVENILE IDIOPATHIC ARTHRITIS (JIA)/JUVENILE RHEUMATOID ARTHRITIS (JRA)

Joint swelling or limitation/tenderness upon range of motion lasting ≥6 weeks and not due to other identifiable cause.

Systemic	Arthritis >1 joints with/or fever >2 weeks and >1 of the following 1. Erythematous rash 2. Hepatomegaly/splenomegaly or both 3. Generalised lymphadenopathy 4. Serositis (pericarditis, pleuritis, peritonitis)
Oligo	Arthritis <4 joints in the first 6 months • Persistent <4 joints for the course of disease • Extended >4 joints after 6 months of disease
Poly	Arthritis >4 joints in the first 6 months • RF—negative • RF—positive

Treatment

NSAIDs, DMARDs, immunomodulators

1. Naproxen—15 mg/kg/day BD
2. Ibuprofen—40 mg/kg/day TDS
3. Methotrexate—0.5–1 mg/kg PO/S/C (give with folic acid)
4. Sulphasalazine—40 mg/kg/day BD
5. Leflunomide—20 mg/kg/day OD

SYSTEMIC LUPUS ERYTHEMATOSUS (SLE)

An episodic, multisystem autoimmune disease characterized by inflammation of blood vessels and connective tissue. Apart from drug-induced SLE, the aetiology remains unknown.

C/F—Mnemonic (MD SOAP BRAIN)

- **M**alar rash
- **D**iscoid lupus,
- **S**erositis (pleuritis, carditis)
- **O**ral ulcer
- **A**rthritis
- **P**hotosensitivity
- **B**one marrow involvement
- **R**enal (nephritis)
- **A**NA positive
- **I**mmunological phenomenon
- **N**eurological involvement

Treatment

NSAIDs, hydroxycholoroquine, steroids, cytotoxic therapy (cyclophosphamide), DMARDs, immunomodulators.

HENOCH-SCHÖNLEIN PURPURA (HSP)

a. Most common small-vessel vasculitis in children
b. More frequent in males than females
c. Typical age of onset 2–7 years
d. History of viral upper respiratory infection several weeks preceding onset of illness

C/F

- Non-thrombocytopenic purpura
- Migratory polyarthritis and/or polyarthralgia

- Abdominal pain
- Glomerulonephritis

Treatment

Supportive/steroids/immunosuppression

Kawasaki Disease

- Fever >5 days
- B/L conjunctival congestion
- Erythema of lips, buccal mucosa, tongue
- Cervical lymphadenopathy
- Polymorphous exanthema
- Erythema of palms and soles (edema followed by desquamation)
- Coronary dilatation

  5 or 4 + coronary dilatation is diagnostic.

Mnemonic—CRASH

- **C**onjunctivitis
- **R**ash
- **A**neurysm
- **S**trawberry tongue,
- **H**and and foot desquamation

Treatment

IVIG/steroids/aspirin/close follow-up.

Proximal Muscle Weakness in

Mnemonic—(MAGNETS)

- **M**etabolic, myasthenia gravis
- **A**drenal (Cushing's syndrome)
- **G**BS
- **N**eoplasm
- **E**lectrolyte imbalance
- **T**hyroid myopathy
- **S**teroid myopathy

Distal Muscle Weakness in

Mnemonic—(MP)

- **M**yotonic dystrophy
- **P**olyneuropathy

DIFFERENCES BETWEEN MYOPATHY AND NEUROPATHY

Features	Myopathy	Neuropathy
Muscle weakness	Proximal (except myotonic muscular dystrophy)	Distal (except juvenile SMA)
DTR	Preserved	Lost
Sensory abnormalities	Not seen	Present
EMG	Low amplitude	High amplitude

RHEUMATIC FEVER

Modified Jones Criteria for Rheumatic Fever

Major Mnemonic— **CANCER**	**C**arditis (clinical/subclinical) **A**rthritis (polyarthritis in low risk, poly/mono-arthritis, polyarthralgia in high risk) Subcutaneous **N**odules **C**horea **E**rythema marginatum
Minor	Fever (≥38.5°C in low risk ≥38°C in high-risk population) Arthralgia (polyarthralgia in low risk Monoarthralgia in high risk) Elevated ESR/CRP/WBC (ESR ≥60 mm/hr in low risk and ≥30 mm/hr in high risk) Prolonged PR interval in ECG
Essential	Evidence of streptococcal infection (ASO titre >333 Todd units, anti-DNAse B, positive throat culture, recent scarlet/streptococcal sore throat, positive RAT for streptococcal)

Low risk papulations is defind as:

1. Incidence of acute RhF <2/1 lakh in school going children.
2. RHD prevalence <1/1000 at any age during one year.

Two major or 1 major + 2 minor + evidence of streptococcal infection is diagnostic of aRhF.

Rheumatic Fever

- Licks the joints
- Bites the heart
- Kicks the brain

DIFFERENCES BETWEEN RHEUMATIC AND RHEUMATOID ARTHRITIS

Features	Rheumatic arthritis	Rheumatoid arthritis
Age	5–15 years	<3 years onwards
Onset	Acute	Chronic
Joints affected	Larger joints	Smaller joints TMJ, IP joints
Symmetry	Asymmetrical	Symmetrical
Pain	Migratory	Non-migratory
Carditis	Common	Rare
ASO titre	Positive	Negative
RA factor	Negative	Positive
Residual effects on joint	Not present	Present (swan neck deformity)
Response to salicylates	In <12–24 hours	Slow
Course	Recovers fast	Chronic course

GENU VALGUS/KNOCK KNEES

- Let the child stand erect with both medial condyles of knee touching each other. If the distance between two malleoli is >5 cm—Genu valgus
- For example—congenital rickets, vit D deficiency

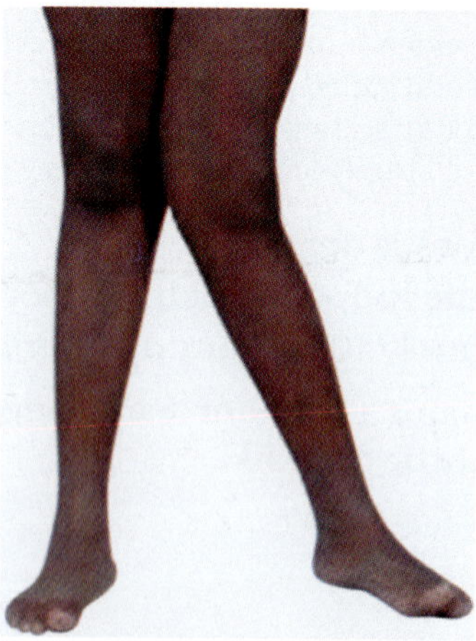

Genu valgus

GENU VARUS

- Let the child stand erect with both medial malleoli touching each other. If the distance between medial condyles of knee is >5 cm—genu varus
- For example—congenital rickets, achondroplasia, renal osteodystrophy
- Both genu valgus and genu varus are physiological up to 2 years of age.

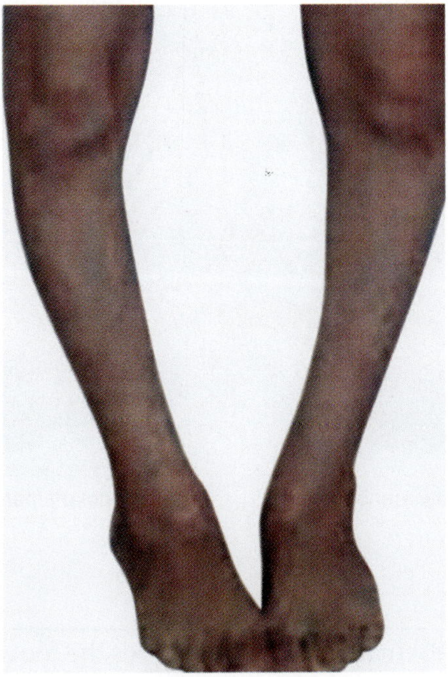

Genu varus

DEVELOPMENTAL DYSPLASIA OF THE HIP (DDH)

- Risk factors includes: **First** (first born), **Female** (80% of all DDH), **Family** history, **Feet** first (Breech)
- Test to do: **Ortolani** goes **in** and **Barlow** pushes **out**
- First do Barlow manoeuvre: Adduct hip while applying gentle downward pressure on knee (may hear pop)—femoral head out.

- Confirm by Ortolani manoeuvre
- Flex knee and hips with index and middle finger to 90°, putting pressure on greater trochanters
- Now abduct thighs with thumbs (may hear clunk)
- Femoral head relocates

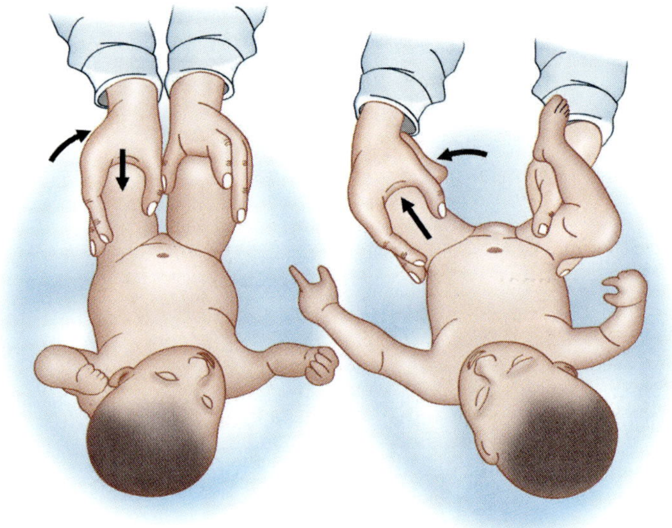

Barlow manoeuvre   Ortolani manoeuvre

CLUB FOOT

Idiopathic, present at birth, and involves the foot and lower leg. M:F 2:1. 50% are bilateral.

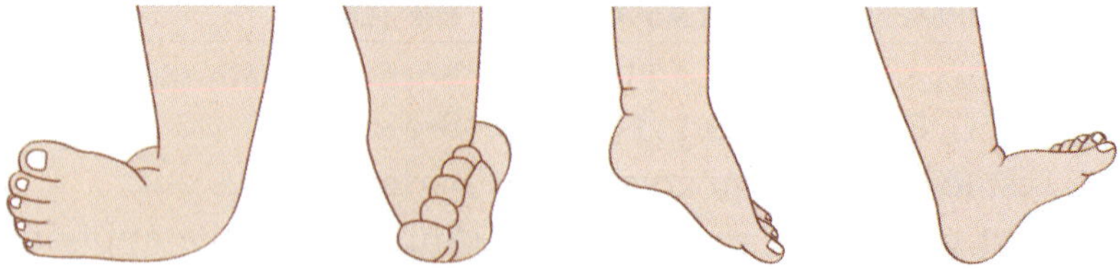

Talipes varus   Talipes valgus   Talipes equinus   Talipes calcaneus

Treatment

Grandma stretching, plaster, brace and sometimes surgery.

Congenital Talipus Equino Varus (Club Foot) CTEV

- Adduction of fore foot
- Inversion of hind foot
- Medial rotation
- Varus deformity
- Equinus deformity (plantar flexion)

PES Planus (Flat Foot)

Absence of longitudinal arch, e.g. cerebral palsy

PES Cavus (Claw Foot)

High longitudinal arch, e.g. polio, syringomyelia

Cubitus Valgus

(Normal carrying angle 3–29°)
Angulation (bowing) of bone (distal part of the forearm points laterally)

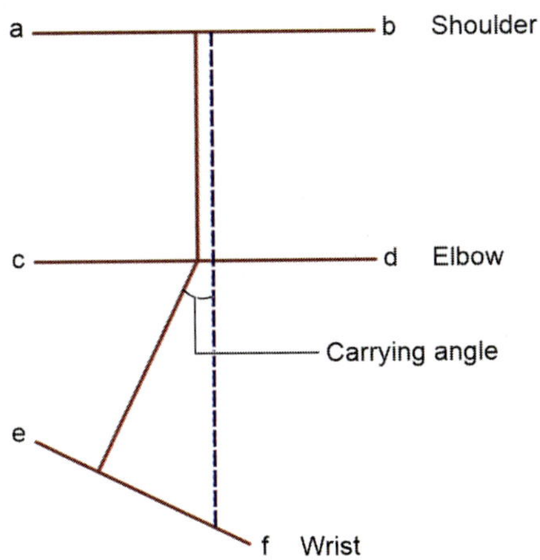

Cubitus Varus

A deformity of the elbow resulting in decreased carrying angle

Rickets

It is disease of growing bone. Defective mineralisation despite normal collagen matrix.

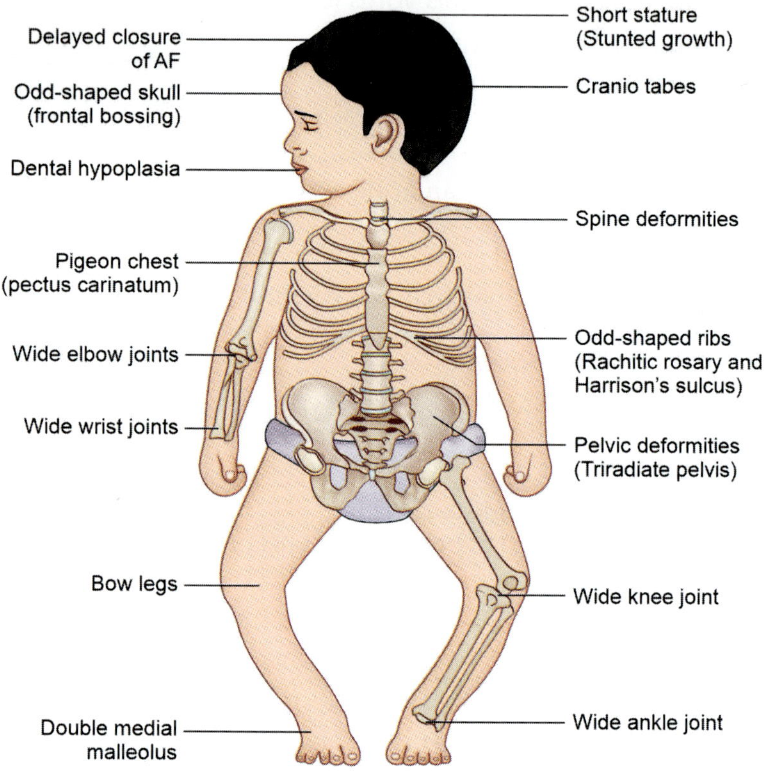

Club foot

Classification of Rickets

1. Vitamin D deficiency rickets
   (Responds to normal dose of vitamin D)
   - Nutritional rickets
   - Calcium deficient rickets
2. Vitamin D dependent rickets
   (Responds to high dose of vitamin D)
   - Type I: Deficiency of 1–α-hydroxylase
   - Type II: Resistance to 1, $25(OH)_2D_3$ (calcitriol)

3. Vitamin D resistant rickets
   (No response to vitamin D)

Hereditory	Renal origin	Oncogenic
(1) X-linked familial hypophosphataemic	RTA	
(2) Idiopathic	Lowe sd	
(3) AR	Galactosaemia	
(4) AD		

Approach to Refractory Rickets

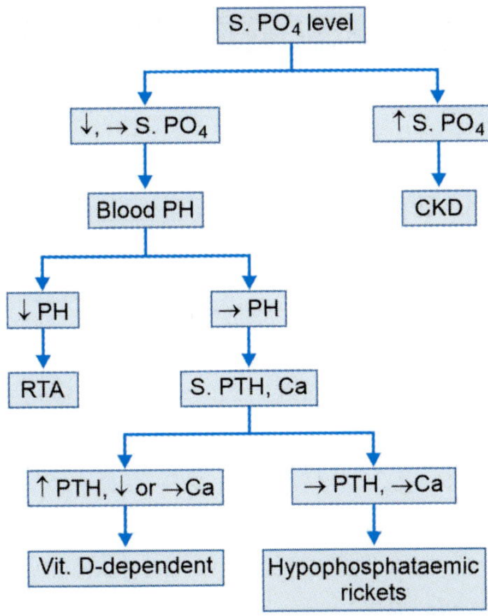

↑ Increase, ↓ Decrease, → Normal

Rachitic Rosary or Costochondral Beading

Prominent knobs of bone at the costochondral joints due to expansion of the anterior ribs ends at the costochondral junction.

Harrison's Sulcus

Indentation of the softened lower rib cage at the site of attachment of diaphragm.

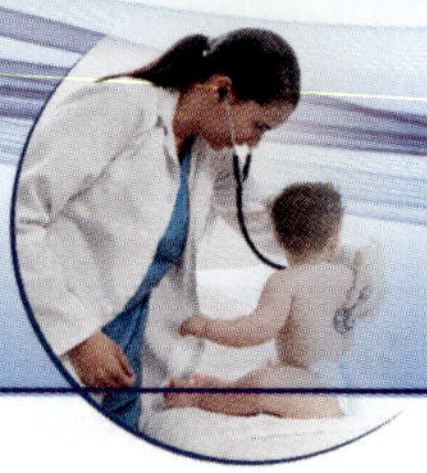

CHAPTER

17

Neonatology

NEONATAL CASE SHEET

Mothers Name:

Age:

Gravida ________ Para ________ Live ________ Abortion ________

NND ________ LMP ________ EDD ____________

Conceived ________ spontaneously/infertility treatment

POG (period of gestation) ________

Ist trimester (12 weeks) ________

IInd trimester (28 weeks) ________

IIIrd trimester (41 weeks) ________

H/o Drug intake   Yes/No

H/o GDM   Yes/No

H/o PIH   Yes/No

Interval b/w ROM (Rupture of membrane) and Delivery—

Vaginal bleeding/Infection ________

Mode of Delivery— Vaginal-assisted

LSCS

Indication—

Date of Birth— Time—

Gestational Age

Singleton/Twin I/II

Sex—M/F

Birth weight—

SGA/AGA/LGA

Resuscitation method: Yes/No

O_2 Blow by

Bag and Mask

Intubation

APGAR: 1″: ______, 5″ ______

Neonatal reflexes: Intact/depressed

Breastfeeding: When started after delivery

Stool/Urine—Passed/Not passed

(Baby should pass stool within 24 hours and urine within 48 hours)

History: Postpartum/family/immunisation/development

Vitals: HR/RR/temperature/colour of skin/pulse oxymetry/CFT

Anthropometry: HC, length, chest circumference

Head to toe examination: Before touching the baby wash your hands properly, dry, warm

Anterior fontanelle (AF) ________

Umbilical cord: 2 arteries, 1 vein

Signs of birth trauma

Congenital anomalies: No/Yes

Look for caput/cephalohematoma, cataract, deformed ears, choanal atresia, cleft lip/palate, fingers, umbilical hernia, imperforated anus, CTEV, DDH, B/L femoral pulses, spine

ASSESSMENT OF GESTATIONAL AGE OF PREMATURE BABY

New Ballard Scoring System

Components—physical maturity, neuromuscular maturity

- Can be used up to 4 days after birth
- Error margin ± 2 weeks

Neuromuscular Maturity

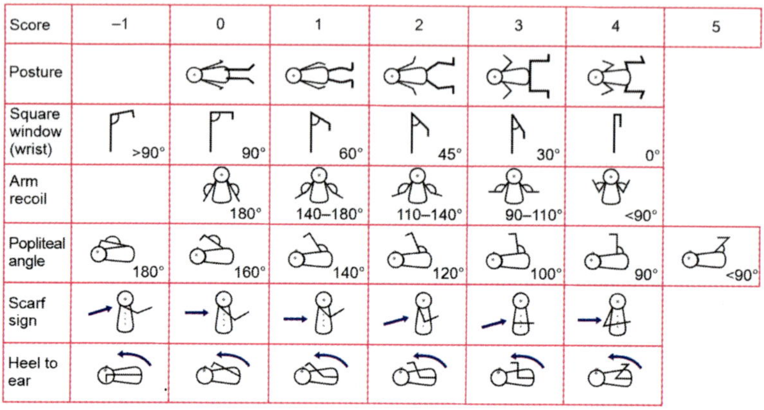

Physical Maturity

Skin	Sticky, friable, transparent	Gelatinous, red, translucent	Smooth, pink, visible veins	Superficial peeling and/ or rash; few veins	Cracking, pale, areas; rare veins	Parchment, deep cracking; no vessels	Leathery, cracked, wrinkled
Lanugo	None	Sparse	Abundant	Thinning	Bald areas	Mostly bald	
Plantar surface	Heel-toe 40–50 mm; –1 <40 mm; –2	>50 mm, no crease	Faint red marks	Anterior transverse crease only	Creases anterior 2/3	Creases over entire sole	
Breast	Imperceptible	Barely perceptible	Flat areola, no bud	Stippled areola, 1–2 mm bud	Raised areola, 3–4 mm bud	Full areola, 5–10 mm bud	
Eye/Ear	Lids fused loosely: –1 tightly: –2	Lids open; pinna flat; stays folded	Slightly curved pinna; soft; slow recoil	Well curved pinna; soft but ready recoil	Formed and firm, instant recoil	Thick cartilage ear stiff	
Genitals (male)	Scrotum flat, smooth	Scrotum empty, faint rugae	Testes in upper canal, rare rugae	Testes descending, few ruage	Testes down, good rugae	Testes pendulous, deep rugae	
Genitals (female)	Clitoris prominent, labia flat	Clitoris prominent, small labia minora	Clitoris prominent, enlarging minora	Majora and minora equally prominent	Majora large, minora small	Majora cover clitoris and minora	

Maturity rating	
Score	Weeks
–10	20
–5	22
0	24
5	26
10	28
15	30
20	32
25	34
30	36
35	38
40	40
45	42
50	44

NEONATAL DEFINITIONS

Neonate/newborn	<28 days
Early neonatal period	<7 days
Late neonatal period	7–28 days
Stillbirth	Fetal death at a GA of >22 weeks or weight >500 g
Perinatal period	22 weeks of gestation to 7 days after birth
Term	37–41 weeks of gestation

Contd.

Preterm	<37 weeks
Post-term	>42 weeks
LBW	Birth weight <2500 g
VLBW	Birth weight <1500 g
ELBW	Birth weight <1000 g
AGA	Birth weight between 10th and 90th centile for GA
SGA	Birth weight <10th centile for GA
LGA	Birth weight >90th centile for GA
Infancy	Birth to 1 year of age

PHASES OF NEONATAL RESUSCITATION (NRP)

- Preparation
- Resuscitation—TABCD
- Post-resuscitation care

PREPARATION

Anticipatory Preparation

Prepare resuscitation kit. Check equipments. Preparation and organize a team. Use pre-resuscitation checklist.

Equipment

1. **Suction:** Meconium aspirator, mechanical suction, suction catheter (10, 12, 14 Fr)
2. **Oxygen source:** Oxygen cylinders with flow meter and tubing, nasal cannula and nasal prongs

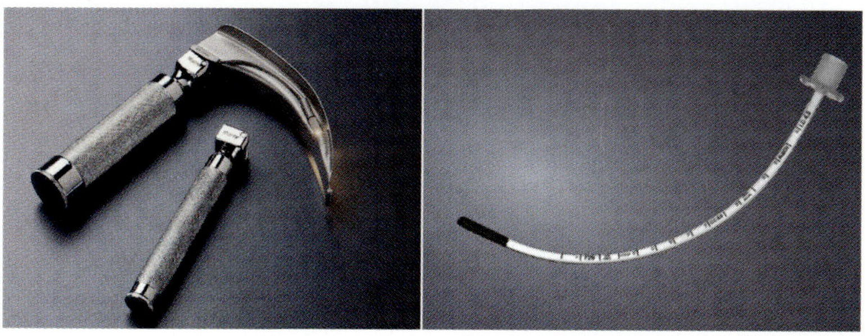

Laryngoscope: Handle, blade, and ET tube

3. **Bag and mask:** Self inflating neonatal resuscitation bags (250 ml, 500 ml), face masks (for term (1) and preterm babies (0))
4. **Intubation:** Laryngoscope with straight blades

Laryngoscope no	Age
Zero	Preterm
1	Term babies
2	1–10 years
3	>10 years

Endotracheal Tubes

Tube size (mm)	Weight (g)	Gestational age (week)
2.5	<1000	<28
3	1000–2000	28–34
3.5	>2000	>34

Old recommendation—to fix at **(6 + weight in kg)**

Example: If baby's wt is 2.5 kg so use 3.5 no ET tube and fix it at 8.5 no (written on tube)

New recommendation: Nasal-tragus length (NTL) + 1

For older children ET size = (Age in years +16)/4
Tube depth from lip/teeth = 3 × ET size
e.g. 4 years old child ET size (4 +16)/4 = 5 no and to fix it
3 × 5 = 15 cm from lower lip
Note: >8 years should use cuffed ET tube

Note: Suction catheter size required in Fr = 2 × ET tube size (for newborn if you are using 3 mm ET for suction you should use 6 Fr size)

5. **Medications:** Epinephrine, normal saline, naloxone/sterile water, vit K
6. Oximeter, EKG monitor, CPAP, exhaled CO_2 monitor

   [to monitor oxygenation use pulse oximeter, for ventilation exhaled CO_2 monitor (end tidal CO_2)]
7. **Miscellaneous:** Stop watch/linen/shoulder roll/gauze/radiant warmer/stethoscope/adhesive tape/syringes/6 Fr feeding tube/umbilical catheter (for <3.5 kg, 3.5 F UC >3.5 kg, 5 F UC)/3-way/gloves, otoscope/ophthalmoscope, cord clamp, sterile blade

8. Observe 5 Cs to prevent sepsis
   i. Clean hands
   ii. Clean surface
   iii. Clean blade
   iv. Clean tie
   v. Clean cord-keep it dry

RESUSCITATION—TABCD

• Thermoregulation	• Wiping/radiant warmer/clothing • Routine care of newborn staying with mother • Warm (skin-to-skin contact is recommended), dry the newborn. • Postpone bath until cord falls off • Measure axillary temperature within 10 minutes of NICU admission
• **A**irway management	• Clear airway by wiping the baby's mouth and nose. (Routine suctioning is not recommended)
• **B**reathing	1. Tactile stimulation 2. Oxygen by nasal prong/hood 3. Bag and mask 4. Chest compression 5. Endotracheal intubation/LMA
• **C**irculation and drugs	1. Adrenaline 2. Naloxone 3. Volume expanders

Initial Steps

- Resuscitation oriented history
  a. What is the expected gestational age?
  b. Is the amniotic fluid clear?
  c. What is our umbilical card management plan?
  d. Are there any additional risk factors?
- At birth, answer 3 questions to determine the need for initial steps at the radiant warmer:
  a. Is the newborn term?
  b. Is the newborn breathing or crying?

c. Does the newborn have good muscle tone?
   If any answer is "No," the newborn should receive initial steps at the radiant warmer. [Positioning → Tactile stimulation → suctioning → repositioning (PSSR)]

The vigorous no meconium-stained newborn need not receive initial steps at the radiant warmer, but may receive routine care (with appropriate monitoring) with his mother.

T: Prevent Heat Loss

Wiping/radiant warmer/clothing

- Routine care of newborn staying with mother: Warm (skin-to-skin contact is recommended), dry the newborn.
- Postpone bath until cord falls off.

A: Clear the Airway/Open the Airway

Clear airway by wiping the baby's mouth and nose. Routine suctioning is not recommended.

- Suctioning following birth (including bulb suctioning with a bulb syringe) should be reserved for babies who have obvious obstruction to spontaneous breathing or who require positive-pressure ventilation.

Suctioning—first mouth (5 cm) then nose (3 cm),
Suction catheter—12 or 14 Fr,
Suction pressure—<50 mm Hg/<100 cm water

B: Initiate Breathing

After clearing the airway as necessary, drying and removing wet linen, repositioning, and stimulating, evaluate respirations and heart rate (not colour).

a. If HR is less than 100 BPM, or if newborn is apnoeic or gasping, begin positive-pressure ventilation (PPV).
b. If HR is more than 100 BPM and respirations are labored, consider CPAP, especially for preterm newborns.

B1: Tactile Stimulation

Gentle back rub

B2: O_2

Resuscitation of term newborns may begin with 21% oxygen (room air); resuscitation of preterm newborns may begin with a somewhat higher oxygen concentration 21–30%.

Evaluation

Breathing/heart rate/ or SpO_2 every 30 seconds

Use pulse oximetry

- HR monitoring—3-**lead EKG monitor for rapid and reliable HR assessment**

Place the oximeter probe on the newborn's right hand or wrist (measure preductal saturation)

Using pulse oximetry, supplemental oxygen concentration should be adjusted to achieve the target values for pre-ductal saturations summarized in the table on the NRP flow diagram. The table is used for both term and preterm babies.

B3: Bag and Mask Ventilation

Self-inflating bag/pressure gauge/oxygen reservoir/face mask/oxygen source with flow meter

Technique

- Keep infant's neck in slight extension (if needed use shoulder roll)
- Select appropriate size mask
- Mask should snuggly fit covering mouth and nose excluding eyes
- Hold the face mask firmly on the face making "C" with thumb and index finger
- Lift the chin slightly making "E" with middle, ring and little finger
- Compress the bag using other hand fingers and release
- Bag-two-three, bag-two three, (press 40–60 times in a minute)

Rate = 40–60/min

Pressure: First breath –30–40 cm H_2O,

Later: 15–20 cm H_2O

Bag + Reservoir + O_2 source = 100%

Bag + Reservoir without O_2 source = 60%

Bag without reservoir and O_2 source = 21%

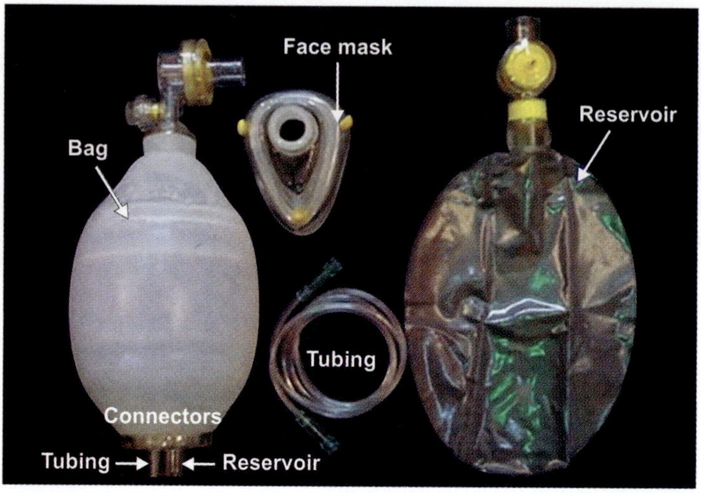

Indication

- Apnoea or gasping respirations
- Heart rate <100 BPM even if breathing
- Persistent central cyanosis and low oxygen saturation, despite free-flow oxygen increased to 100%.

Note: T piece resuscitator or free flow inflating bag (anaesthesia bag) can maintain PEEP better than a self inflating bag with a PEEP.

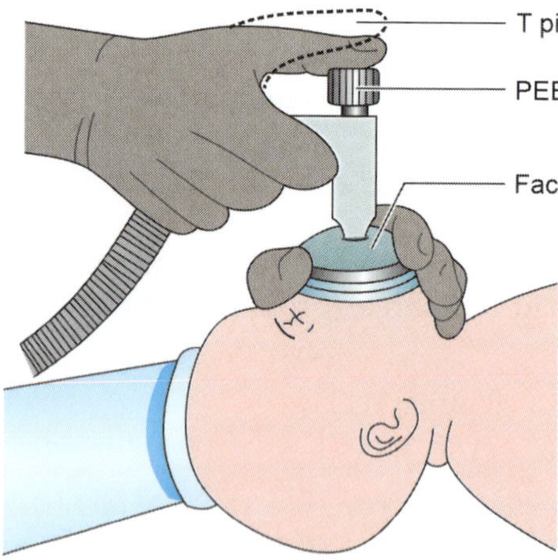

T piece resuscitator

Use **MR SOPA** to help you remember the ventilation corrective steps in order:

M: Adjust the mask on the face.

R: Reposition the head to ensure an open airway. Re-attempt ventilation, if not effective.

S: Suction the mouth and nose

O: Ventilate with the baby's mouth slightly open and lift the jaw forward. Re-attempt ventilation, if not effective.

P: Gradually increase pressure every few breaths, (cautiously, and to a maximum of 40 cm H_2O)

A: Consider airway alternative (endotracheal tube or laryngeal mask airway)

C/I for bag and mask ventilation is—
CDH (congenital diaphragmatic hernia)

Signs of improvement

- Increasing heart rate
- Spontaneous respirations
- Increasing SpO_2

B4: Chest Compression (CC)

Establishing effective ventilations is the highest priority in neonatal resuscitation. Do not start chest compressions without first establishing effective ventilation (defined by audible bilateral breath sounds and chest movement).

- Chest compressions are indicated if after 30 seconds of PPV with 100% of oxygen, the heart rate is: Below 60 beats/min
- **Discontinue:** Once the heart rate is >60 beats/min
- **Pressure:** Dept 1/3rd of AP diameter of the chest
- **Rate:** 90 compressions and 30 breaths/min. (1 and 2 and 3 and bag–1 and 2 and 3 and bag.....)
- Area on sternum just below line drawn between nipples
- Technique: **2-thumb technique is still recommended**

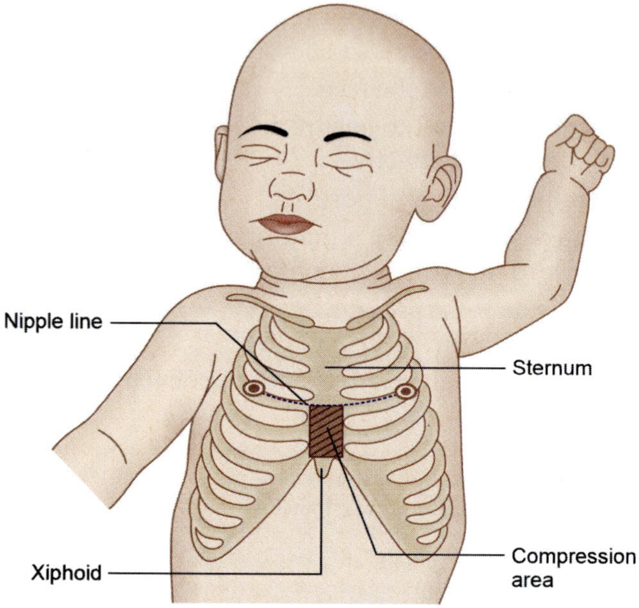

Landmark of chest compression

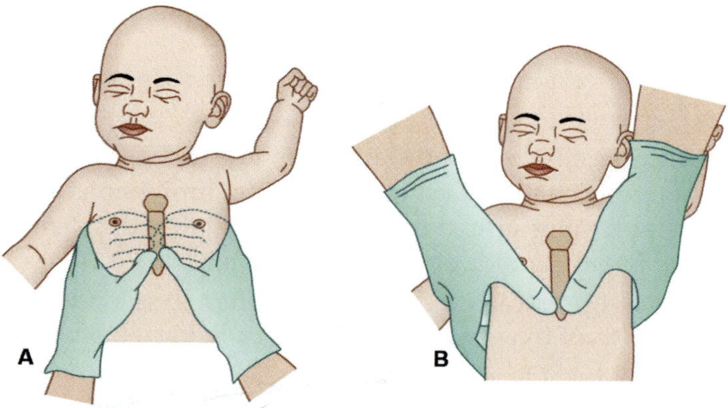

Thumb technique of chest compression administered from (A) Foot end; (B) Head end

Note: In children chest compression the depth of 2 inches (5 cm) (1/3rd of AP diameter)
When only one resuscitator is available 30 CC followed by 2 breaths

When two resuscitators are available

- <8 years 15 CC followed by 2 breaths
- >8 years 30 CC followed by 2 breaths

Note: Intubated child need to receive 10 breaths/min without any interruption for CC.

B5: Endotracheal Intubation

The intubation procedure ideally should be completed within 30 seconds (not 20 seconds). Do not administer free-flow oxygen during the intubation procedure to an apneic newborn.

Indications

- Prolonged positive pressure ventilation if required.
- Bag and mask ventilation is ineffective.
- Tracheal suctioning/medications
- Diaphragmatic hernia

Signs of correct tube position

- Chest rise with each breath
- Equal breath sounds over both lung fields
- No gastric distension with ventilation
- Vapour condensing on inside of tube during exhalation
- Carbon dioxide detector will change colour (or reads more than 2–3% during exhalation)—capnography
- X-ray confirmation

  Note: If intubation is not successful or feasible, laryngeal mask airway (LMA) should be used.
- Spontaneously breathing preterm infants <32 weeks gestation at high risk of RDS should be supported with CPAP of 5 cm H_2O using T-piece as soon as respiratory distress is noted.
- Infants needing positive pressure ventilation are to be provided with PIP and PEEP using T-piece device. Initial settings on the device being 15/5. If prompt improvement in heart rate or chest movement is not obtained, then higher pressures to achieve effective ventilation may be used.

C: Circulation and Drugs

Immediate cannulation/umbilical line/intraosseous cannulation (1–2 cm below and just medial to the tibial tuberosity).

C1: Epinephrine

It is indicated when the heart **rate remains below 60 BPM after 30 seconds of effective assisted ventilation** (preferably via Endotracheal tube) and at least another 60 seconds of coordinated chest compressions and effective ventilation.

Dose: Epinephrine administration (IV parameters unchanged; **note new dose for intratracheal epinephrine).**

a. Recommended concentration: 1:10,000 (0.1 mg/ml)
b. Recommended route: Intravenous (umbilical vein). Consider endotracheal route ONLY while IV access being obtained
c. Give rapidly—as quickly as possible.
d. Recommended IV dose: 0.2 ml/kg (0.02 mg/kg) of 1:10,000 solution in a 1-ml syringe. Follow IV administration of epinephrine with 3 ml of normal saline. Slow over 5–10 min.
e. Recommended intratracheal dose: 1 ml/kg of (0.1 mg/kg) 1:10,000 solution using PPV breaths to distribute in the lungs.
f. Check the newborn heart rate about 1 minute after administering epinephrine (longer if given endotracheally). *Epinephrine dose may be repeated every 3–5 minutes.*

C2: Naloxone

Indication

- Respiratory depression
- Recorded narcotic administration within 4 hours of delivery.
- Dose: 0.1 mg/kg IV, IO, ET, IM
- "Insufficient evidence to evaluate safety and efficacy" of *naloxone and risks of complications*

NRP Flow Diagram

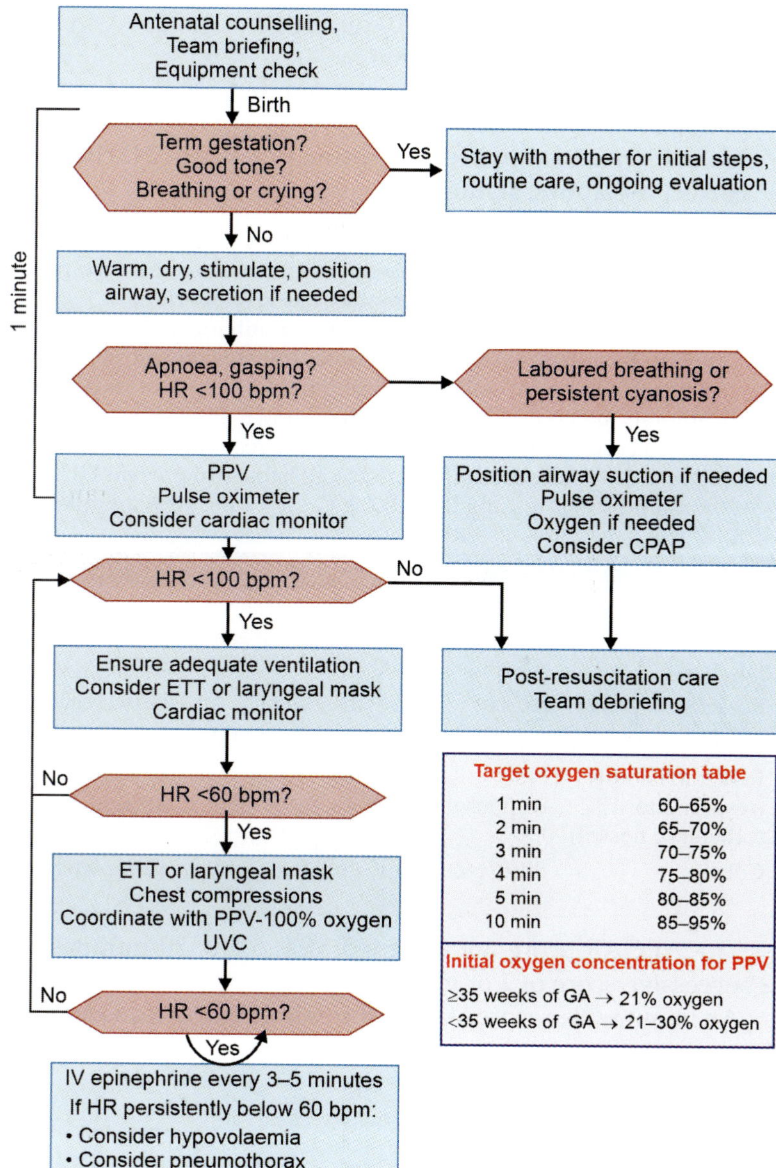

Target oxygen saturation table	
1 min	60–65%
2 min	65–70%
3 min	70–75%
4 min	75–80%
5 min	80–85%
10 min	85–95%

Initial oxygen concentration for PPV

≥35 weeks of GA → 21% oxygen
<35 weeks of GA → 21–30% oxygen

Note: Consider cessation around 20 minutes after death

C3: Volume Expanders

Whole blood/normal saline—10 ml/kg IV
Indication—signs of hypovolaemia.

- Ringer's lactate **no longer recommended** for management of hypovolaemic shock
- **No evidence to support the routine practice of $NaHCO_3$ to correct metabolic acidosis**

- **Cord clamping:** Delayed cord clamping for 1–3 minute for both term and preterm infants who do not require resuscitation at birth. DCC must be done even if the mother has HIV infection
- **Cord milking is not recommended:** Cord milking is an alternate method for rapidly achieving placental transfusion and involves milking 20 cm length of the umbilical cord two to three times before clamping the cord. Cord milking has shown similar benefits as delayed cord clamping but is currently not recommended
- Vitamin K should be administered to all babies (to prevent HDN) 0.5 mg IM <1000 g, 1 mg IM >1000 g (1 ml = 1 mg vit K ampule)

APGAR SCORE

Sign	0	1	2
HR	Absent	<100	>100
Respiratory effort	Absent	Slow irregular	Good/crying
Muscle tone	Limp	Some flexion of limbs	Active motion
Reflex irritability (response to catheter in nostril)	No response	Grimace	Cough or sneeze
Colour	Blue/pale	Body pink/extremities blue	Completely pink

The APGAR score are assigned at 1, 5, 10, 20 minutes till 2 successive score of 7 or greater.

An infant with a score of <4 requires immediate resuscitation.

Mnemonic: APGAR

Activity (muscle tone)
Pulse rate (HR)
Grimace (reflex irritability)
Appearance (colour)
Respiratory effort

MANAGEMENT OF INFANT BORN THROUGH MECONIUM-STAINED LIQUOR

- Every delivery is an emergency.
- Need two persons for resuscitation.
- If there is meconium-stained liquor, prepare yourself.
- Intrapartum suctioning of the mouth and nose (after delivery of the head and before delivering the shoulders) is no longer recommended.
- First step is to decide whether baby is vigorous (good cry/HR >100/minute, good tone) or not.

For nonvigorous baby

- Place the baby under radiant warmer.
- Residual meconium in the mouth and posterior pharynx should be removed by suctioning under direct vision using a laryngoscope.
- Neonates born through meconium-stained amniotic fluid and who are non-vigorous at birth, should be placed a radiant warmer and PPV should be initiated if needed. **Routine intubation for tracheal suction is no longer recommended.**
- Intubation and suction of the airway may be used as needed for ensuring oxygenation and ventilation.

NEONATAL REFLEXES

Reflex	Onset	Disappearance
Palmar grasp	32 weeks	3 months
Plantar	Birth	9 months
Rooting	32 weeks	3 months
Moro	32 weeks	3–4 months
Asymmetrical TNR	36 weeks	3–5 months
Symmetrical TNR	4–6 months	9 months
Landau	9 months	24 months
Parachute	9 months	Throughout life

TNR, tonic neck reflex

Moro (startle) reflex

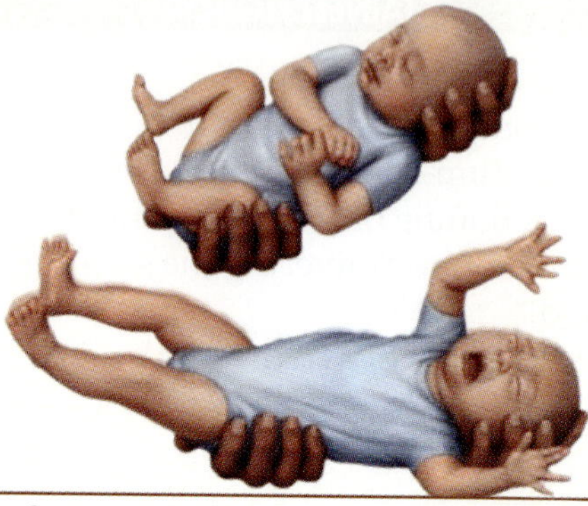

Asymmetrical tonic neck reflex (ATNR)

Onset ~ 36 weeks gestation **Integrates by ~ 3–5 months**

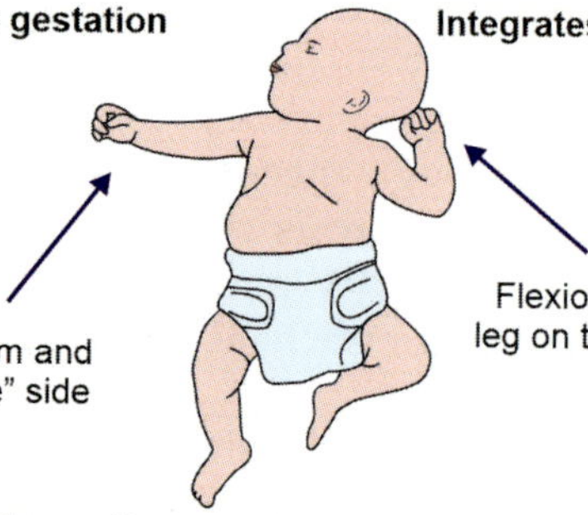

Extension of arm and leg on the "face" side

Flexion of arm and leg on the "skull" side

Importance: Promotes hand-eye coordination

Symmetrical tonic neck reflex (STNR)

Onset ~ 4-6 months **Integrates by ~ 9 months**

Test # 1: Place in crawling position and flex the head

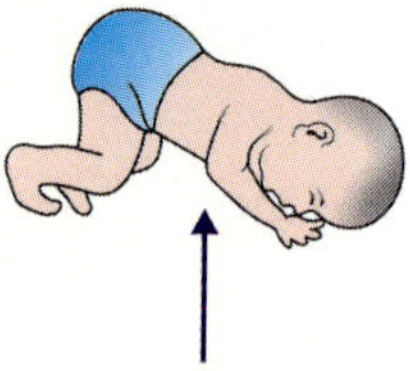

Arms flexed and legs extended

Test # 2: Place in crawling position and extend the head

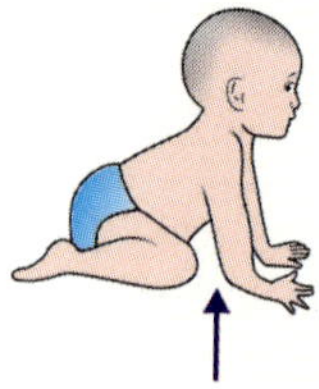

Arms extend and legs bend

Tip: Whatever the top half of the body does, the bottom does the opposite

NORMAL VARIATIONS IN NEWBORN

- Erythema toxicum
- Milia
- Mongolian spot
- Stork bites
- Peeling of skin
- Subconjunctival haemorrhages
- Cradle cap
- Breast engorgement
- Vaginal bleeding/discharge
- Hymenal tags
- Physiological phimosis
- Skin dimples/sinuses
- Epstein pearl—palatal/prepucial
- Natal teeth

ASSESSMENT FOR SEVERITY OF RESPIRATORY DISTRESS (DOWNE SCORE)

Parameter	Score 0	1	2
RR	<60	60–80	>80
Cyanosis	No	Cyanosis at room air	Cyanosis with >40% O_2
Retraction	Nil	Mild	Mod to severe
Grunt	Nil	Audible with stethoscope	Audible without stethoscope
Air entry	Good	Decreased	Barely audible
Prematurity	>34 weeks	30–34 weeks	<30 weeks

Score: <5 mild, 5–8 moderate, >8 severe

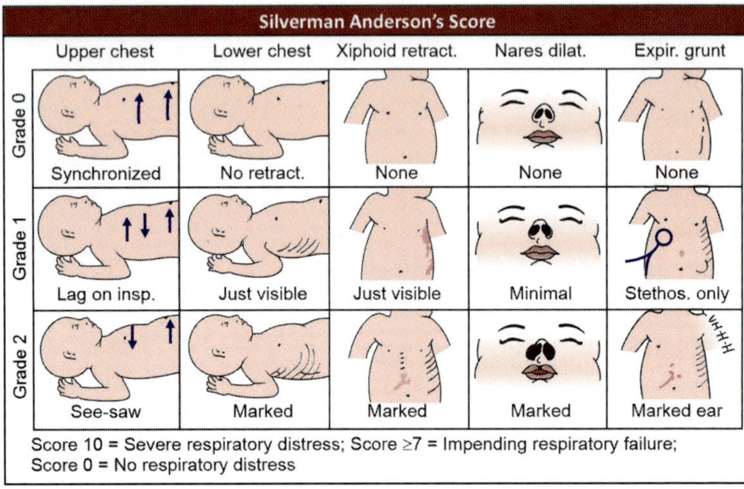

BABY-FRIENDLY HOSPITAL INITIATIVE (BFHI)

Critical management procedures:

1a. Comply fully with the international code of marketing of breast-milk substitutes and relevant world health assembly resolutions.

1b. Have a written infant feeding policy that is routinely communicated to staff and parents.

1c. Establish ongoing monitoring and data-management systems.

2. Ensure that staff have sufficient knowledge, competence and skills to support breastfeeding.

Key clinical practices:

3. Discuss the importance and management of breastfeeding with pregnant women and their families.
4. Facilitate immediate and uninterrupted skin-to-skin contact and support mothers to initiate breastfeeding as soon as possible after birth.
5. Support mothers to initiate and maintain breastfeeding and manage common difficulties.
6. Do not provide breastfed newborns any food or fluids other than breast milk, unless medically indicated.
7. Enable mothers and their infants to remain together and to practice rooming in 24 hours a day.

8. Support mothers to recognise and respond to their infants' cues for feeding.
9. Counsel mothers on the use and risks of feeding bottles, teats and pacifiers.
10. Coordinate discharge so that parents and their infants have timely access to ongoing support and care.

Points of Good Latching

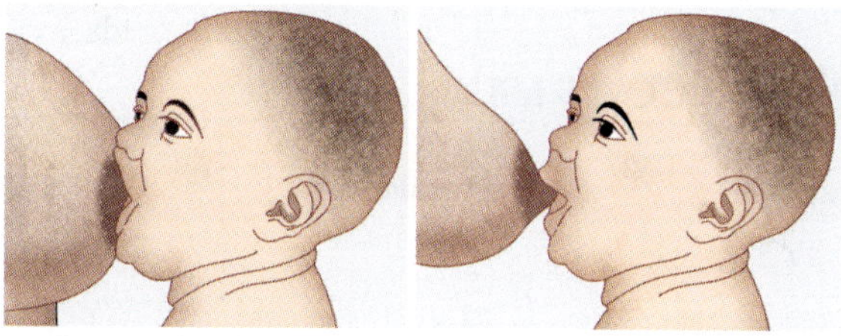

Correct latch on Incorrect latch on

- Baby's month is wide open
- Chin of the baby touches the breast
- Nipple and most of the areola is inside the baby's month
- Lower lip is turned outward
- Mother feels no pain or discomfort

Note: Rooting, sucking, swallowing reflex help the baby

BREASTFEEDING: BENEFITS (MNEMONIC: ABCDEFGH)

BF should start as soon as possible (ASAP)

For Infants

- **A**llergic condition reduced
- **B**est food for infant
- **C**lose relationship with mother
- **D**evelopment of IQ, jaws, mouth

For Mother

- **E**conomical
- **F**itness: quick return to pre-pregnancy body shape
- **G**uards against cancer: breast, ovary, uterus
- **H**aemorrhage (postpartum) reduced

Note: Prolactin—milk producing hormone; Oxytocin—milk ejection hormone

DRUGS CONTRAINDICATED DURING BREASTFEEDING (MNEMONIC—BREAST)

- **B**enzodiazepines/bromocriptine
- **R**adioactive isotope
- **E**rgotamine
- **A**ntiepileptic (ethosuximide)/antipsychotic (lithium)
- **S**ex hormones
- **T**etracycline

HUMAN MILK VS COW'S MILK

Constituent	Human milk	Cow's milk
Water	88%	88%
Calories	71 kcal	67 kcal
Protein (g/10 ml) Casein	1.1 0.4	3.3 2.7
Fats (g/100 ml) % PUFA	3.8 3	3.7 2
Carbohydrate (g/100 ml)	7	4.8
Minerals (g/100 ml)	0.2 iron though less but better absorbed	0.8 less iron and copper
Vitamins	Poor source of Vit D/K/C	Rich in vitamin B
Digestibility	Better	Poor
Renal solute load	79 (mOsmol/L)	221
Protective substance	Ig, bifidus factors, lactoferrin, antibodies	Not present

PHASES OF BREAST MILK

Colostrum	<4 days	More antibodies, vitamins and proteins, less in fat
Transitional milk	4–14 days	More fat, calories less immunoglobulin and protein

Contd.

Mature milk	>14 days	More fat, proteins and calories, less minerals
Foremilk	At the start of feed	Watery, rich in protein, sugar and minerals. Satisfies babies thirst
Hind milk	At the end of feed	Rich in fat content Satisfies babies hunger

Caput succedaneum—Ill-defined margins, disappear, by 1 week
Cephalhaematoma—defined margins, disappear by 6 weeks

Kangaroo Mother Care

Kangaroo mother care (KMC) refers to care of stable preterm or LBW infant by placing the infant in skin-to-skin contact with the mother or any other care givers.

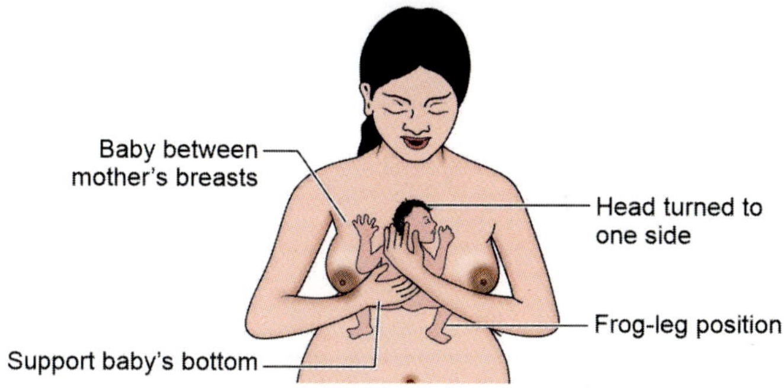

World Breastfeeding Week

- An annual celebration held every year from 1st to 7th August
- To highlight the benefits of breastfeeding for mother and baby
- Supported by WHO/UNICEF/Ministry of Health and others.
- 2022 theme—Step up for Breastfeeding—Educate and Support
- 2023 theme—Enabling Breastfeeding—Making a Difference for Working Parents
- 2024 theme—Closing the gap—Breastfeeding Support for All

JAUNDICE IN THE NEWBORNS

Jaundice is the most common morbidity in the first week of life, occurring in 60% of term and 80% of preterm newborn.

Jaundice in neonates is visible in skin and eyes when total serum bilirubin (TSB) concentration exceeds 5–7 mg/dl. In contrast to adults >2 mg/dl.

Increased TSB concentration in neonate results from 3 mechanisms:

1. Increased production from degradation of red cells
2. Decreased clearance by the immature hepatic mechanisms
3. Reabsorption by enterohepatic circulation (EHC).

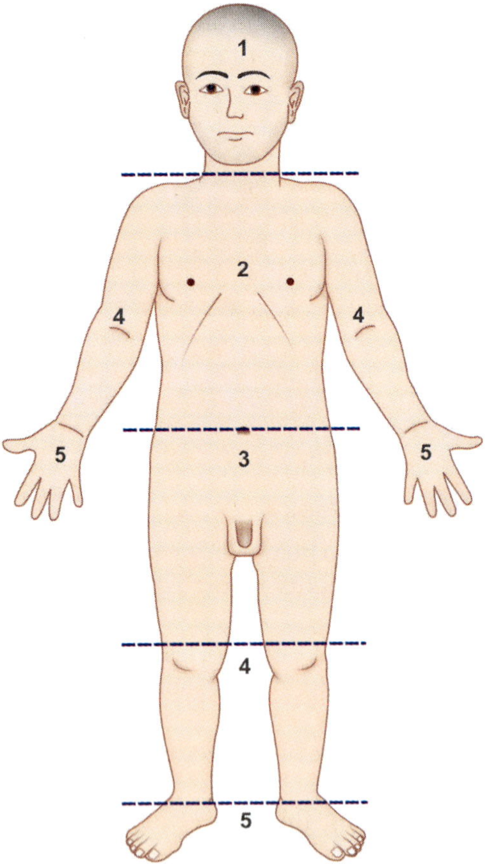

Kramer's scale

PATHOLOGICAL JAUNDICE

- Appear <24 hours
- Increase of bilirubin >5 mg/dl/day
- Persists >14 days
- Direct bilirubin >2 mg/dl or 20% of total bilirubin
- Signs of acute bilirubin encephalopathy or kernicterus

Example: Haemolysis—blood group incompatibility, enzyme deficiencies such as G6PD, extravasated blood—cephalhaematoma

Treatment: Breastfeeding, blue light phototherapy, exchange transfusion

Kramer's scale in predicting hyperbilirubinaemia in healthy full term infant

Dermal zone	Bilirubin (mg/dl)
1	5
2	10
3	12
4	15
5	>15

Modified Sarnat and Sarnat Staging for Hypoxic-ischemic Encephalopathy

Mnemonic: SARNAT

	Stage I	Stage II	Stage III
Seizure	Absent	Common	Uncommon
Autonomic function			
HR	Normal	Bradycardia	Variable
RR	Regular	Periodic	Apnoic attack
Pupil	Mydriasis	Miosis	Dilated and fixed
Reflex	Normal	Exaggerated	Absent
Neuromuscular	Flexion	Flexion	Intermittent decerebration
Activity	Hyperalert	Lethargic	Comatose
Tone	Normal	Hypotonia	Flaccid

Neonatal Thyroid Screening

- ↑ S.TSH, ↓ S.FT_4 levels
- Ultrasound neck/thyroid gland
- Antithyroid antibodies
- Radionuclide scan
  (Also evaluate mothers TFT/ATAb)

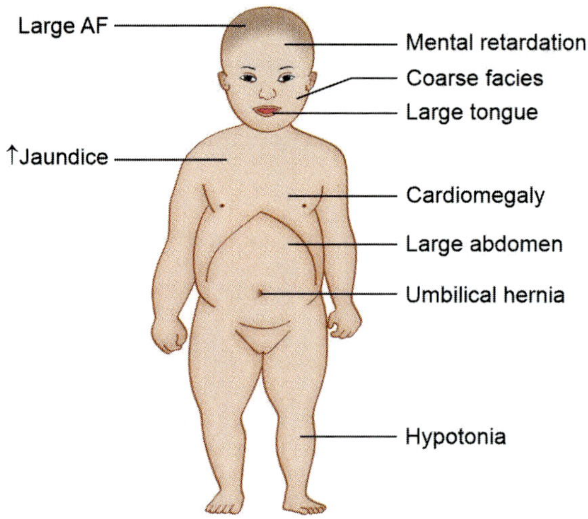

Features of congenital hypothyroidism

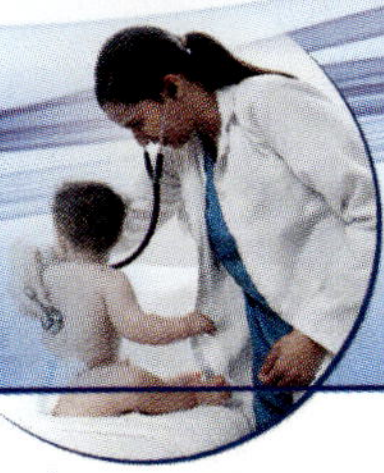

CHAPTER

18

Drugs/Formulary

COMMONLY USED PAEDIATRIC DRUGS

Drug	Indication	C/I	Dosage
Antipyretic, NSAIDs			
Paracetamol	Analgesic/ antipyretic/ NSAIDs	Hepatic failure, renal failure	10–15 mg/kg/dose (oral) 5 mg/kg/dose (IV)
Ibuprofen	Analgesic/ antipyretic/	NSAID allergy, peptic ulcer disease	5–10 mg/kg/dose q6–8h orally For PDA closure in Preterm babies- 10 mg/kg IV/PO followed by 5 mg/kg IV OD × 2 days (total 20 mg/kg)
Diclofenac			0.5–1 mg/kg/dose orally
Mefenamic acid	Analgesic/ antipyretic/ Dysmenorrhoea	Aspirin allergy, peptic ulcer disease	5–8 mg/kg/dose SOS PO
Naproxen	JRA/JIA Juvenile rheumatoid arthritis	Advanced renal disease, peptic ulcer disease	10–20 mg/kg/day q8–12h PO
Aspirin (Acetyl salicylic acid)	Acute rheumatic fever	Avoid empty stomach	90–120 mg/kg/day q6 h oral

Contd.

Drug	Indication	C/I	Dosage
Antacids			
Ranitidine	H_2 blocker-GERD, Antacid		1–4 mg/kg/dose q12h PO
Pantoprazole	PPI		<40 kg 20 mg OD >40 kg 40 mg OD PO
Antibiotics			
Amoxicillin	Gram-positive and gram-negative cocci	Hypersensitivity to penicillin gp	30–50 mg/kg/day in 3–4 divided doses (oral) 100–300 mg/kg/day in 3–4 divided doses (IV)
Erythromycin	Macrolides antibiotic-Treating gram-positive infection in penicillin allergic children, atypical pneumonia, pertussis		30–50 mg/kg/day q6h orally
Amikacin	Gram-negative organism	Ototoxic nephrotoxic	15–20 mg/kg/day in 2–3 divided doses, slow IV infusion over 1 hour
Gentamicin inj	Gram-negative infections	Myasthenia gravis	5–7.5 mg/kg/day IV/IM BD
Cefaclor	Cephalosporin antibiotics	Hypersensitivity to cephalosporin	20–40 mg/kg/day q8–12h orally
Cefoperazone with sulbactum sodium	ESBL organisms	Hypersensitivity to cephalosporin	80–160 mg/kg/day IV q6–12 h
Cefotaxime	Cephalosporin antibiotics	Hypersensitivity to cephalosporin	50 mg/kg/dose IV q6–8 h

Contd.

Drug	Indication	C/I	Dosage
Cefpodoxime	Covers both gram-positive and gram-negative bacteria		10 mg/kg/day q12h orally
Ceftazidime	*Pseudomonas aeruginosa*		50 mg/kg/dose IV q 6–8 h
Ceftriaxone		Hypersensitivity to cephalosporin and penicillin	50–75 mg/kg/day IV/IM q 12–24 h for typhoid 100 mg/kg/day IV q 12 h For meningitis
Cefuroxime			100–150 mg/kg/day IV/IM q 6–8 h 20–30 mg/kg/day q12h orally
Cephalexin (Sporidex)			25–100 mg/kg/day q8h orally
Ciprofloxacin			10–20 mg/kg/day IV/orally divided into two doses
Cloxacillin	First line drug for *Staphylococcus aureus*		50–200 mg/kg/day IV/PO q4h
Co-trim-oxazole (Septran)	Trimethoprim + sulfamethoxazole	<6 weeks Hyper-sensitivity to sulfa drugs, G-6-PD deficiency	8 mg/kg/day of TMP IV/PO Q12H
Cefixime	URTI/UTI/ Acute bacillary dysentery/ enteric fever	Penicillin or cephalosporin hypersensitivity reactions	10 mg/kg/day BD oral For enteric fever 20 mg/kg/day BD
Ofloxacin	Fluoroquinolones antibiotics		15 mg/kg/day q12h PO 5–10 mg/kg/day q12h IV

Contd.

Drug	Indication	C/I	Dosage
Metronidazole	Anti-protozoal		10 mg/kg/dose t.d.s. PO
Penicillin G Benzathine (Penidure)	Secondary prophylaxis against Rheumatic fever		<6 years 0.6 mega units IM 3 weekly >6 years 1.2 mega units IM 3 weekly
Piperacillin with tazobactam	Broad spectrum antibiotic gram-positive and gram- negative aerobic/anaerobic bacteria		300–400 mg/kg/day q6–8h IV
Imipenem/ Cilastatin	Extended spectrum beta -lactamase producing microorganisms (ESBL)	Use with caution in seizure disorder	60–100 mg/kg/day of imipenem q6h IV
Meropenem	ESBL		60 mg/kg/day q8h IV for neonatal meningitis 40 mg/ kg/dose q8h IV
Azithromycin	Atypical pneumonia	<6 weeks	10 mg/kg/d OD × 3 days
Colistin	Gram-negative bacteria including *Pseudomonas, Enterobacter and Klebsiella*	Nephrotoxic	50,000–75000 IU/ kg/day q8h IV
Doxycycline	Lyme disease, *brucellosis, rickettsia, Chlamydia*	<8 years of age, pregnancy and lactation	2–5 mg/kg/day q12h PO
Linezolid	Vancomycin resistant entero-cocci, MRSA		10 mg/kg/dose q12h IV
Vancomycin	Penicillin resistant staphylococci, pneumococcal infection		40–60 mg/kg/ day q6h slow IV infusion over 1 hour

Contd.

Drug	Indication	C/I	Dosage
Antifungal			
Fluconazole	Candidiasis, cryptococcal meningitis		12.5–25 mg/kg/day OD oral/slow IV infusion over 1 hour
Clotrimazole	Topical use for oral and vaginal candidiasis		
2% Ketoconazole shampoo	Dandruff		3 times a week × 8 weeks
Antiviral			
Acyclovir	Herpes simplex	Renal failure	20 mg/kg/dose q6h × 5 for varicella (oral) 10 mg/kg/dose slow IV over 1–2 hours in HSV encephalitis q8h × 21 days
Amphotericin B (Liposomal)	Severe fungal infection, candidaemia, *Aspergillosis*	Reduced renal and hepatic toxicity than conventional Amphotericin B	3–5 mg/kg IV infusion with 5% dextrose over 2 hours once daily
Antiparasitic			
Albendazole (Zentel, bendex)	Pinworms/ roundworms/ hookworms/ tapeworms/ *H. nana*/ neurocysticercosis	Ocular and intraventricular cysticercosis	<2 years = 200 mg single dose >2 years = 400 mg single dose (repeat dose after 2 weeks in case of round worms), pinworms (For taeniasis, strongyloidosis and *H. nana* 400 mg OD for 3 days) (For giardiasis 400 mg OD for 5 days) (For neurocysticercosis 15 mg/kg BD × 7 days started on 3rd day of steroid)

Contd.

Drug	Indication	C/I	Dosage
Mebendazole	Antihelminthics		100 mg BD × 3 days
Di-ethyl-carbamazine citrate (DEC)	Filariasis/ tropical eosinophilia		Filariasis– 6 mg/kg/d q8h × 3 wks Tropical eosinophilia-10 mg/kg/d q8h × 3 weeks
Ivermectin	Scabies, lice, visceral larva migrans	<6 years	0.2 mg/kg single dose
Niclosamide	*Taenia saginata, Taenia solium*		1g empty stomach followed by another dose after one hour. Give a brisk purgative after 2 hours of last dose. <6 years 0.5 g
Antihistaminics			
Cetrizine		Avoid in <6 months of age	<5 years 2.5–5 mg HS orally >5 years 5 mg HS orally
Fexofenadine	Non-sedative antihistamine		<5 years 30 mg bid, 5–12 years 60 mg bid, >12 years 120 mg OD orally
Hydroxyzine (Atarax)	Urticaria	Acute porphyria	2 mg/kg/day q6h PO
Steroids			
Dexame-thasone	Hib meningitis, CAH, cerebral oedema	Head injury	For cerebral oedema and Hib meningitis –0.5 mg/kg/day IV/IM q 6 h For congenital adrenal hyperplasia (CAH) 0.5–1 mg/kg/day oral

Contd.

Drug	Indication	C/I	Dosage
Hydro-cortisone	Status asthmaticus, Acute adrenal insufficiency		For status asthamaticus—10 mg/kg IV loading dose, 5 mg/kg/dose q6h IV For Acute adrenal insufficiency 50 mg/m^2/day IV initially followed by 100 mg/m^2/day
Prednisolone	Nephrotic syndrome, Rheumatic carditis, SLE, CAH, Bronchial asthma	Obesity, Hypertension, Diabetes mellitus	1–2 mg/kg/day q6–8h oral after meals
Antispasmodic			
Dicyclomine	Antispasmodic	<6 months of age	0.5 mg/kg/dose SOS orally
Hyoscine (Buscopan)	Antispasmodic Intestinal and biliary colic	Glaucoma	6–12 years 10 mg q8h oral 10–20 mg IV/IM SOS
Anti-epileptics			
Diazepam	Status epilepticus/ Febrile seizure	Myasthenia gravis, acute narrow angle glaucoma	0.3–0.5 mg/kg/dose IV/oral/PR
Carbamaze-pine/ Oxcarbaze-pine	Partial tonic-clonic seizure/ postherpetic neuralgia	Patient on MAOI/ porphyria	10–30 mg/kg/day BD/TID
Phenobar-bitone	Neonatal seizures/ Tonic-clonic seizure	Porphyria/ Hepatic and renal disease	20 mg/kg loading dose 5 mg/kg/day OD/BD Maintenance dose
Phenytoin	Tonic-clonic seizures/ generalized seizure/trige-minal neuralgia	Porphyria/ Heart block	20 mg/kg loading dose 5 mg/kg/day OD/BD Maintenance dose

Contd.

Drug	Indication	C/I	Dosage
Valproate	Broad spectrum for majority of epilepsy	Hepatic disease	10–60 mg/kg/day BD/TID
Levetiracetam	Add on therapy for refractory seizures		10–60 mg/kg/day BD/TID
Clobazam (Frisium)	Febrile seizure prophylaxis	Myasthenia gravis	0.25–1 mg/kg/day orally OD/bid
Antiemetics			
Domperidone (Domstal)	Reflux oesophagitis Acute nausea and vomiting	Prolactinaemia/ GI haemorrhage	0.2–0.4 mg/kg/ dose
Ondansetron (Emeset)	Selective 5HT3 Receptors-Antiemetic	Liver dysfunction	<4 years 2 mg 4–11 years 4 mg >12 years 8 mg PO SOS 0.15–0.45 mg/kg/ dose IV SOS
Promethazine theoclate (Avomin)	Motion sickness	<2 years of age, sleep apnoea	0.5 mg/kg/dose SOS PO
Antihypertensive			
Captopril	ACE inhibitor Anti-hyper-tensive	Aortic stenosis, ARF, B/L Renal artery stenosis	0.5–5 mg/kg/day q8–12h orally
Enalapril	ACE inhibitor Anti-hyper-tensive	Aortic stenosis, ARF, B/L Renal artery stenosis	0.08-0.6 mg/kg/day q12–24h orally
Amlodipine	Calcium channel blocker-anti hypertensive		0.1–0.5 mg/kg/day q12–24h orally
Losartan	ARBs--anti-Hypertensive	<6 years of age	1 mg/kg/day OD orally

Contd.

Drug	Indication	C/I	Dosage
Propanolol	Beta blocker		For hypertension 0.5–1 mg/kg/day q6–12h oral For cyanotic spell/ arrhythmia— 2–6 mg/kg/day q6–8h oral For migraine prophylaxis <35 kg 10–20 mg t.d.s., >35 kg 20–40 mg t.d.s PO
Furosemide (Lasix)			1–2 mg/kg/dose IV/oral
Miscellaneous			
Digoxin	CCF		0.02 mg/kg stat, 0.01 mg/kg at 8 and 16 hours, then 0.01 mg/kg OD from next day (Total dose of rapid digitalization is 0.04 mg/kg orally)
Desmopressin (DDAVP)	Nocturnal enuresis	Severe hypo-natraemia, seizure, water intoxication	Intranasal spray 10–20 μg/day divided into two doses
Deferiprone (Kelfer)	Oral iron, chelating agent thalassaemia, haemolytic anaemia		50–100 mg/kg/day q6–12h orally
Desferoxa-mine	Iron chelating agent S. ferritin >1000 is a indication to start chelation therapy	ARF	For chronic iron overload—20–40 mg/kg/day subcutaneous administered over 8–12 hours, using infusion pump
Dextro-methorphan	Antitussive		1 mg/kg/day orally q6–8h

Contd.

Drug	Indication	C/I	Dosage
Cypro-heptadine	Appetite stimulant, Skin allergy, Prophylaxis of migraine	Glaucoma, urinary retention, asthma, neonates	0.25–0.5 mg/kg/day q8–12h orally
Triclofos (Pedicloryl)	Sedative		1 ml/kg maximum 15 ml
Ursodeoxy cholic acid (UDCA)	Direct hyperbili-rubinaemia	Severe hepatic failure, complete obstruction of biliary tract	5 mg/kg/dose tds PO
Kayexalate	Potassium exchange resin		1 g/kg/dose PO/PR
Lactulose	Laxative		1 ml/kg/dose PO SOS
Montelukast	Asthma		<5 years 4 mg 5–12 years 5 mg >12 years 10 mg HS PO
Racecadotril (Enough sachets)	Anti-diarrhoeal		1.5 mg/kg/dose t.d.s PO
Tranexamic acid			25 mg/kg/dose t.d.s PO
Prazosin	Scorpion bite		0.03 mg/kg/dose q3–5h PO
Baclofen	Relieve muscle spasticity due to spinal or cerebral origin, e.g. cerebral palsy		0.75–2 mg/kg/day q6h oral Maximum dose 40 mg <8 years 60 mg >8 years
Carnitine	Myopathy, IEM		50–100 mg/kg/day q8–12h orally
Atomoxetin (Axepta)	ADHD	<6 years of age	0.5–1.2 mg/kg/day OD/bid PO
Imipramine	Nocturnal enuresis		>6 years 25 mg HS PO

THYROXIN—SINGLE ORAL DOSE, EMPTY STOMACH IN THE MORNING

Age	μg/kg/day
Neonate	10–15
<1 year	7.5
1–3 years	5
4–10 years	4
>10 years	2–3

NTEP GUIDELINES FOR TREATMENT OF TUBERCULOSIS

Revised National Tuberculosis Control Program (RNTPC) has been changed to National Tuberculosis Elimination Program (NTEP).

Instead of regimen based on type of patient NTEP recommends regimen based on drug susceptibility to TB so for all

- New microbiologically confirmed pulmonary TB
- New clinically diagnosed pulmonary TB
- New microbiologically confirmed extra-pulmonary TB
- New clinically diagnosed extra-pulmonary TB
- Previously treated TB (recurrent, treatment after loss to follow up, treatment after failure)

The available regimens are:

Treatment groups	Drug regimen
RS-TB	2 HRZE (IP) + 4 HR (CP)
(H) Mono/poly dug resistant RS-TB	6–9 LfxRZE (no separate IP/CP)
Shorter oral bedaquiline containing MDR/RR-TB	4–6 LfxCfzZEH^hEtoBdq (IP) + 5LfxCfzZE(CP)
Longer oral MDR/XDR-TB	18 LfxCfzBdqLzdCs (no separate IP/CP)

IP—Intensive phase, CP—Continuation phase
RS—Rifampicin sensitive, RR—Rifampicin resistant
MDR—Multi drug resistant, XDR—Extensively drug resistant

First line Drugs

H-Isoniazid: 10–20 mg/kg, R-Rifampicin: 15 mg/kg
Z-Pyrazinamide: 25 mg/kg, E-Ethambutol: 20 mg/kg

Second Line Drugs

Grouping of anti-TB drugs and steps for designing longer MDR-TB regimen			
	Drug	**Abbreviation**	**Dosage**
Group A (include all 3 drugs)	1. Levofloxacin or Moxifloxacin 2. Bedaquilline 3. Linezolid	Lfx Mfx Bdq Lzd	15 mg/kg 15 mg/kg 200 mg/400 mg per day-wt based 10–15 mg/kg
Group B Add 1 or 2	4. Clofazimine 5. Cycloserine	Cfz Cs	2–5 mg/kg 15–20 mg/kg
Group C Add to complete the regimen when drugs from group A and B cannot be used	6. Ethambutol 7. Delamanid 8. Pyrazinamide 9. Meropenem 10. Amikacin or Streptomycin 11. Ethionamide or 12. P-aminosalicylic acid	E Dlm Z Mpm Am S Eto PAS	25 mg/kg 50 mg BD X 24 weeks for 6–11 years, 100 mg BD X 24 weeks for 12–17 years 35 mg/kg 20–40 mg/kg IV TDS 15–20 mg/kg IV/IM OD 15–20 mg/kg IV/IM OD 15–20 mg/kg 200 mg/kg BD

TREATMENT OF MALARIA

I. Low Risk Area for Resistance Except *P. falciparum*

Chloroquine 25 mg base/kg over 3 days orally (250 mg tab contains 150 mg of base)

WHO regime	• 10 mg base/kg stat dose followed by • 5 mg base/kg 6 hours later • 5 mg base/kg 24 hours later • 5 mg base/kg 48 hours later
National Malaria Eradication Programme	• 10 mg base/kg stat dose followed by • 10 mg base/kg 24 hours later • 5 mg base/kg 48 hours later

Primaquine—needed to prevent relapse

15 mg tab contain 15 mg of base primaquine

P. Vivax—0.25 mg base/kg for 14 days

II. High Risk Area for Resistance and *P. falciparum*

Plasmodium falciparum in India is chloroquine resistant

Artemisinin combination therapy (ACT)

Artesunate 50 mg tablet	Day 1 4 mg/kg	Day 2 4 mg/kg	Day 3 4 mg/kg
Sulphadoxine+ Pyrimethamine 500+25 mg tablet	Single dose on day 1 25/1.25 mg/kg		
Primaquine 7.5 mg or 15 mg tablet		Single dose on day 2 0.25 mg base/kg	

III. Mixed Infection

ACT + Primaquine 0.25 mg base/kg once daily for 14 days

HIV TREATMENT (ANTIRETROVIRAL THERAPY—ART)

Three groups of drugs for treatment of AIDS:

1. Nucleoside reverse transcriptase inhibitors (NRTI): Zidovudine (AZT), Lamivudine (3TC), Didanosine (DDI)
2. Non-nucleoside reverse transcriptase inhibitors (NNRTI): Nevirapine (NVP), Efavirenz (EFV)
3. Protease inhibitors: Indinavir, ritonavir

ART Regimen in children
2NRTI + 1 NNRTI (AZT + 3TC + NVP/EFV)

WHO Classification of HIV-associated Clinical Disease

Classification of HIV associated clinical disease	Clinical stage
Asymptomatic	1
Mild	2
Advanced	3
Severe	4

Note: To protect fetus of the affected mother-start zidovudine from 14 weeks of gestation, give IV AZT peripartum.

Important

Management of a newborn of a HIV-infected mother

- Nevirapine 2 mg/kg as single dose within 72 hours of birth, or
- Zidovudine 4 mg/kg orally twice a day for 6 weeks or both

Post-exposure prophylaxis for healthcare personal
AZT 300 mg + 3TC 150 mg bid × 4 weeks.

- IV fluids

	Na mEq/L	K mEq/L	Cl mEq/L	Dx g/L	Fluid of choice
DNS	154	–	154	50	>5 years maintenance fluids
1/2 DNS	77	–	77	50	<5 years maintenance fluids
NS	154	–	154	–	Resuscitation fluid
Isolyte-p	25	20	22	50	In newborn
RL	130	4	109	–	In bum

Calculation of Drops/Minute

- Macro drip/IV drip (1 ml = 16 drops)

$$\frac{\text{ml/hr}}{4} = \text{drops/min}$$

- Micro drip/paedia drip (1 ml = 60 drops)
  ml/hr = drops/min

Calculation of Maintenance IV Fluids

Based on child's current weight

Holliday-Segar Formula
1st 10 kg = 100 ml/kg/day
11–20 kg = 1000 + (50 ml/kg/day)
>20 kg = 1500 + (20 ml/kg/day)

Note: For hypovolemic shock

Give 20 ml/kg (NS or RL) over 20–30 min
↓Reassess
If shock persists
↓
Repeat boluses twice over 1 hour
(maximum of 60 ml/kg)

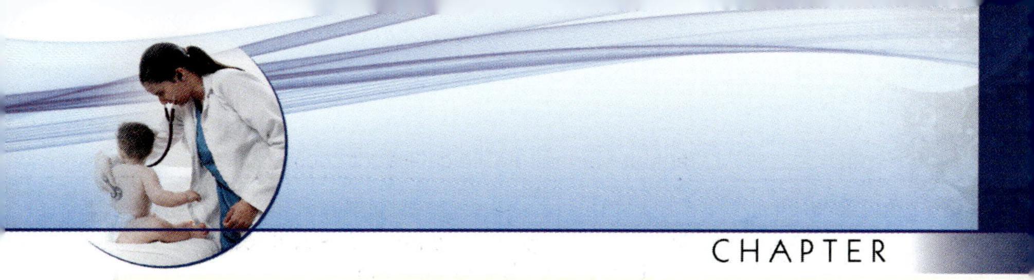

CHAPTER

19

Emergency Paediatrics

PAEDIATRIC ASSESSMENT TRIANGLE (PAT)

Appearance	Work of breathing	Circulation to skin	Interpretation
Normal	Normal	Normal	Stable
Normal	Abnormal	Normal	Respiratory distress
Abnormal	Abnormal	Normal	Respiratory failure
Abnormal	Normal	Abnormal	Shock
Abnormal	Normal	Normal	CNS/metabolic disturbance
Abnormal	Abnormal	Abnormal	Cardiopulmonary failure

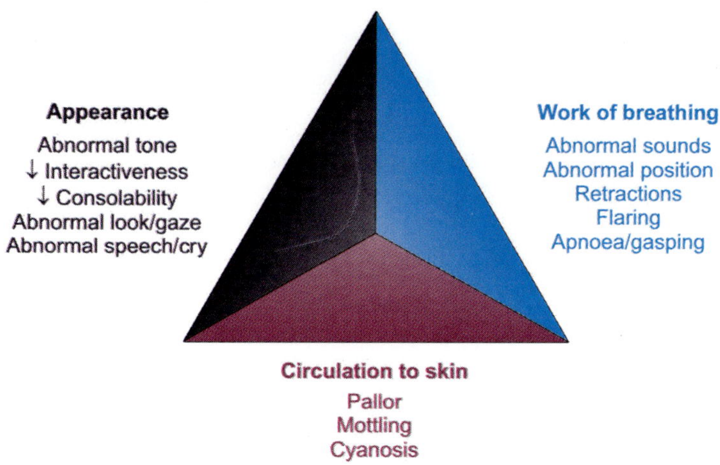

Pediatric Basic Life Support Algorithm for Healthcare Providers—Single Rescuer

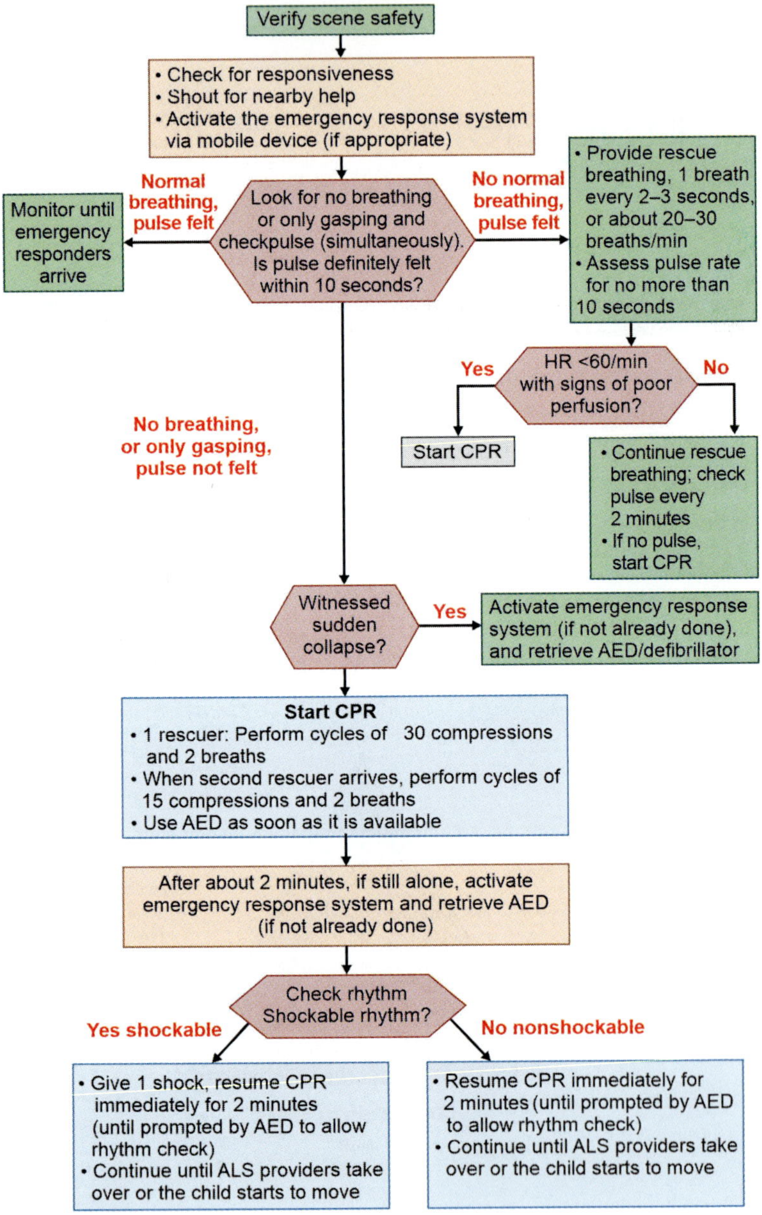

aediatrics/ALS Algorith

Paediatric cardiac arrest algorithm

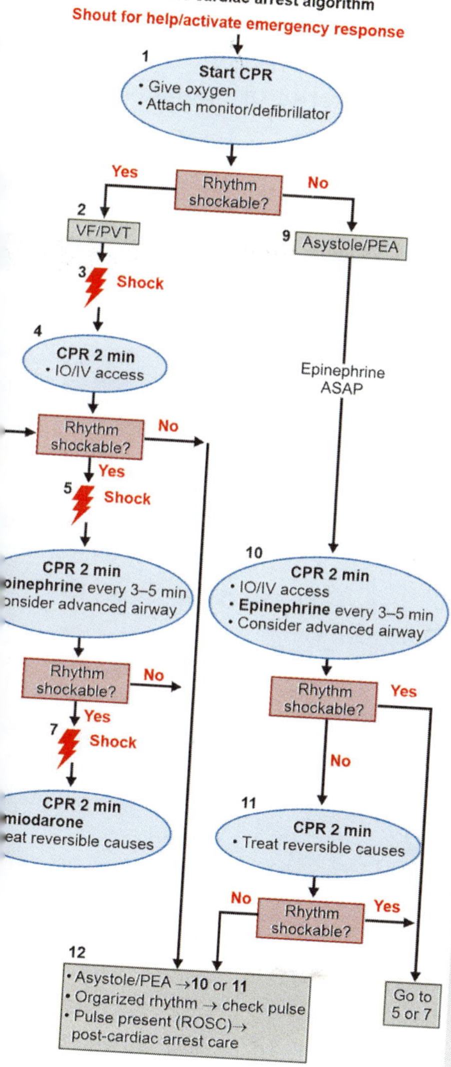

Doses/details

CPR quality

- Push hard (≥1/3 of anterior-posterior diameter of chest) and fast (at least 100/min) and allow complete chest recoil
- Minimize interruptions in compressions
- Avoid excessive ventilation
- Rotate compressor every 2 minutes
- If no advanced airway, 15:2 compression ventilation ratio, if advanced airway, 8–10 breaths per minute with continuous chest compressions

Shock energy for defibrillation

First shock 2 J/kg, second shock 4 J/kg, subsequent shocks ≥4 J/kg, maximum 10 J/kg or adult dose

Drug therapy

- **Epinephrine IO/IV dose:** 0.01 mg/kg (0.1 ml/kg of 1:10 000 concentration). Repeat every 3–5 minutes. If no IO/IV access, may give endotracheal dose: 0.1 mg/kg (0.1 ml/kg of 1:1000 concentration)
- Amiodarone IO/IV dose: 5 mg/kg bolus during cardiac arrest. May repeat up to 2 times for refractory VF/pulseless VT

Advanced airway

- Endotracheal intubation or supraglottic advanced airway
- Waveform capnography or capnometry to confirm and monitor ET tube placement
- Once advanced airway in place give 1 breath every 6–8 seconds (8–10 breaths per minute)

Return of spontaneous circulation (ROSC)

- Pulse and blood pressure
- Spontaneous arterial pressure waves with intra-arterial monitoring

Reversible causes

– Hypovolaemia
– Hypoxia
– Hydrogen ion (acidosis)
– Hypoglycaemia
– Hypo-/hyperkalaemia
– Hypothermia
– Tension pneumothorax
– Tamponade, cardiac
– Toxins
– Thrombosis, pulmonary
– Thrombosis, coronary

AUTOMATED EXTERNAL DEFIBRILLATOR (AED) PAD SIZE

- <1 year 4.5 cm, >1 year 8 cm
- One pad/paddle is placed to the right of the sternum ju below the clavicle, and the other is centred lateral to t normal cardiac apex in the anterior or midaxillary line (ju left to left nipple)
- Defibrillation is the treatment of choice to revert ventricu fibrillation (start with 2 joules/kg can go up to 4 joules/k

EMERGENCY DRUGS

Drug	Indication	Dosage
Adrenaline/ Epinephrine	Bradycardia Asystole Pulseless arrest	0.1 ml/kg/dose of 1:10 can repeat after 3 minu IV
Atropine	Bradycardia Primary AV block	0.02 mg/kg/dose IV
Adenosine	Supraventricular tachycardia	0.1 mg/kg IV may repe 0.2 mg/kg after 2 min
Amiodarone	Ventricular tachycardia Ventricular fibrillation	5 mg/kg IV/IO
Dopamine (40 mg/ml)	Shock, CCF	5–20 µg/kg/minute as IV infusion
Dobutamine (50 mg/ml)	Shock, CCF	2–20 µg/kg/minute as IV infusion
$NaHCO_3$	Metabolic acidosis Hyperkalaemia	1–2 mEq/kg IV bolu
Calcium Gluconate (10%)	Hypocalcaemia Hyperkalaemia	1 ml/kg slow IV inf
Lidocaine	Ventricular tachycardia Ventricular fibrillation	1 mg/kg IV/IO Followed by infusi 20–50 µg/kg/min
Naloxone	Opioid poisoning	0.1 mg/kg, IV/IO/

mg/100 ml of dobutamine or dopamine solution

$$= \frac{6 \times \text{wt in kg} \times \text{dose } (\mu g/kg/min)}{\text{Fluid infusion rate } (ml/hour)}$$

Note:
- Never mix dopamine or dobutamine with sodium bicarbonate
- Never mix phenytoin with glucose containing fluids
- Never mix calcium with sodium bicarbonate

STATUS EPILEPTICUS

Seizure lasting for >20 minutes or generalized recurrences without recovery of consciousness in-between

LMD (lorazepam 0.1 mg/kg, midazolam 0.2 mg/kg, diazepam 0.3 mg/kg) IV are the first line of drugs.

ORAL HYPOGLYCAEMIC AGENTS

Category	Example
Sulphonyl ureas	Tolbutamide, glipizide
Biguanides	Metformin
Alpha-glucosidase inhibitors	Acarbose
Thiazolidinediones	Pioglitazone
Meglitinides	Repaglinide

INSULIN

Fast acting (insulin analogue)	Lispro, aspart
Short acting (soluble, regular)	Regular insulin
Intermediate acting	Isophane (NPH), lente
Long acting	Ultralente
Longest acting	Glargine, detemir, deglu

Research is going on inhaled and oral insulin therapies.

Diagnostic Criteria for Diabetes Mellitus Type 1

Clinical Feature of Unexplained Weight Loss, Polydi and Polyuria, Polyphagia Plus

1. Fasting blood glucose (FBS) >126 mg/dl
2. Random blood glucose (RBS) >200 mg/dl

3. Post blood glucose (PPBS) (2 hours after giving 75 g glucose) OGTT PPBS >200 mg/dl
4. Hae A1c (HbA1c)
   Hb

DIABE CIDOSIS (DKA)

Criter nosis of DKA

- Hy mia (blood glucose >200 mg/dl)
- Me dosis (PH <7.3, HCO_3 <15 mEq/L)
- Ke d ketone >1.5 mmol/L or urine ketone >2+)

IV f ur (to be given over 48 hours)

$$= \frac{[8 \times \text{maintenance fluid for 24 hours}) - \text{bolus given}]}{47\ \text{hours}}$$

Not of regular insulin mix with 500 ml of NS if give n at rate 1 ml/kg/hr will deliver 0.1 unit of insu

HC o Correct Acidosis is C/I in DKA

C × [(S.Na) + (BUN/2.8) + (Glucose/18)]

- blood glucose is equivalent to 18 mg/dl
- Cl contains 2 mEq of potassium

BURN

1s epidermis

2n dermis + part of dermis

3r dermis + Dermis including blood vessels and ne

- nes is not applicable for children.
- of age head –19%, both lower limbs 14% each. ghly deduct 1% from head and add 0.5% for nbs for each year.

Depth classifications of burn injury

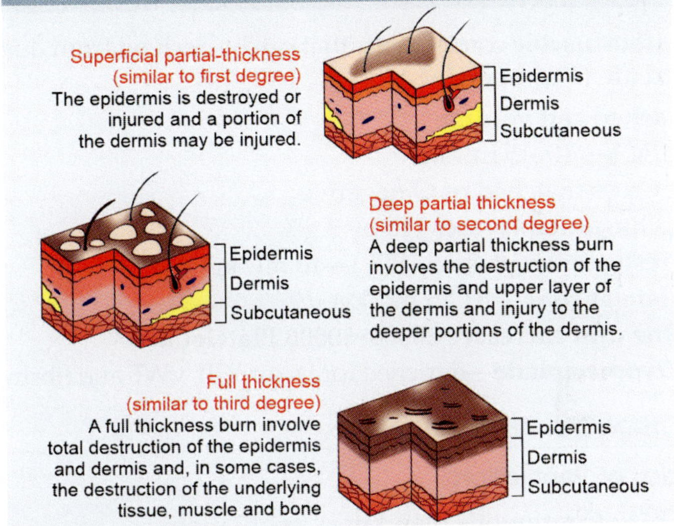

Parkland Formulas

- 4 × wt in kg × % TBSA burn + maintenance fluid = total volume of fluid to be given over 24 hours.
- Half fluid to be given over 8 hours rest over 16 hours.
- Reassess after 24 hours

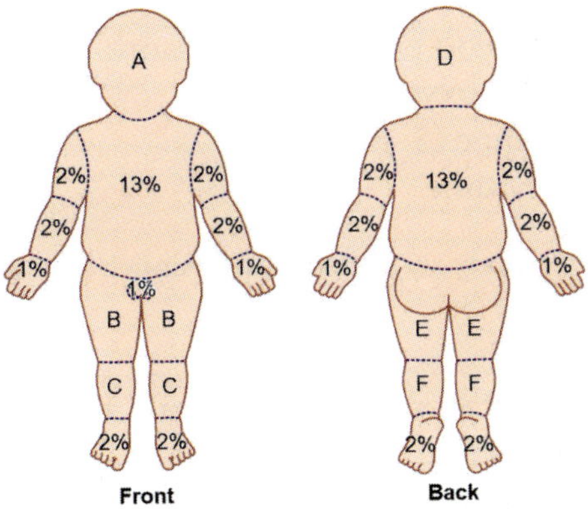

Areas	By age in years			
	0	1	5	10
Head (A/D)	10%	9%	7%	6%
Thigh (B/E)	3%	3%	4%	5%
Leg (C/F)	2%	3%	3%	3%

BLOOD TRANFUSION

The transfusable components that can be derived from donated blood are (4 components)

1. **Packed cell volume**
   - PCV—10–15 ml/kg
   - Cross matched or O negative
   - One unit increases Hb by 3 g%
2. **Fresh frozen plasma** (FFP)—10 ml/kg
3. **Platelet conc**—10–15 ml/kg
   One unit increases 20000–50000 Platelet mm^3
4. **Cryoprecipitate**—enriched for factor VIII, vWF and fibrinogen

MECHANICAL VENTILATION

Modes of Ventilation

- **CMV:** Continuous mandatory ventilation
- **IMV:** Intermittent mandatory ventilation
- **SIMV:** Synchronized intermittent mandatory ventilation
- **CPAP:** Continuous positive airway pressure

Parameters

- **PIP:** Peak inspiratory pressure
- **PEEP:** Positive end expiratory pressure
- **FiO_2:** Fractional oxygen
- **VT:** Tidal volume (6–10 ml/kg)
- **Ti:** Inspiratory time

Foreign body suspected—do Heimlich manoeuvre.

POISONING

Emesis is not indicated in case of alkali, acid or hydrocarbon poisoning.

- Miosis—morphine, organophosphorus
- Mydriasis—dhatura, atropine

Lizards/spiders/centipede/millipede found in India are usually non-poisonous

Datura Poisoning/Tricyclic Antidepressants Overdose (Amitriptyline/Imipramine)

- C/F—Red as beet, dry as a bone, blind as a bat, mad as hatter, hot as hare.
- Rx—Physostigmine 0.02 mg/kg

Organophosphorus Poisoning

- C/F—DUMBBELLS (Diarrhoea, Urination, Miosis, Bronzchorrhea, Bronchospasm, Emesis, Lacrimation, Secretion, and CCC (Coma, Confusion, Convulsions)
- Rx—Atropine 0.02 mg/kg
  Pralidoxime 25 mg/kg

Scorpion Sting

Prazocin can be used.

Snakes

Viper: Nephro—Cardiovascular toxic

Cobra: Neuro—Muscular toxic

Krait: Neuroparalysis

Sea Snake—Myotoxic

Treatment

Right Protocol

Reassure

Immobilise

Go to

Hospital

Tell to doctor

Antivenin –10 vial of polyvalent antisnake venom (against 4 major species) reconstitute with 240 ml of NS and give slowly over 2 hours after test dose, repeat till signs of envenomation disappear (maximum 30 vials)

ANTIDOTE

Drug	Antidote
Acetaminophen	N-acetyl cysteine
Amphetamines	Chlorpromazine
Atropine/belladona poisoning	Physostigmine
Benzodiazepines (Diazepam)	Flumazenil
Carbon monoxide	Oxygen
Cyanide	Amyl nitrite
Ethylene glycol/methanol	Ethanol
Hg, Lead	BAL
Arsenic	EDTA
Heparin	Protamine sulfate
Iron	Desferoxamine
Isoniazid	Pyridoxin
Methemoglobinaemia	Methylene blue
Morphine	Naloxone
OP poisoning	Atropine Pralidoxime
Scorpion bite	Prazosin
Warfarin	Vitamin K
Digoxin	Digoxin specific antibody fragments

Partial TPN (for Newborn)

Isolyte-P	250 ml
25% Dx	75 ml
AA sol.	150 ml
$NaHCO_3$	18 ml
KCl	5 ml
MVI	2 ml
Total	500 ml

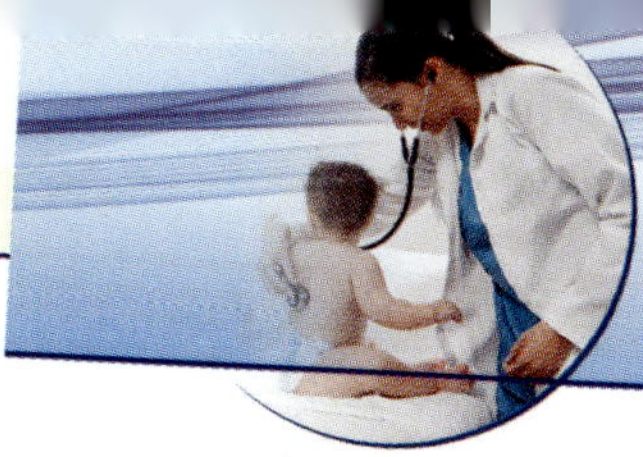

APTER 20

OSCE and AETCM

ATTITUDE, ETHICS AND COMMUNICATION MOD (AETCOM)

Objective is to teach empathy, ethics, decisioraking, moral reasoning and communication.

Competency 4.9 A/B: The student should bele to: Identify, discuss and defend medico-legal, socio-cultu, professional and ethical issues pertaining to medical neglige/malpractice.

OBJECTIVE STRUCTURED CLINICAL EXAMIMION OSCE

Objective, structured, uniformed, broad-bas format to assess the candidate on multiple aspects of the subct.

Conducting the OSCE

- Make a proper blue print
- Design and prepare the stations well in dvance
- Print all the stations and checklists
- Prepare answers for response stations
- Allocate the area where exam to be conducted
- Collect all the equipment/furniture required
- Select the observers and brief them
- Decide the patients to be taken and prepare them
- Prepare a station map of the OSCE with proper arrows
- Brief the students before the exam
- Ensure someone keeps the time

The OSCE usually consists of 4–10 stations that the candidate has to attend by rotation. Each station has one or more tasks for the can e to complete in a fixed time. The stations consist of questio problems and usually cover the following topics:

1. Case es.
2. Interp ion of laboratory reports.
3. Interp ion of radiological investigations, ultrasonograms, CT sca r MRIs.
4. Interp ion of ECGs.
5. Clinica otographs.
6. Observ tations—at these stations, an examiner observes the acti of the candidate while performing a task. The task given m be one of the following:
   a. A sit ion in neonatal resuscitation.
   b. A sit ion in paediatric basic life support.
   c. Clini examination of a system.
   d. Anth ometry and derivation of indices of growth and nutrit .
   e. Hand ashing steps
   f. Couns ling—includes counselling parents to use a particul r drug device (e.g. use of MDI with spacer), regardin mmunization, breast feeding, or regarding a child's chr ic/terminal illness.
7. Biomedical wa e management.

Note: *Internal and xternal examiners will be provided with a key which is their guide e for assessment.*

Observe Station

In observed station content rather than the style is assessed, marks are awarded for each point covered by the candidate including introducing oneself and establishing rapport, taking permission and using sanitizer prior to uncovering and before examining a patient, covering a patient after having completed the examination and thanking the parent and the child before leaving.

GENERAL FORMAT FOR COUNSELLING A PARENTS

Dear (Parent's Name)

I understand that facing a chronic illness in your child is a challenging journey, and I am here to offer my support and guidance. It is completely normal to feel a range of emotions, and I want you to know that I am here to help you navigate through them.

Acknowledging Emotions

I want to acknowledge the emotional weight that comes with managing a chronic illness. Your feelings of concern, confusion, and even frustration are valid. I'm here to listen and support you through this.

Understanding the Diagnosis

Let us take some time to discuss your child's diagnosis thoroughly. I want to ensure that you have a clear understanding of the condition, its trajectory, and the various treatment options available.

Collaborative Treatment Plan

We will work collaboratively to develop a treatment plan tailored to your child's unique needs. This may involve medical interventions, lifestyle adjustments, and ongoing monitoring. Your input is invaluable in shaping the best approach for your child.

Open Communication

Communication is key in our journey together. I encourage you to share your thoughts, concerns, and any changes you observe in your child's health. Regular check-ins will allow us to assess progress and make any necessary adjustments to the treatment plan.

Building a Support System

Navigating a chronic illness is not a solitary journey. I can connect you with support groups and resources where you can connect with other parents facing similar challenges. Sharing experiences can provide a sense of community and valuable insights.

Empowering Your Role

As a parent, your role is instrumental in your child's care. Your love, understanding, and advocacy play a crucial part in their well-being. While I am here to provide guidance, your active involvement is essential.

Holistic Well-being

In addition to medical care, we will consider the holistic aspects of your child's life. Together, we can explore strategies to ensure they thrive emotionally, socially, and academically despite the challenges posed by the chronic illness.

Remember, you are not alone in this journey. We are a team, and I am committed to supporting both you and your child every step of the way.

If there is anything specific you would like to discuss or if you have questions, please do not hesitate to reach out.

SAMPLE OSCE

1. **Elicit deep tendon reflex and tell the root values**
   Key (each point gives one mark)
   i. Establishes rapport. Introduces himself/herself. Asks for a female attendant. Use sanitizer. Explain the procedure. Taken consent .
   ii. Correct technique: Exposure of limb, positioning of limb, identifying the tendon, use of knee hammer.
   iii. Elicited bicep/triceps/supinator/knee/ankle reflex
   iv. Knows root values of each
   v. Cover the exposed area, thank mother/attender and the child.
2. **You have recently diagnosed a 3-year-old male child to be suffering from beta thalassaemia. Counsel the parents about the further management.**
   Key (each point gives one mark)
   i. Establishes rapport. Introduces himself/herself. Asks for a female attendant.
   ii. States that based on history, examination and investigations, a diagnosis of thalassaemia has been made.

iii. Explains the need for blood transfusions and hepatitis/ Pneumococcal/varicella/influenza vaccinations and need to maintain the Hb above 9 g/dl.
iv. Explains that cure can be achieved by bone marrow transplantation from a sibling.
v. Asks if mother has any doubts and encourages her to ask questions. Thank mother and ask if she has any other queries.

3. Measure BP of a 13 years old male child

Check list—record BP					
S. No.	**Skill component**	**Marks**	**Correct**	**Wrong**	**Missed**
1	Procedure explained/ consent taken/ sanitizer used	0.2			
2	Position the child	0.2			
3	Select cuff size/check BP apparatus	0.2			
4	Palpate brachial artery	1			
5	Tie the cuff	0.5			
6	Palpatory method	1			
7	Auscultatory method	1			
8	Record the BP	0.5			
9	Recheck BP	0.2			
10	Remove cuff/put back instrument/ thanking child	0.2			

4. Assess children <2 months or >2 months to 5 years using IMNCI guidelines and stratify risk

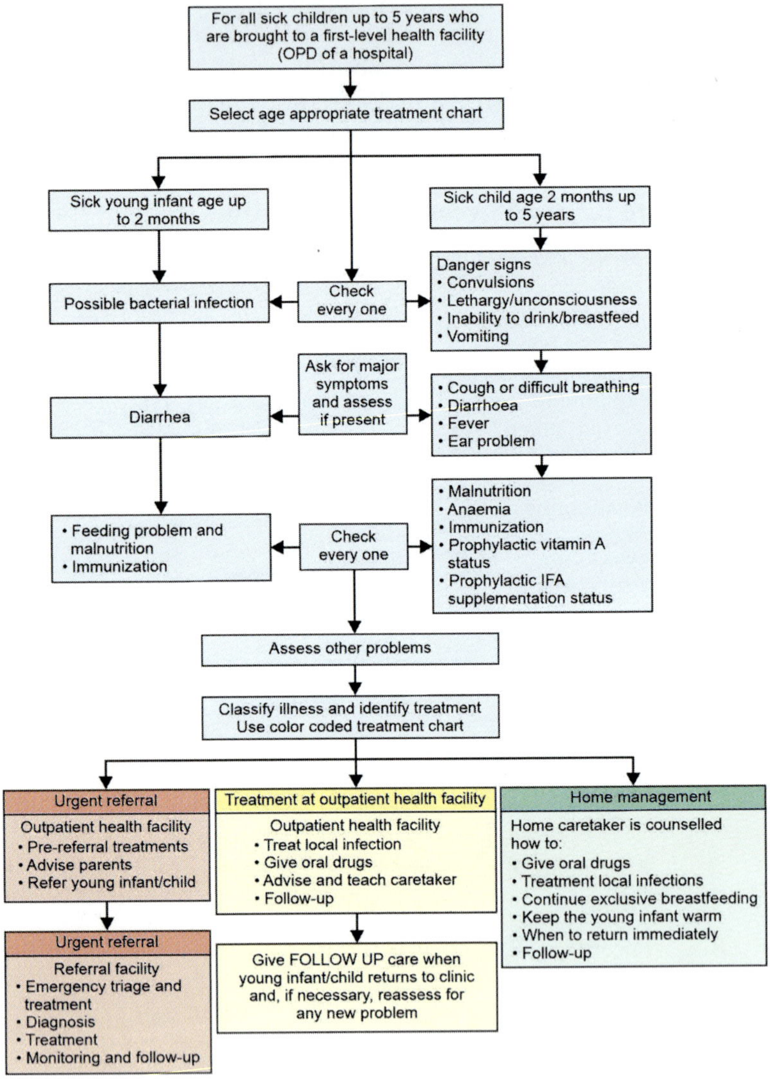

5. Obtain informed consent from a parents of an 8-year-old female child suffering from severe respiratory distress whom you are going to admit in your hospital

Informed Consent Form for Paediatric Admission

Patient Information

Patient Name: ______________________________

Date of Birth: ________________ Sex________________

Parent/Guardian Name: ______________________________

Relationship to Patient: ______________________________

Medical Procedure

I, the undersigned, hereby grant my informed consent for the admission and necessary medical procedures to be performed on my child, ______________________, under the care of Dr. __________________, a licensed paediatrician.

Nature of Admission

The purpose of this admission is to assess, diagnose, and treat the medical condition affecting my child. This may include but is not limited to medical examinations, diagnostic tests, medication administration, and any required medical interventions.

Risks and Benefits

I understand that there may be risks associated with the medical procedures, including but not limited to potential side effects, complications, or unforeseen reactions to treatment. The potential benefits include the improvement of my child's health and well-being.

Alternatives

I have been informed of any alternative treatments or procedures, including the option of outpatient care, and I understand the potential risks and benefits associated with these alternatives.

Explained in my Language

The treatment modalities, risks and benefits have been explained to me in my local language which 1 understand.

Confidentiality

I understand that my child's medical information will be kept confidential in accordance to the applicable healthcare privacy laws.

Voluntary Consent

I acknowledge that my consent is voluntary, and I have had the opportunity to ask questions regarding the nature and purpose of the admission. I am satisfied with the explanations provided.

Withdrawal of Consent

I understand that I have the right to withdraw my consent at any time, and I will be informed of the consequences of such withdrawal.

Emergency Situations

In the event of a medical emergency where immediate treatment is necessary to protect the life or health of my child, I authorize the medical team to proceed with necessary interventions without obtaining additional consent.

Contact Information

I have been provided with contact information to address any concerns or questions related to my child's care.

Consent Validity

This consent form is valid for the duration of the admission and related medical procedures.

Date:_______________

Parent/Guardian Signature_______________

Witness signature_______________

Doctor signature_______________

6. **A 6-year-old boy weighing 16 kg has recently been diagnosed as having type I diabetes. He has to be started on insulin at 1 U/kg/day.**
   i. Show calculations of regular and lente insulin therapy he should receive.
   ii. What counselling would you give regarding possible complication of insulin therapy?

iii. This child was advised a diet having low glycemic index. What is glycemic index of a food?
iv. What base line investigations would you do at start of treatment

Answer

i. Total insulin dose: 16 × 1 = 16 units/day. A-combination of regular and lente (1:2) insulin subcutaneously in 24 hours.
2/3 before breakfast and 1/3 before dinner.
ii. Counsel for hypoglycemia and its treatment. Counsel for need for compliance.
iii. Glycemic index is a measure of rise of blood sugar after a particular type of food is eaten in comparison with glucose which is 100. Low glycemic index food should be taken more as green vegetables, kidney beans, eggs, nuts, meat.
iv. Base line investigations-fundus examination, serum lipid profile, thyroid function tests, KFT, urinalysis, HbA1c, FBS, PPBS.

7. **A term female baby is born by emergency LSCS. Amniotic fluid was not stained with meconium. The baby is born limp and is not crying. Resuscitate with the provided mannequin and equipment. You can ask vital signs of the baby whenever appropriate.**
   i. Mention your intention to handwash, dry and wear gloves.
   ii. Check the equipment: Radiant warmer, oxygen source, suction, ambu bag—if time is available. If not, mention your intention to have done so prior to baby's birth.
   iii. Perform all basic steps within 30 seconds in correct order provide warmth, PSSR—positioning, suctioning, stimulation, repositioning, give oxygen if required.
   iv. Evaluate and ask for vitals—examiner says HR 90/min.
   v. Assembling bag and mask after choosing appropriate size mask, position baby neck in slight extension, use shoulder roll if needed.
   Position mask and provide appropriate ventilation (rate and rise—40–60/min). Say out loud: squeeze-two-three-squeeze.

vi. Evaluate vitals-examiner says HR 50/min.
vii. Mention your intention to have an assistant to provide bag and mask ventilation during chest compressions.
viii. Chest compression-two finger technique, depth 1/3 of AP diameter of the chest ratio 1:3, check pulses. Say out loud: One-and two-and three-and squeeze-and evaluate HR decide about medication (Epinephrine).

8. i. What all national program for child and maternal health you know?
ii. Tell the recent IMR/NNR/U5MR/5–24 MR/MMR?
iii. Define, calculate and interpret demographic indices—birth rate, death rate, fertility rates/IMR/NNR/MMR.

i. **National programs in India**
- Reproductive, Maternal, Newborn, Child Plus Adolescent Health (RMNCH + A)
- *Navjaat Shishu Suraksha Karyakaram* (NSSK)
- *Janani Shishu Suraksha Karyakaram* (JSSK)
- *Rashtriya Bal Swasthya Karyakam* (RBSK)
- *Rashtriya Kishor Swasthya Karyakam* (RKSK)
- Child nutrition programs
  1. Umbrella Integrated Child Development Services Scheme
  2. Mid-day Meal Programme
  3. Anaemia Mukt Bharat/Intensified National Iron Plus Initiative (iNIPI)
- Facility based Integrated Management of Neonatal and Childhood Illness(F-IMNCI)
- India Newborn Action Plan (INAP)
- Intensified Mission Indradhanush (IMI)
- Control of Diarrheal Disease Programme
- Revised National Tuberculosis Control Programme
- Acute Respiratory Infection Control Programme
- National School Health Programme
- National Mental Health Programme
- Child Health Screening and Early Intervention Services—4Ds

ii. Indicators of child health (2020 NHS data)
- IMR 28/1000 live birth
- NNR 20/1000 live birth

- U5MR 32/1000 live birth
- 5–24 MR 13/1000
- MMR 97/100000 live birth

iii.

$$\text{Birth rate} = \frac{\text{No. of live births during the year}}{\text{Mid year population}} \times 1000$$

$$\text{Death rate} = \frac{\text{No. of deaths during the year}}{\text{Mid year population}} \times 1000$$

$$\text{Infant mortality rate (IMR)} = \frac{\text{No. of infant deaths during the year}}{\text{No. of live births during the year}} \times 1000$$

$$\text{Maternal mortality rate (MMR)} = \frac{\text{No. of maternal deaths during the year}}{\text{No. of live births during the year}} \times 100{,}000$$

$$\text{General fertility rate (GF rate)} = \frac{\text{No. of live births during the year}}{\text{Mid year female population in the age group of } (15-49)} \times 1000$$

$$\text{Neonatal mortality rate (NMR)} = \frac{\text{No. of infant deaths less than 29 days during the year}}{\text{No. of live births during the year}} \times 1000$$

9. **You are provided with black/blue/yellow/red plastic bin and used blood stained cotton swab, syringe wrappers, used indwelling IV cannula, waste food material, glass IV bottles. How will you dispose them?**

Medical waste—colour coding		
Yellow	Anatomical waste soiled waste	Blood, dressings, cotton swabs
Red	Infections waste	IV set cannula, catheter, urine bags
Blue	Medicines	Unused, IV drugs, glass bottle
Black	Municipal waste	Food, non-medical waste
White	Sharp	Blades, scalpel, needles

10. Demonstrate steps of hand-washing.

Step 1

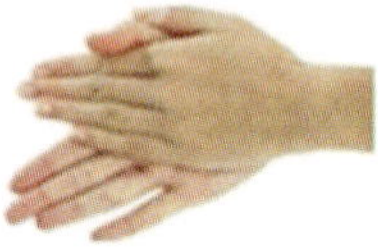

Rub palms together

Step 2

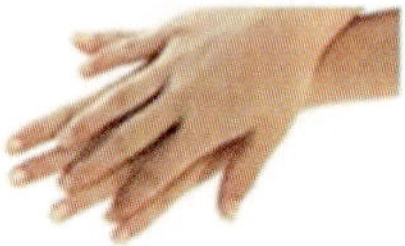

Rub the back of both hands

Step 3

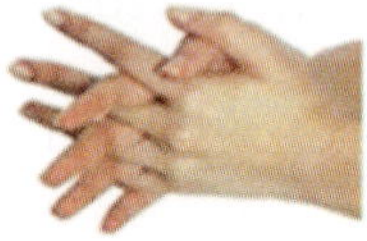

Interface fingers and rub the hands together

Step 4

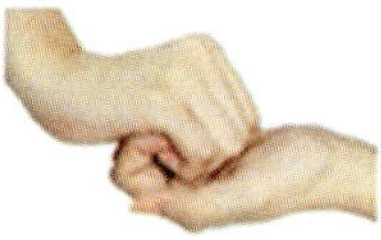

Interlock fingers and rub the back of fingers of both hands

Step 5

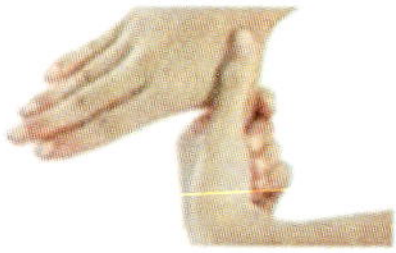

Rub thumb in a rotating manner followed by the area between index finger and thumb

Step 6

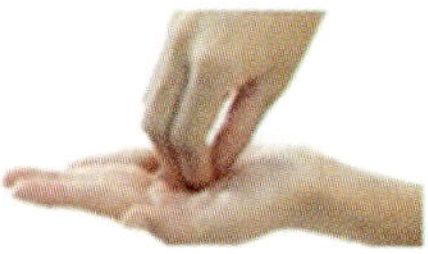

Rub fingertips on palm for both hands

Step 7

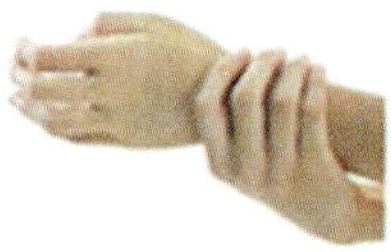

Rub both wrists in a rotating manner, rinse and dry thoroughly

Hand-washing steps

11. i. Interpret peripheral smear haemogram, and iron panel.

ii. Propose a management plan for iron deficiency anaemia

S. Fe – 30 mg/dl

Transferrin saturation –10%

S. Ferritin – 15 ng/ml

TIBC – 600 μg/dl

i. Red blood cells are microcytic and hypochromic with anisocytosis, poikilocytois and increased red cell distribution width (RDW) (normal 13–64%), mean corpuscular volume (MCV) (normal 86–94 fl) and mean corpuscular hemoglobin concentration (MCHC) (normal 32–34 g/dl) are reduced.

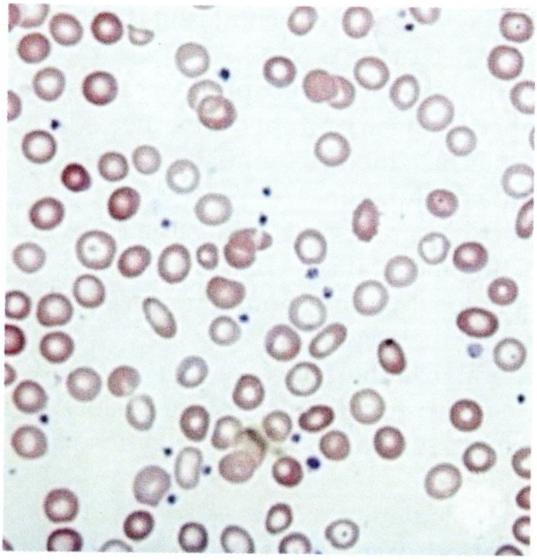

Total RBC Count is Decreased

(Note in thalassemia total RBC count is increased)

Iron panel	Noral values
S. Iron	60–170 μg/dl
Transferrin saturation	20–30%
S. Ferritin	15–300 ng/ml (Boys) 15–200 ng/ml (Girls)
Total irion binding capacity	250–400 μg/dl

In iron deficiency anaemia *S. Iron* ↓, transferrin saturation ↓, S ferritin ↓, Total iron binding capacity↑
Interpretation—iron deficiency anamia (IDA)

ii. **Management plan for IDA**
   1. Treat treatable cause, e.g. bleeding, caeliac disease
   2. Dietary advice—diet rich in iron
      Nuts and seeds, dried fruits, green leafy vegetables, legumes, meat, eggs, liver, sea foods, dark chocolates,
   3. Deworming—worm infestation is the common cause of IDA. Albendazole <2 years 200 mg; >2 years 400 mg (repeat after 2 weeks)
   4. Oral iron therapy
      3–6 mg/kg/day of elemental iron (ferrous sulfate), once a day for 3–6 months
      - Syrup/tablets of iron preparation should be taken empty stomach or in-between meals.
      - Side effect includes nausea/vomiting/abdominal pain/constipation
      - Counsel parents regarding black colour stool after starting medication—that is normal
      - Reticulocyte count should increase within 3 days after starting therapy
   5. Parenteral iron therapy
      - Iron sucrose preparation infuse slow IV mixed with normal saline once a day—total dose to be given over 5–7 days
      - Dose calculation
        Total dose (mg) = (target Hb – observed Hb) × weight (kg) × 2.4 + [15 × wt (kg)]
   6. Blood transfusion
      - PCV/PRBC 10–15 ml/kg
      - Rarely needed only in emergency
   7. Close follow up, ensure compliance
   8. In younger children one of the common cause of IDA is excess cow/buffalo milk intake [due to cow milk protein allergy which could cause anemia (occult blood loss), constipation and recurrent wheeze]

9. Child with anemia not responding to iron therapy should get high performance liquid chromatography (HPLC)/ hemoglobin electrophoresis
   Thalassemia → ↓HbA, ↑HbF
   Sickle cell anemia → ↑HbSS

12. i. Elicit, document and present a history pertaining to disease of the genitourinary tract

ii. Perform and interpret the common analytes in a urine report

iii. Identify external markers of kidney disease

iv. What imaging study you recommend in a child with genitourinary tract disease

i. Symptoms and sings of genitourinary tract disease
   1. Malnutrition/failure to thrive/growth retardation
   2. Polyuria/polydipsia/oliguria
   3. Enuresis/bed wetting
   4. Haematuria/recurrent UTI/poor urinary stream
   5. Abdominal swelling/mass/pain
   6. Facial puffiness/pedal oedema/anasarca
   7. Hypertension/skin rash

ii. Complete urinary examination (CUR or urine R/E)

Test	Normal range
Physical	
Colour	Pale yellow
Appearance	Clear
pH	5.0–8.0
Specific gravity	1.001–1.030
Chemical	
Albumin	Nil
Ketones	Nil
Sugar	Nil
Blood	Negative
Bile salt	Nil
Leukocyte esterase/nitrite	Negative
Bile pigment	Nil

Contd.

Test	Normal range
Microscopy	
Pus cells	0–5/HPF
Epithelial cells	0–5/HPF
RBC	0/HPF
Crystals	0/HPF
Others	0/HPF

Note: First-morning, mid stream clean catch specimen should be collected for urine routine and culture.

iii. See figure below.

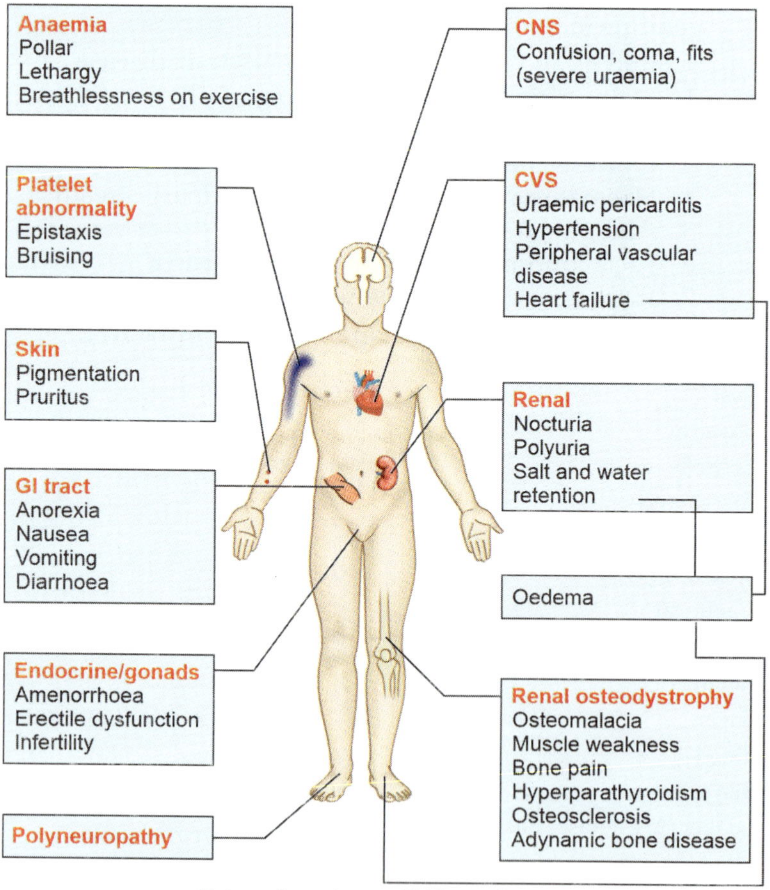

External markers of kidney disease

iv. 1. X-ray—Erect abdomen
   2. Ultrasonography—USG-KUB/Doppler
   3. Micturating cytosurethrography (MCU)—To diagnose VUR/PUV
   4. CT abdomen/KUB—contrast/noncontrast
   5. DMSA scan (dimercaptosuccinic acid scan)—as DMSA attains high conc. In the cortex, it is used for evaluating renal parenchyma (structure of kidney)
   6. DTPA scan (diethylenetriamine pentaacetate scan)—as DTPA is freely filtered—used for evaluating perfusion and function of kidney
   7. MAG-3 scan (mercaptoacetyl triglycine scan)—used for evaluating renal structure and function both.

13. Recognise and interpret signs of physical abuse in a child—

Types of child abuse

1. Physical abuse
2. Emotional abuse
3. Sexual abuse
4. Child neglect
5. Child labour
   - Signs of child physical abuse (see figure on page 222)
   - Management—confidentiality is utmost important.
     - Medical
     - Psychological support
     - Medicolegal procedure

14. Counsel/educate a sick child's parent for referral
Mnemonic—REFERRAL

- **R**eview the need for referral
- **E**mpathize with parents
- **F**acilitate discussion with the parents and specialist
- **E**ducate the parents about the benefits in their language
- **R**esolve doubts take informed consent

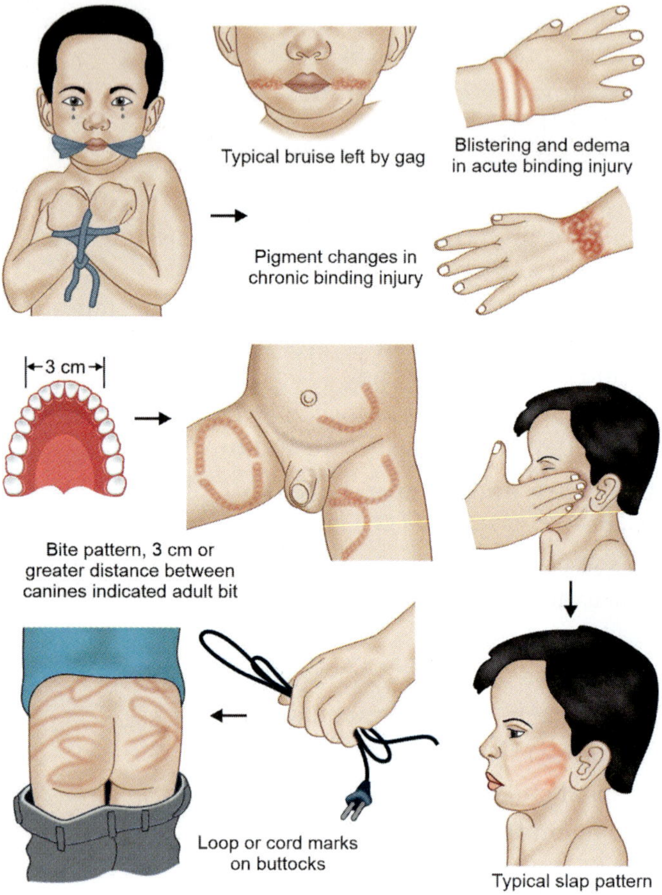

Signs of physical child abuse

- **R**einforce follow up
- **A**lternative remedy
- **L**ist all the medical records test reports

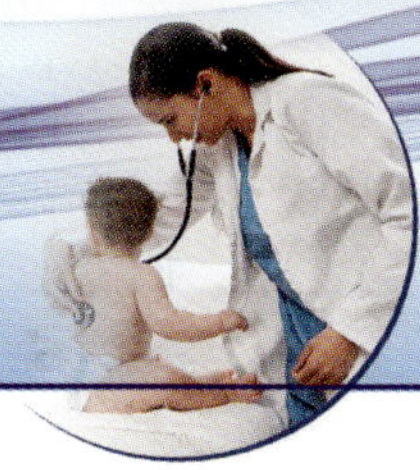

CHAPTER

21 Procedures and Instruments

LUMBAR PUNCTURE

Most common space used in children → L_3–L_4, L_5–S_1

INDICATIONS

- Suspected CNS infection
- Leukemia after diagnosis to rule out CNS leukaemia
- Pseudotumor cerebri
- Neonatal sepsis
- Spinal anaesthesia

Therapeutically:

1. To inject drugs for CNS leukaemia—methotrexate
2. To inject amphotericin for fungal infection

CONTRAINDICATIONS

- Intracranial space-occupying lesion
- Hydrocephalus
- Unequal pupils, irregularity of pulse, BP, respiration
- Papilloedema
- Infections of the skin over lying the LP site
- Focal seizures and focal deficits
- Thrombocytopenia

COMPLICATIONS

- Tonsillar herniation with sudden collapse and cardio-respiratory arrest
- Introducing infection into CSF space
- Post-LP headache
- Traumatic tap

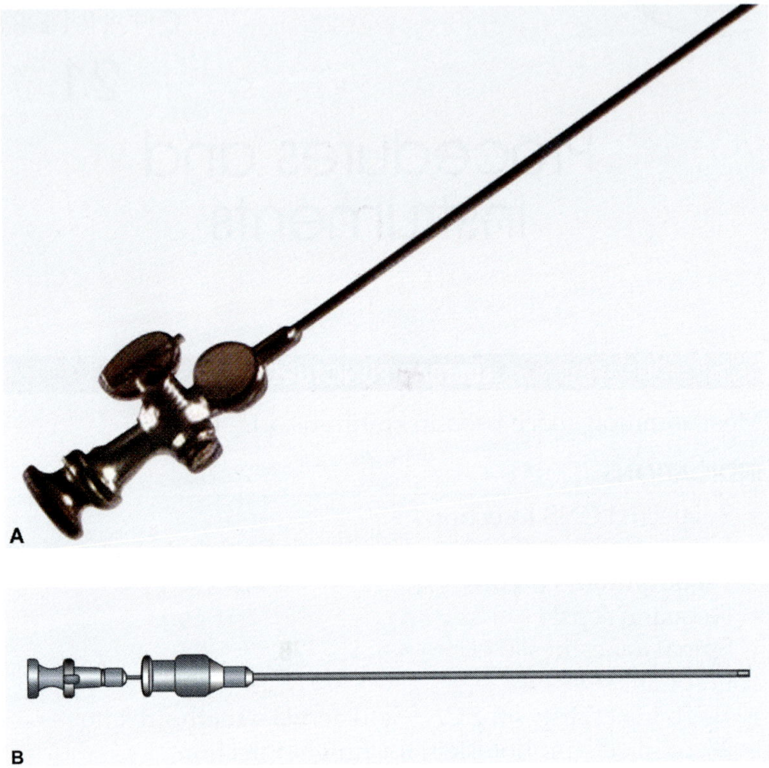

Lumbar puncture needles

How to interpret traumatic LP?
Every 500 RBC/mm^3 will have 1 WBC and there is a rise of 1 ml/dl of protein for every 1000 RBC/mm^3.

Normal CSF Values

- Colourless
- Cells WBC <5/mm^3 for children and up to 10 in newborn
- Protein 10–40 mg/dl in children and up to 120 mg/dl in newborn
- Glucose 60% or 2/3rd of blood glucose level
- No RBCs are seen.

CSF Values in Various Diseases

Condition	Cells	Sugar	Proteins	Specific features
Normal	<5 all L	2/3rd of random blood sugar	<40 mg/dl	Nil
Pyogenic meningitis	↑ N > L	<2/3rd of random blood sugar	↑	Culture positive
Tuberculous meningitis	↑ L > N	Low	↑↑↑	Cob web coagulum AFB culture
Viral encephalitis (AES)	↑	Normal	↑	Viral studies, In mumps sugar is low, In herpes RBC will be there

N: neutrophil, L: lymphocytes, ↑ Increased

NASOGASTRIC TUBE/INFANT FEEDING TUBE

- Estimate length of tube needed by extending the tubing from the tip of the child's nose to the ear lobe and then to the xiphoid process.
- Neonates—size 5–8 French
- Young children—size 12–16 French

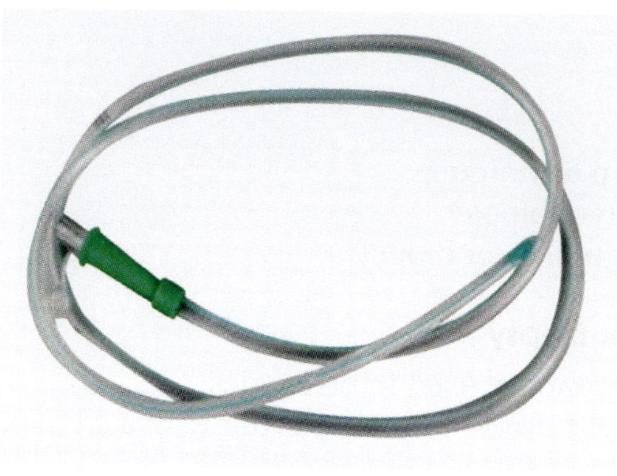

Nasogastric tube

- Uses:
  - **Diagnostic:** Internal bleeding/poisoning/gastric analysis (TB) /TEF.
  - **Therapeutic:** Nasogastric feeding/intestinal obstruction/ administration of drugs

LIVER BIOPSY NEEDLE

In a liver biopsy, a needle is inserted through the rib cage or abdominal wall and into the liver to obtain a sample for examination.

Indications

- Investigation of obscure hepatomegaly
- Chronic hepatitis
- Chronic or recurrent conjugated hyperbilirubinaemia
- Investigation of portal hypertension
- Diagnosis of Wilson's disease
- Diagnosis of metabolic or storage disorders

Contraindications

- Prolonged PT/aPTT
- Platelet counts of less than 40,000/mm^3
- Hydatid disease of the liver
- Pyogenic abscess of the liver
- Biliary tract infection
- Angiomatous malformation of the liver
- Ascites

Types

- Menghini technique
- Trucut liver biopsy
- Transjugular liver biopsy

Trucut Liver Biopsy

- Most commonly used in pediatrics
- Instrument used—a trucut needle with a 2 cm notch and cutting.
- Sleeve

Complications

- Local pain
- Infection
- Subcapsular and intrahepatic haematoma
- Intrathoracic and intraperitoneal bile leaks
- Pneumothorax
- Penetration of other abdominal organ
- Arteriovenous fistula.

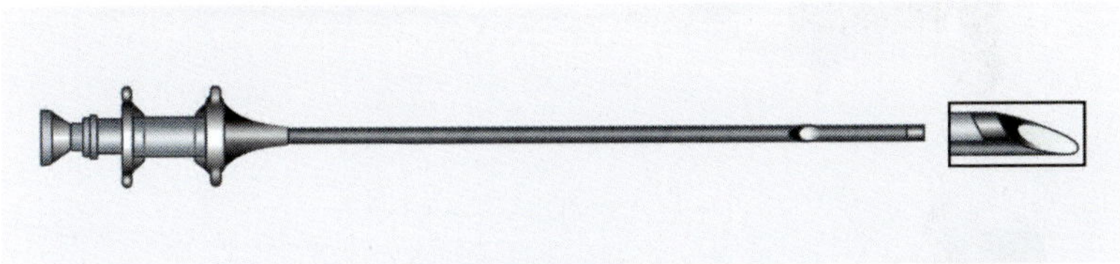

Liver biopsy needle

BONE MARROW ASPIRATION

INDICATIONS

- Malignancies
- Bone marrow failure syndromes
- Aplastic anaemia
- Fanconi's anaemia
- Haemolytic anaemia
- ITP
- Storage disorders

SITE

Posterior superior iliac spine.

PARTS OF NEEDLE

Needle/lock/inner stylet

COMPLICATIONS

- Incomplete penetration of the bony cortex
- Penetration of the posterior cortex
- Blockage of the needle by marrow
- Infection
- Necrosis and sloughing of the skin at site.

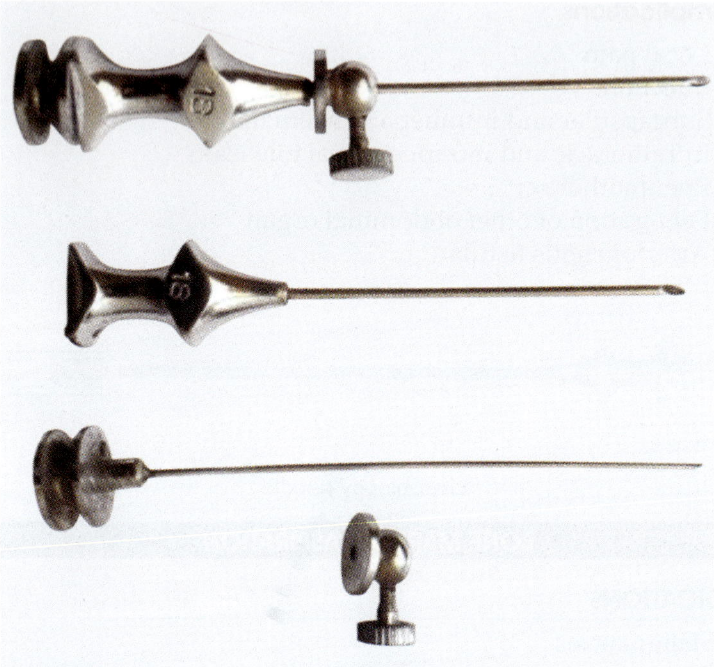

Bone marrow needles

RESPIRATORY DEVICES

NEBULISERS

A nebuliser is a device that generates an aerosol vapour of the medicine.

Parts of Nebuliser

- Compressor/oxygen source
- Mouthpieces and masks
- Tubing
- Medication chamber
- Outlet connection
- Inlet connection
- Jet
- Cap
- Baffle plate
- Filter

Principle of Nebulisation

Nebulisers produce a poly-disperse aerosol where most of the drug released is in particles 1–5 μm in diameter. They use compressed air for automisation.

Nebulisation time: 10–20 minutes
Dose: 0.02 ml/kg of salbutamol, max 1 ml.
Add normal saline to make a volume of total of 5 ml.

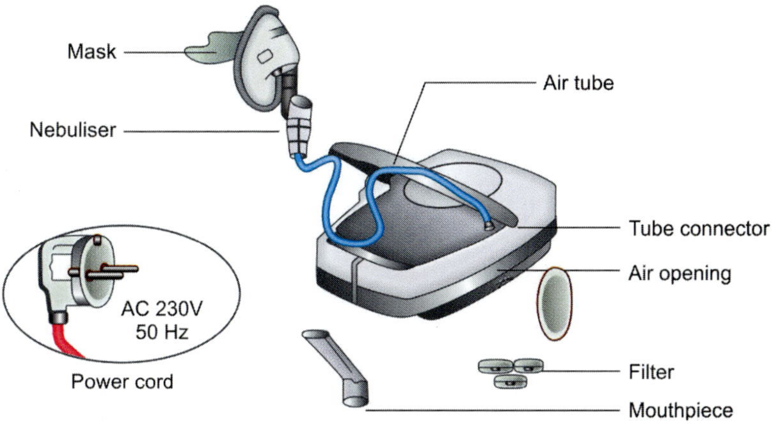

Parts of nebuliser

METERED DOSE INHALER (MDI)

An MDI is a device, which delivers a fixed amount of medication in aerosol form each time it is activated. It can be used for exacerbation and maintenance therapy.

<4 years to be used with mask and spacer
4–12 years to be used with spacer
>12 years without spacer

How to use an MDI?

Steps

1. Shake the inhaler well before use (3 or 4 shakes)
2. Remove the cap
3. Breathe out, away from your inhaler

4. Bring the inhaler to your mouth. Place it in your mouth between your teeth and close your mouth around it.
5. Start to breathe in slowly. Press the top of your inhaler (at start of inspiration) once and keep breathing in slowly until you have taken a full breath—press and breath coordination.
6. Remove the inhaler from your mouth, and hold your breath for about 10 seconds, then breathe out.
7. If you need a second puff, wait 30 seconds, shake your inhaler again, and repeat steps 3–6. After you have used your MDI, rinse out your mouth and record the number of doses taken.

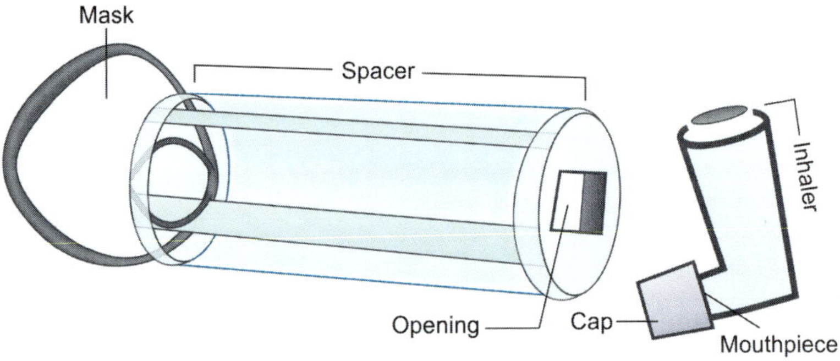

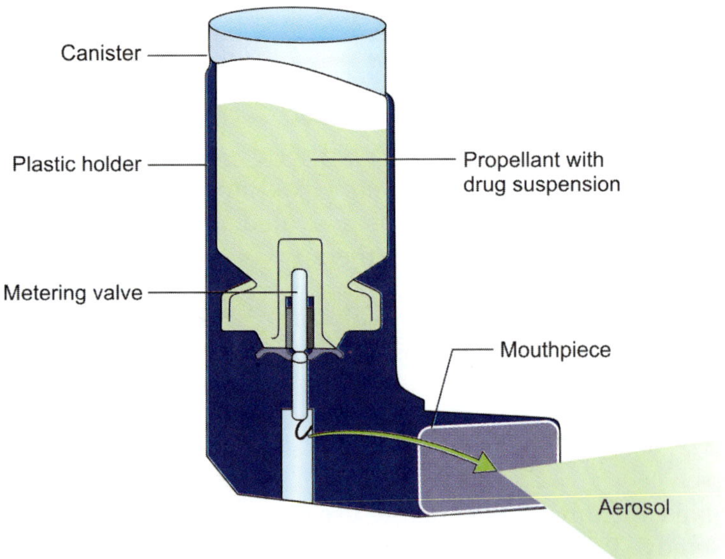

Metered dose inhaler

DRY POWDER INHALER (DPI)

These are breath activated device like rotahaler. Used >4 years

PEAK EXPIRATORY FLOW RATE (PEFR)

Children >5 years

- Indication:
  - To recognize an impending attack of wheezing
  - To know the prognosis/compliance of asthma
- The marker of the mini flow meter is slided to zero. Child is asked to stand up and take a deep breath. The mouthpiece of the flow meter is then taken in the mouth and lips are tightly closed over it. Child is asked to exhale out with max effort and force. The procedure is repeated 3 times and the highest reading is recorded.
  - Green zone—PEFR >80%,
  - Yellow zone—PEFR 50–80%
  - Red zone—<50%.
- Baseline PEFR value

For male {2.96 × height (in cm)}—110
For female {3.43 × height (in cm)}—178

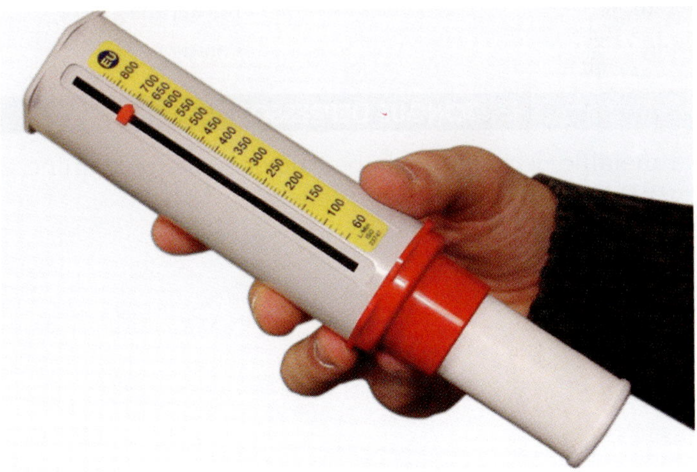

Mini flow meter

TUBERCULIN SYRINGE

It is a 1 cc syringe with a white piston (plastic syringes) or metal piston (glass syringes).

USES

- To administer PPD for Mantoux test
- To administer BCG vaccine/fIPV
- To administer test doses, e.g. penicillin
- Provocative testing—to test atopy
- Insulin injection in DM.

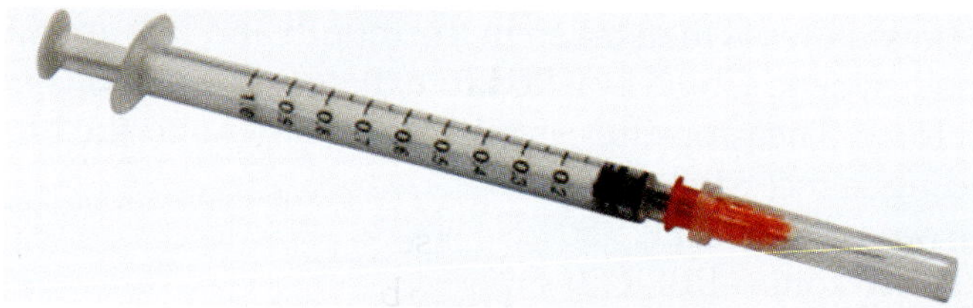

Tuberculin syringe

Interpretation of Mantoux Test

Induration size	Result
<5 mm	Negative
5–10 mm	Borderline
>10 mm	Positive

TONGUE DEPRESSOR

It is a metallic/wooden L-shaped device use to examine gag reflex/pharynx/oral cavity and tonsils.

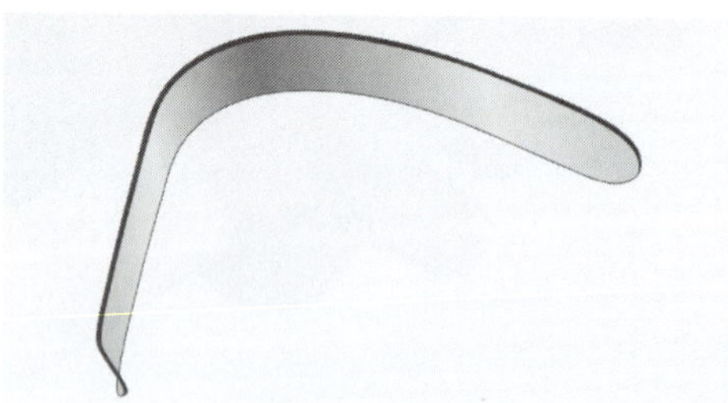

Tongue depressor

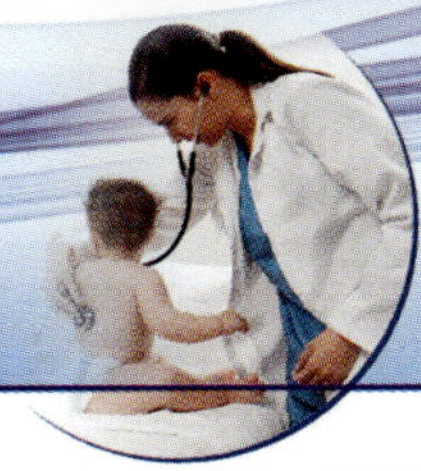

CHAPTER 22

X-ray

CHEST

In newborn infants, it is advisable to get AP view.

- After the patient is able to sit or stand unsupported PA view is advisable.
- Decubitus films are useful in case of **pleural effusion.**
- Remember the thicker the part the brighter it appears in X-ray.
- Assume child is facing you whether its AP/PA view

Mnemonic

RIPE ABCDEFG

- **R**otation
- **I**nspiration
- **P**osition
- **E**xposure
- **A**irways
- **B**ones
- **C**ardiac
- **D**iaphragm
- **E**xtrathoracic tissues
- **F**ields and fissures
- **G**reat vessels

Comment on

1. **Exposure:** Normal exposure—one should be able to see the spine with **intervertebral disc space up to T_3/T_4** beyond that indicates overexposed film.
2. **View:**
   - PA/lateral/AP view
   - Generally PA view is taken for heart and lung.
   - If the scapular shadow is overlying the lung field it is an AP film
3. **Positioning/rotation**
   - In a properly positioned PA X-ray medial ends of clavicles are at equal distance from the spinous process

- Look for rotation of film which is judged by shape and position of clavicle or comparing the position of the anterior ends of the lower ribs on both the sides.

4. **Inspiratory/expiratory film:** Mid inspiratory films are satisfactory. If the right diaphragmatic dome is projected at the level of the 6th rib anteriorly and the 9th to 10th rib posteriorly, a satisfactory inspiratory film has been made. If you could count more than 7 rib anteriorly s/o hyperinflated lung.
5. **Soft tissue and bony cage:** Look for any soft tissue or bony cage abnormalities look for subcutaneous emphysema, crowding of ribs, etc.
6. **Position of trachea:** Normally slightly shifted to right (due to aortic arch).
7. **Mediastinum and hilum:** 2/3rd of the heart shadow is left of midline and 1/3rd to the right.
   Right hilum is 1–2 cm lower than left.
   - Look for hilar and mediastinal shadows (? lymph nodes)/ mediastinum shift
8. **Heart:** Look for cardiomegaly/shift/pericadial effusion. Look for cardio-thoracic ratio if its more than 0.55 its suggestive of cardiomegaly.
   - Obliteration of left cardiac border **(silhouette sign)** suggests collapse/consolidation of lingular segment of left lung.
   - Obliteration of right cardiac border **(silhouette sign)** suggests collapse/consolidation of right middle lobe.

   Note:
     - In CHD with **L-R shunt** there would be cardiomegaly (LVH) with plethoric lung fields.
     - In TOF with **R-L shunt** there would be cardiomegaly-RVH (boot-shaped heart) with oligaemic lung fields.
9. **Lung fields:** Lung parenchyma is divided into upper/middle and lower zones by horizontal lines drawn from 2nd and 4th ribs. Abnormalities in each zones are described in the forms of **opacities, hyperinflation, collapse,** etc.
10. **Diaphragm:** Normally right diaphragm is higher than the left.
    Congenital diaphragmatic hernia: Coils of air filled small bowel in one side of hemithorax with part of missing diaphragm and mediastinal shift to the other side.

11. **Costophrenic angles:** Clear/fuzzy obliteration of costophrenic angles suggest pleural effusion or pleural thickening
12. **Broncho-vascular marking**
13. **Great vessels:** Comment on SVC/IVC/ascending aorta/aortic arch/PA/atrial appendages

    Pneumothorax: Condition represents of air in the pleural cavity causing an area of peripheral lucency which leads to a collapse of the underlying lung.

    The condition can be differentiated from emphysema by the total absence of bronchovascular marking in the area of lucency.

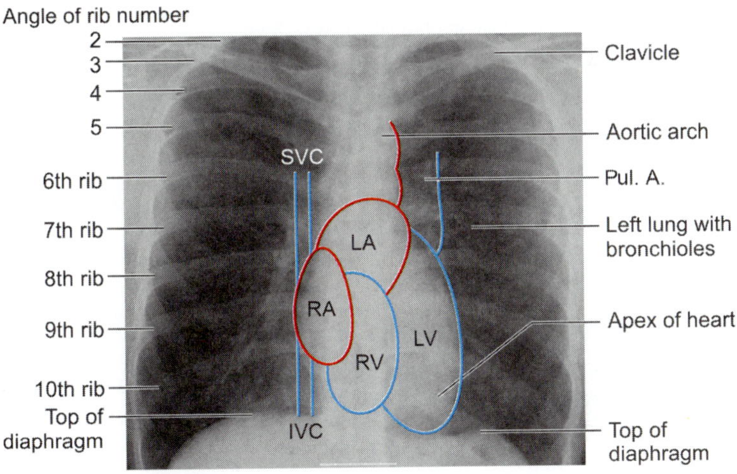

Schematic diagram of chest X-ray: PA view

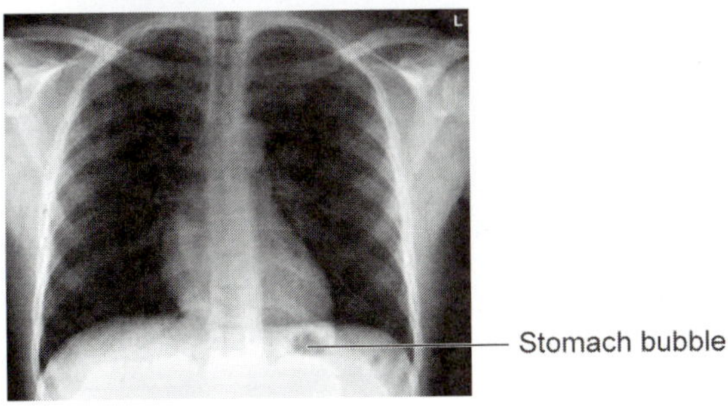

Mid inspiratory, normally exposed well-positioned chest X-ray: PA view

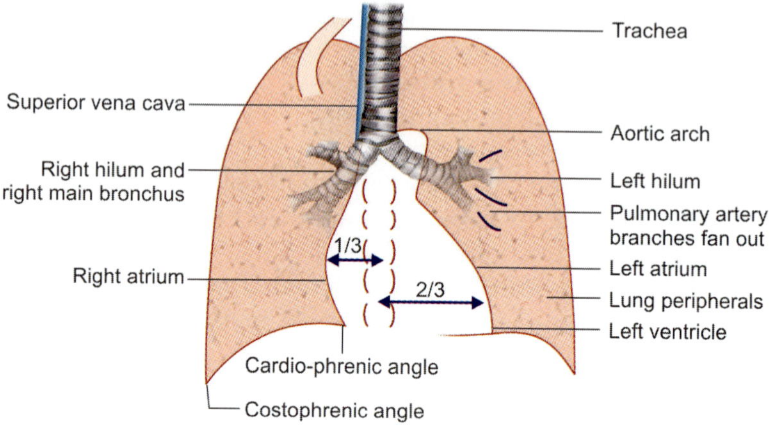

Schematic diagram of chest X-ray PA view defining heart and mediastinum

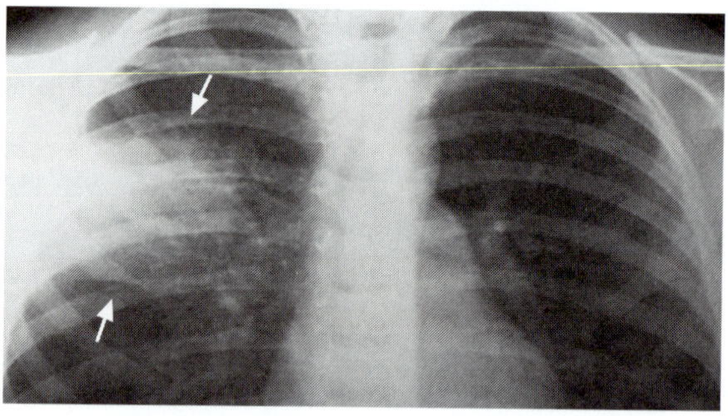

Right middle lobe pneumonia

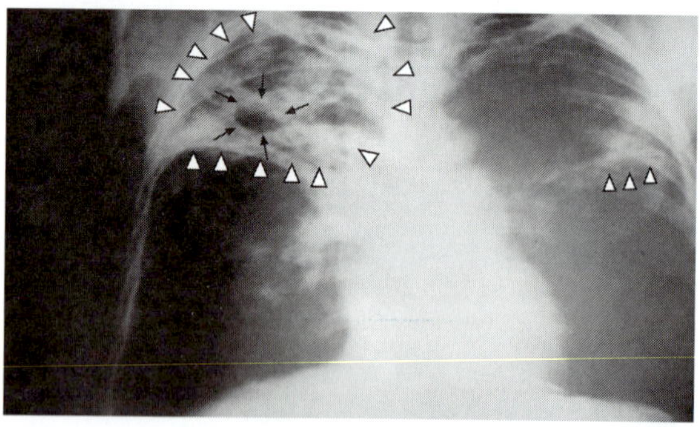

Cavity in right upper lobe in pulmonaryTB

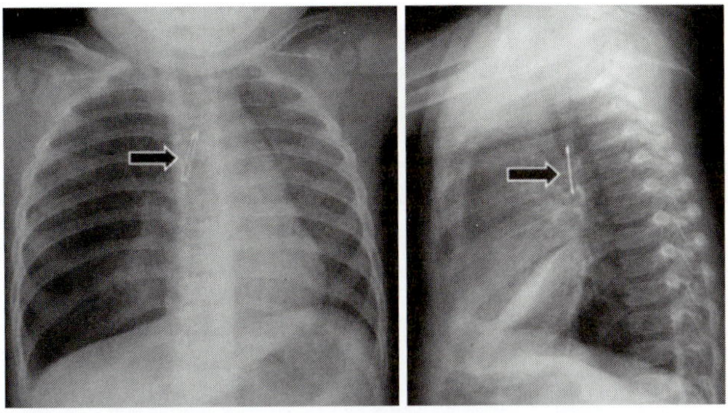

X-ray of tracheobronchial foreign body aspiration

TRACHEO-OESOPHAGEAL FISTULA

- 5 types of TEF are recognised
- In most common type (80%) the upper part of the oesophagus ends blindly and the lower part is connected to the trachea by a fistula.
- Maternal polyhydramnios and single umbilical artery gives a clue.

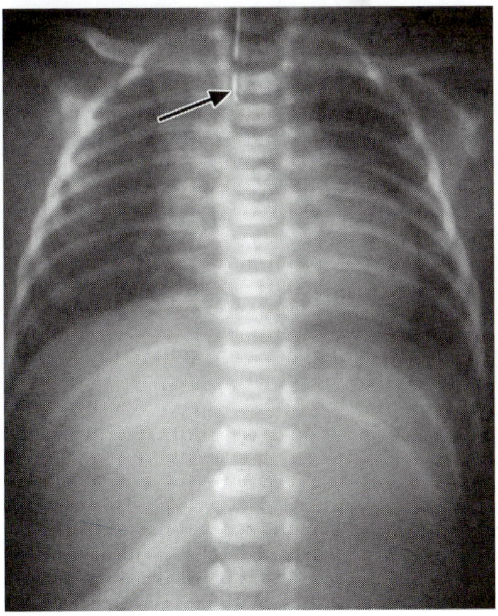

Chest X-ray PA view with coiled NG tube s/o TEF

Lateral Neck X-ray

- Croup—steeple sign (subglottic narrowing)
- Epiglottitis—thumb print sign (enlarged epiglottis)

X-RAY ABDOMEN

Gas under the diaphragm with multiple air fluid levels s/o peritonitis—**intestinal perforation/NEC.**

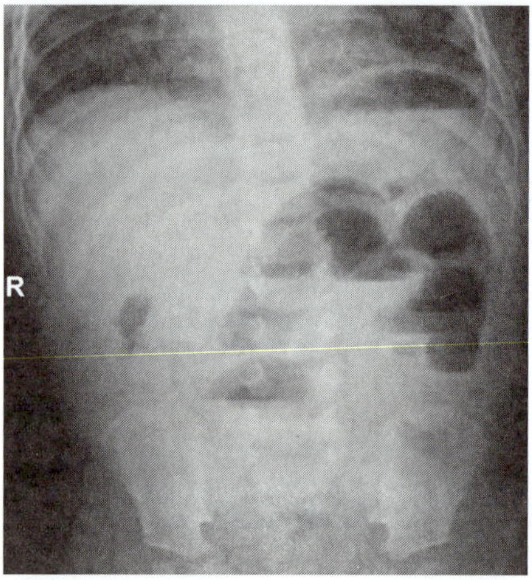

Multiple air fluid level in the intestine s/o intestinal obstruction

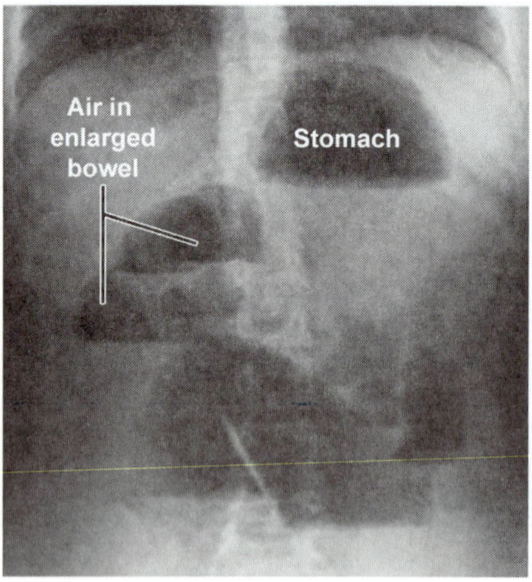

X-RAY BONES

For upper/lower limb fracture the most common view taken is AP/lateral view (schematic diagram is shown below):

- Look carefully epiphysis/diaphysis/metaphysis/soft tissue
- Normally the sum diameter of cortex of both the sides is equal to that of the medulla.

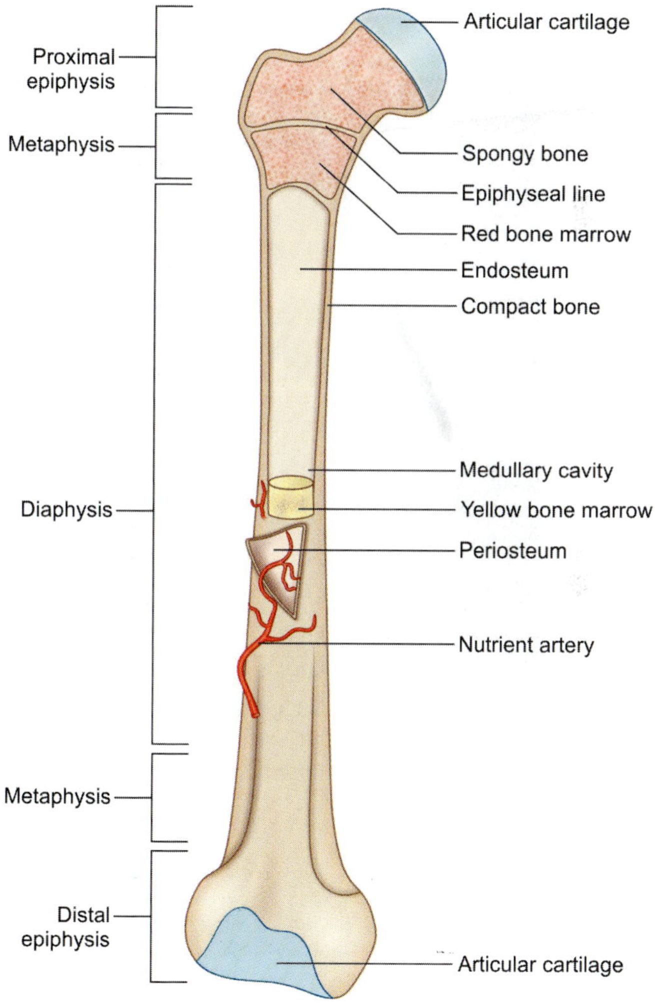

Schematic diagram of X-ray femur: AP view

RICKETS

- Increased distance between epiphysis and metaphysis
- Cupping/fraying (blurring)/splaying (widening) of the margins at the end of the bone (metaphysis).
- Fracture of the bone
- Deformities—bending of the bones/rickety rosary/bossing of the skull
- Rarefaction

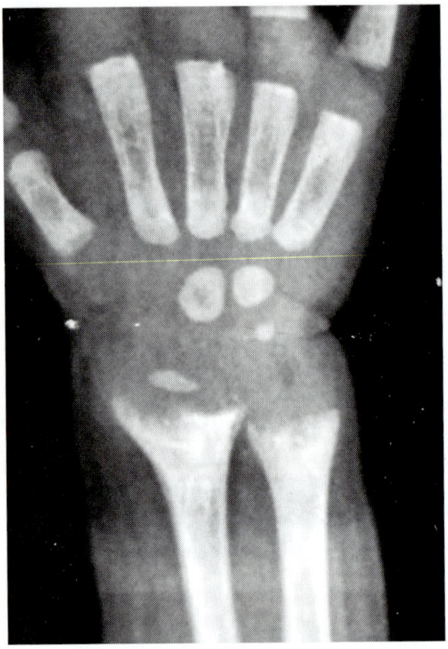

AP view of wrist X-ray suggestive of rickets

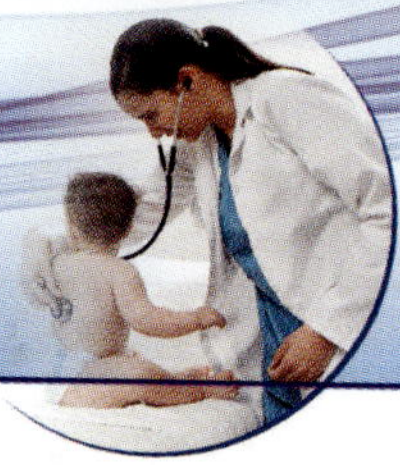

CHAPTER

23

Electrocardiogram (ECG or EKG)

Graphical representation of heart electrical activity (generated due to cardiac muscle depolarization and repolarization) on a voltage *vs* time graph by electrode placed on the skin.

ECG helps to detect abnormalities of cardiac conduction, arrhythmias, hypertrophy of heart chambers, ischaemic events, electrolyte abnormalities.

ELECTRICAL CONDUCTION OF HEART

Consist of:

- **Sino atrial node (SA node):** Lies in the wall of RA near the opening of SVC
- **Atrioventricular node (AV node):** Lies in the base of RA near coronary sinus (on the AV valve)
- **Bundle of His:** Originates from AV node and passes into interventricular septum
- Right and left bundle branches
- Purkinje fibres

Electrical impulse arises in pacemaker cells of SA node (Pacemaker of heart) travels through wall of atria and internodal fibres and reaches AV node.

SA node activation causes contraction of both atria **(Atrial depolarization)**.

From AV node impulses travel along bundle of His and goes to right and left bundle branches and finally spreads diffusely

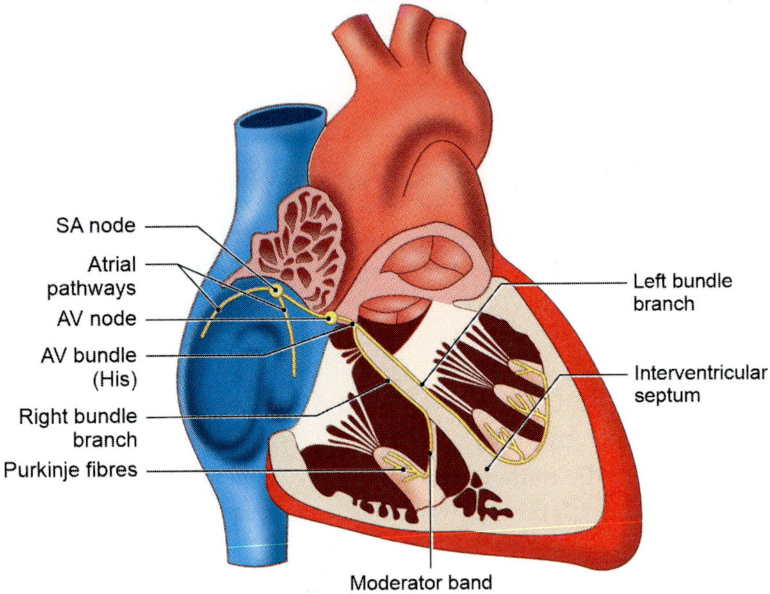

to the ventricular myocardium through Purkinje fibres causes contraction of both ventricle **(Ventricular depolarization).**

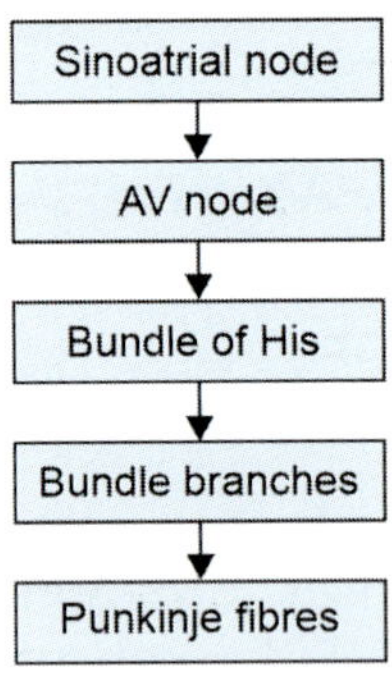

ECG is Taken by 12 Leads (10 Electrodes)

- 3 Limb leads (bipolar)— I, II, III
- 3 Augmented leads (unipolar)—aVL, aVR, aVF
- 6 Chest leads (unipolar)—V_1, V_2, V_3, V_4, V_5, V_6

12 lead ECG placement

Types of electrodes

Limb electrodes

There are **4** electrodes placed on the **limbs:**

Lead wires
Right arm
Left arm
Right leg
Left leg

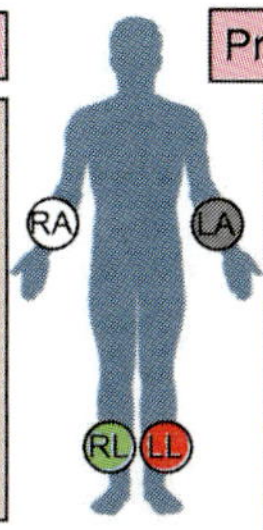

Precordial electrodes

There are **6** electrodes placed on **chest:**

Lead wires
V_1
V_2
V_3
V_4
V_5
V_6

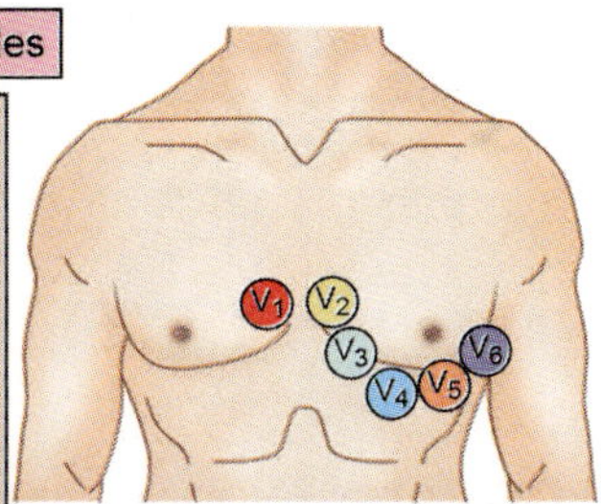

Electrode/ lead wire	Position	Color
RA	Right arm	White (clouds)
RL	Right leg	Green (grass)
LA	Left arm	Black (smoke)
LL	Left leg	Red (fire)

Electrode/ lead wire	Position	Color
V1	4th ICS, right of sternum	Red (ride)
V2	4th ICS, left of sternum	Yellow (your)
V3	Between V_2 and V_4	Green (green)
V4	5th ICS, mid clavicular line	Blue (bike)
V5	5th ICS, ant. axillary line	Orange (on)
V6	5th ICS, mid axillary line	Purple (parvement)

Note: Limb leads and augmented leads measure electrical activity of heart in vertical plane.

Chest leads measure electrical activity of heart in transverse (anteroposterior) plane.

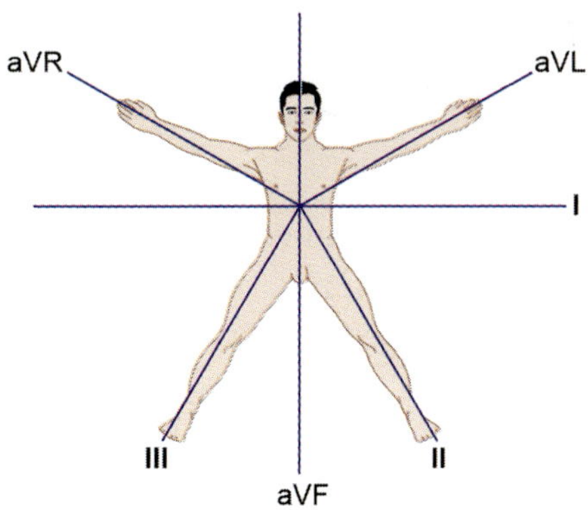

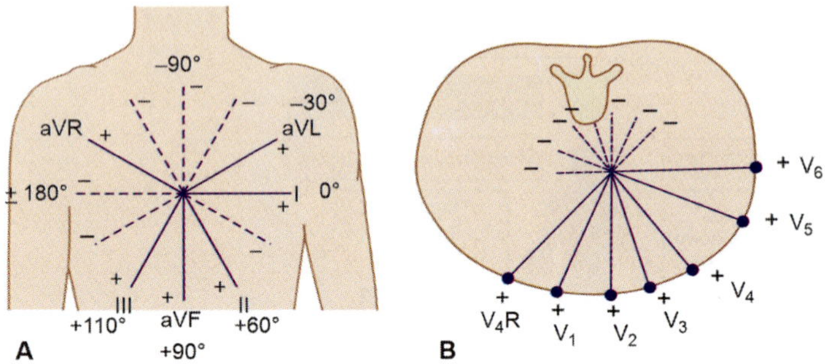

ECG Paper/Graph

- **Vertical axis:** Amplitude in mm
- **Horizontal axis:** Duration in seconds

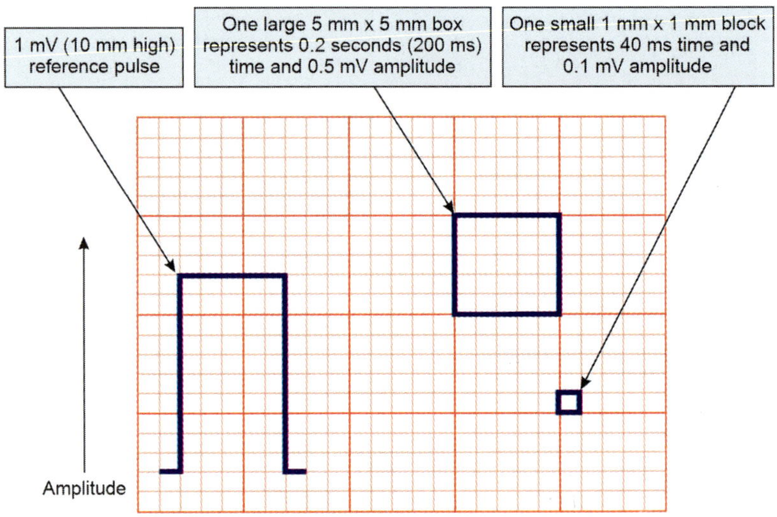

1 small square/box = 1 mm × 1 mm = 0.04 sec × 0.1 mV
1 large square/box = 5 mm × 5 mm = 0.2 sec × 0.5 mV
(1 large box has 5 × 5 small box)
Standard paper speed is 25 mm/sec
(that is, in 1 sec 5 big box/25 small box passes away)

- Normal ECG taken for 10 seconds

Normal ECG has mainly 5 waves PQRST, 2 intervals (PR and QT interval) and 2 segments (PR and ST segment)

Each wave and segment corresponds to a certain event of cardiac cycle.

P wave: Represent atrial depolarization

QRS complex: Represent ventricular depolarization

- *Q wave:* Represent ventricular septal depolarization
- *R wave:* Represent main ventricular depolarization
- *S wave:* Represent last phase of ventricular depolarization at the base of heart

T wave: Represent ventricular repolarization

(sometime **U wave** immediately after T wave also seen which represent late phase of ventricular repolarization)

Note: Atrial repolarization merges with the QRS complex hence not seen.

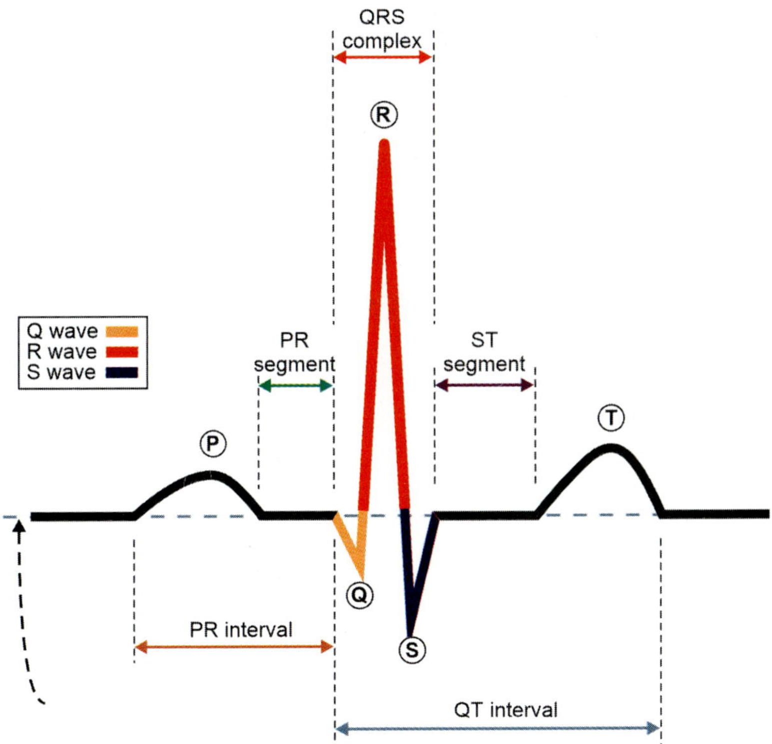

PR segment (from end of P wave to the start of Q wave)—represent time signal travel from SA node to AV node
ST segment (from end of S wave to the start of T wave)—represent the plateau in the myocardial action potential, this is when ventricles contract.
PR interval (from start of P wave to the start of Q wave)—atrial repolarization + time signal travel from SA node to AV node
QT interval (from start of Q wave to the end of T wave)—ventricular depolarization+ repolarization.

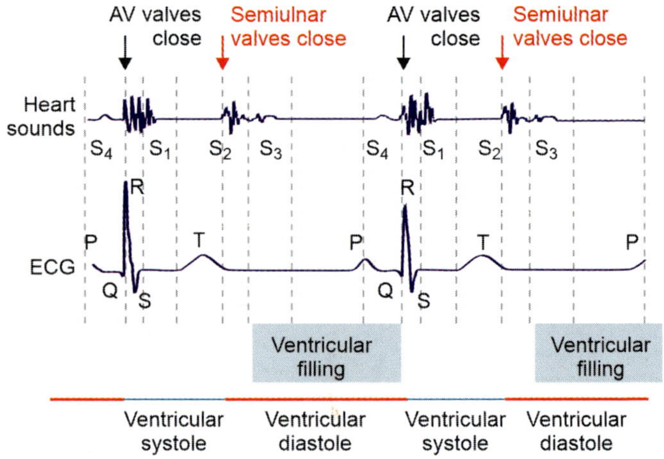

What to Read in ECG: 10 Steps

1. Rhythm
2. Rate
3. Axis
4. P wave
5. PR interval
6. Q wave
7. QRS complex
8. ST segment
9. T wave
10. QT interval

1. Rhythm

First step is to check rhythm in rhythm strip (Lead II)

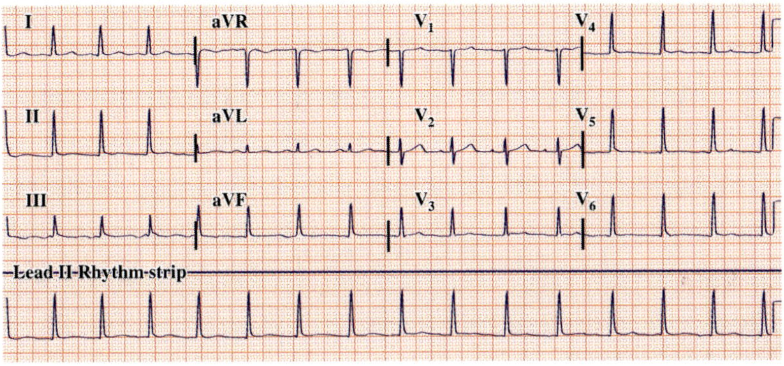

Is it regular or irregular? if irregular is it regularly irregular or irregularly irregular?

Normal sinus rhythm—regular rhythm

- RR interval equal
- P wave before each QRS complex

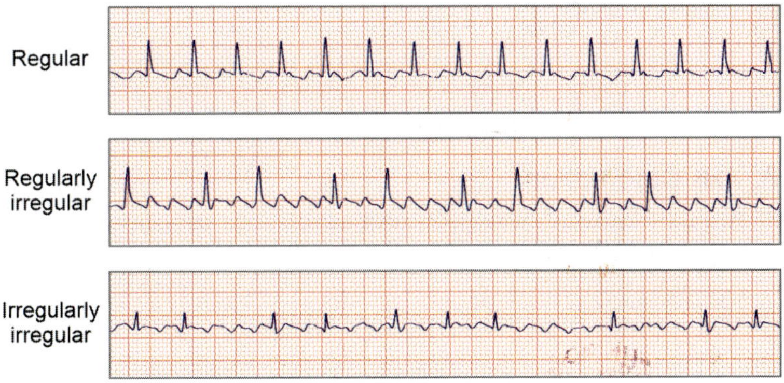

Regularly irregular:

- Unequal RR interval with set pattern
- Seen in 2nd degree (type 2) heart block-missed/drop beat

Irregularly irregular:

- Unequal RR interval with no set pattern
- Seen in atrial fibrillation

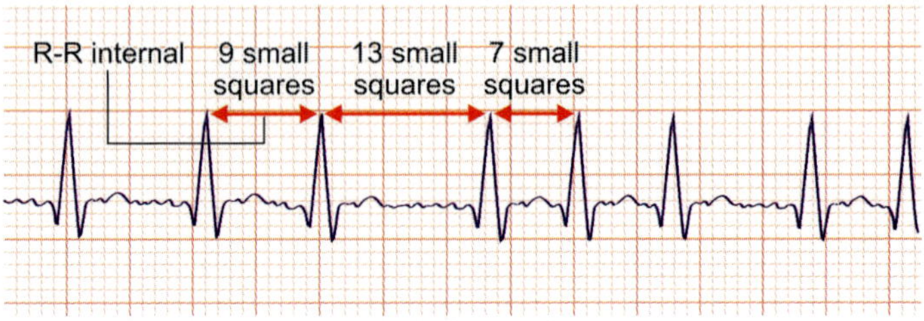

Irregularly irregular

2. Rate

Check rate in rhythm strip (Lead II)

If regular rhythm

Rate = 300/no. of big box between 2 R wave

If irregular rhythm

Rate = no. of R wave in 6 sec (30 big box) × 10

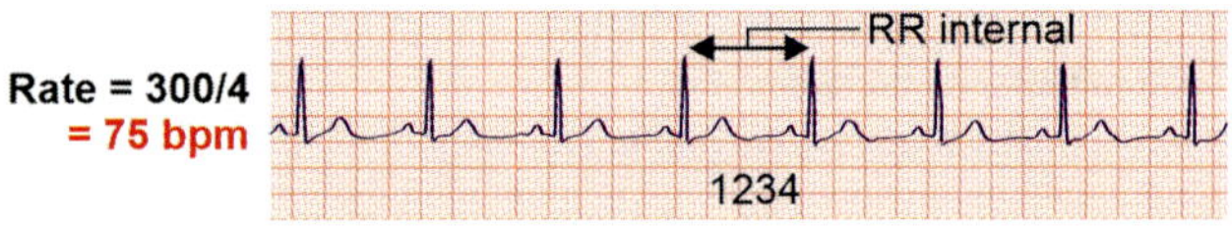

Irregular rhythm = No. of R waves in 6 sec x 10

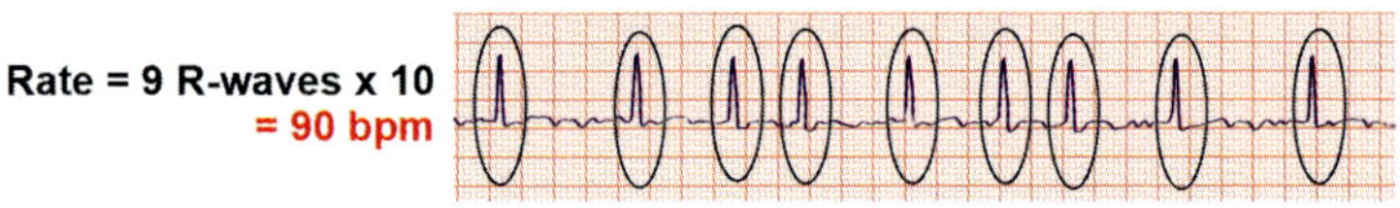

3. Axis Calculation

- In Lead I and aVF (height of R wave – depth of S wave)
- Normal axis of heart: –30* to + 110* (always compare with age matched values)
- Mnemonic—RAD Returns, LAD leaves

I	↓	↑
avF	↑	↓
	RAD	LAD

Note: RAD s/o RVH and LAD s/o LVH

4. P wave

Look in lead II and V_1

- Duration <0.12 sec
- Amplitude <2.5 mm in lead II
  <1.5 mm in lead V_1

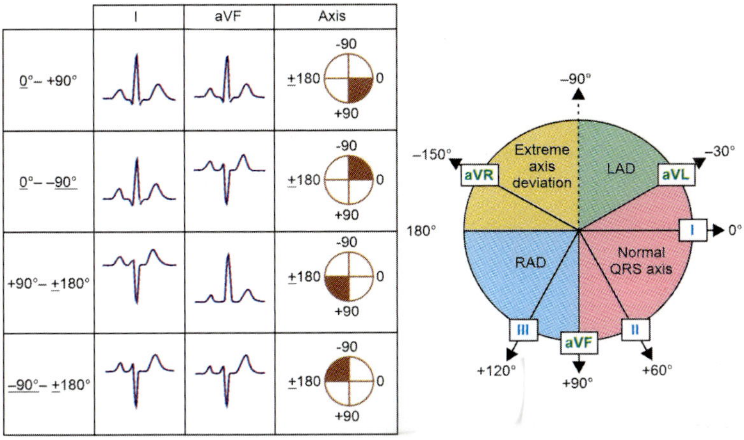

In all leads P wave is upright except

- In lead aVR—inverted P wave
- In V_1 lead—biphasic P wave
- If P wave duration >0.12 sec in lead II (P mitrale)—LAH (as in MS)
- If P wave amplitude >2.5 mm in lead II (P pulmonale)— RAH (as in PS)
- Absent P wave—SA node block, AF

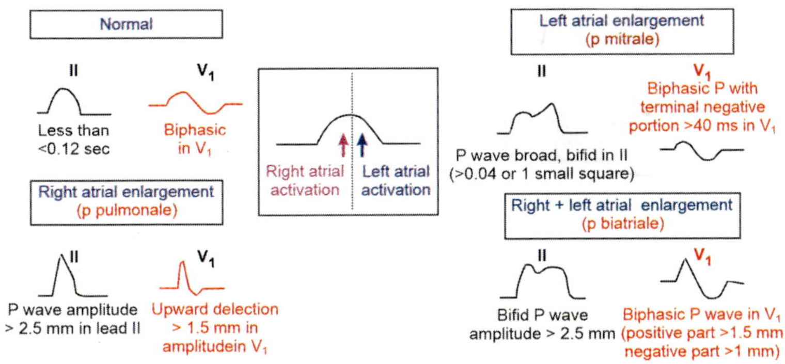

5. PR interval

Read in lead II

- Normal duration—0.12–0.20 sec
- Short PR interval <0.12 sec as seen in Wolf-Parkinson-White (WPW) syndrome

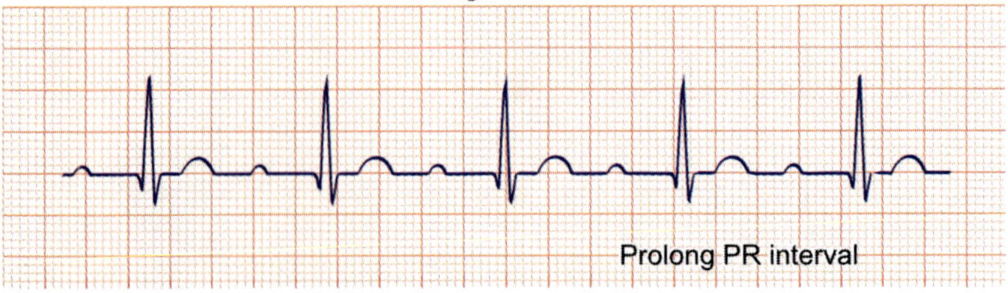

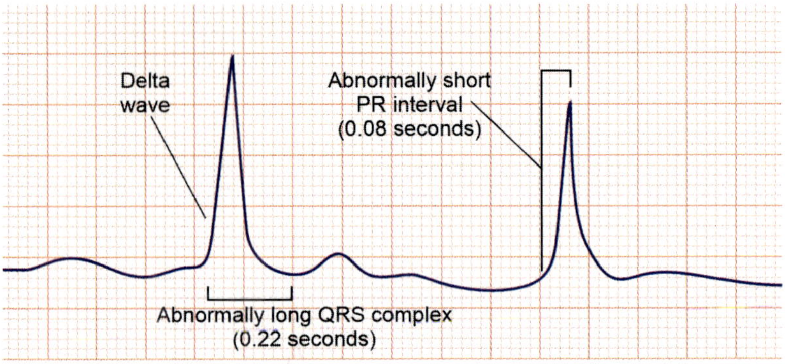

- Prolong PR interval >0.20 sec as seen in 1st, 2nd or 3rd degree heart block, Hyperkalemia, ASD, digitalis toxicity, rheumatic myocarditis.

6. Q wave

- <0.04 sec and <25% of QRS complex, read in V_1 to V_3
- Pathological if (seen in old or recent MI)
  >2 mm deep

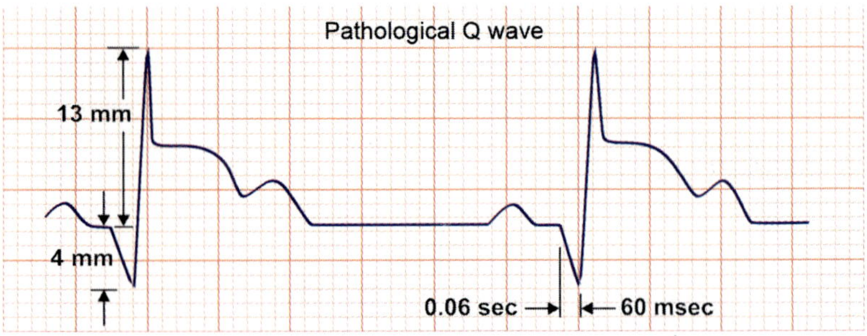

>1 mm wide (>0.04 sec)
>25% of QRS complex depth

7. QRS complex (0.08–0.12 sec)

- Narrow QRS complex <0.08 sec—PSVT, AF
- Broad QRS complex >0.12 sec—VT, Torsades de pointes, Bundle branch block

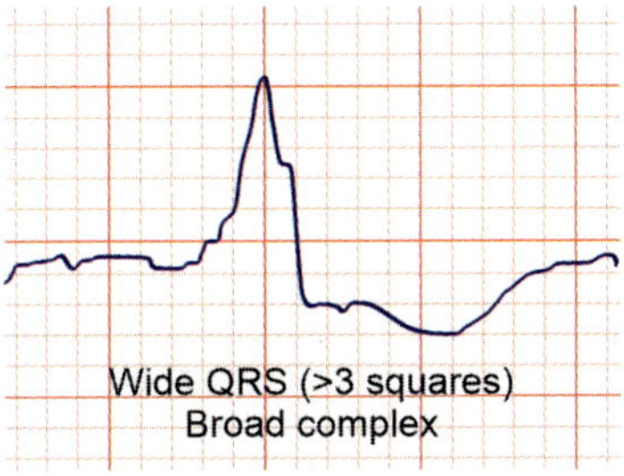

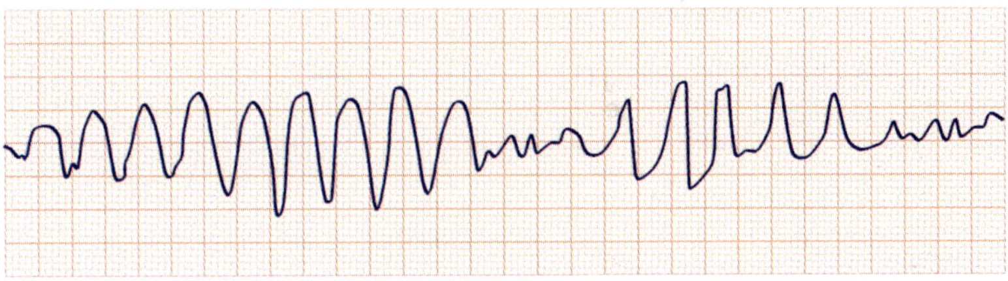

Ventricular tachycardia: Torsades de Pointes

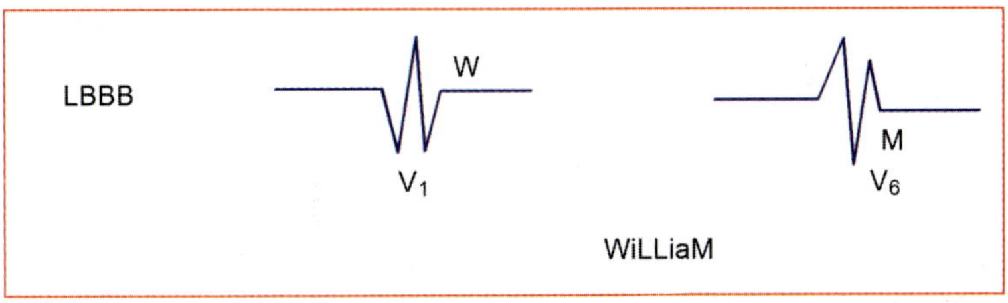

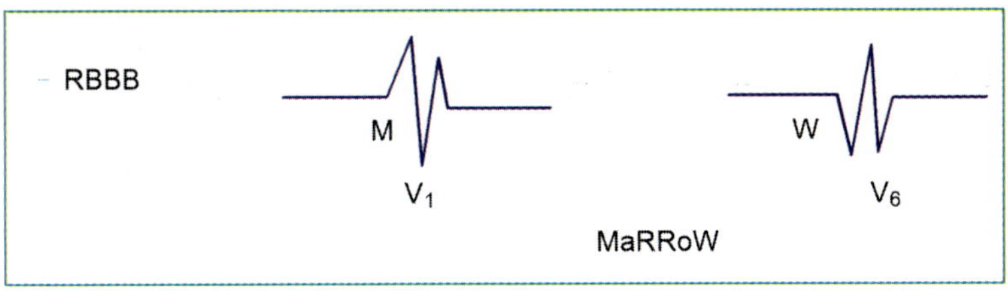

8. ST segment

Elevation of ST segment seen in
Myocardial infarction—(convex shape)
(ST segment elevation in particular lead suggest site of infarction)

- Lead II/III/aVF—inferior wall MI (supplied by right coronary artery)
- Lead I/aVL/V_5/V_6—lateral wall MI (supplied by left circumference coronary artery)
- Lead aVR/V_1/V_2—septal wall MI
- Lead V_3/V_4—ant wall MI (supplied by left coronary artery)

Hyperkalaemia
Pericarditis—(concave shape)
Depression of ST segment seen in: Chronic stable angina, NSTEMI

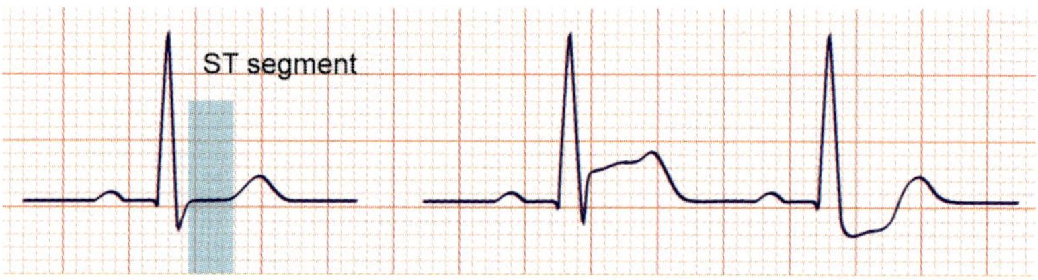

Normal ST elevation ST depression

9. T wave

(<5 mm in limb lead and <10 mm in chest lead)
Tall T wave (look in lead V_5) if:

- R wave >T wave its hyperacute T wave—MI
- T wave >R wave its tall-tented T wave—hyperkalaemia

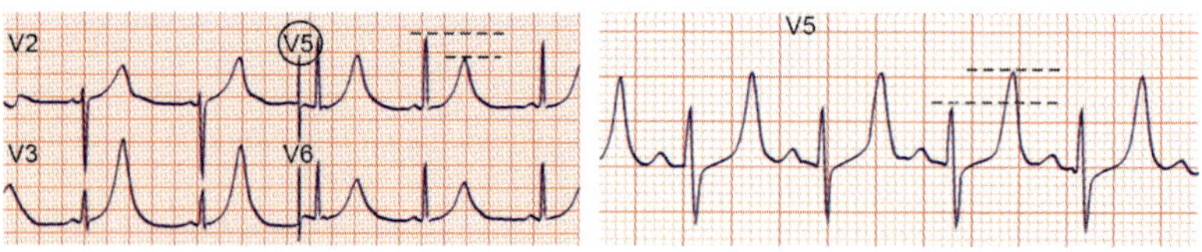

Hyperacute T wave Tall tented T wave

T wave inversion

- STEMI/NSTEMI
- Hypokalaemia

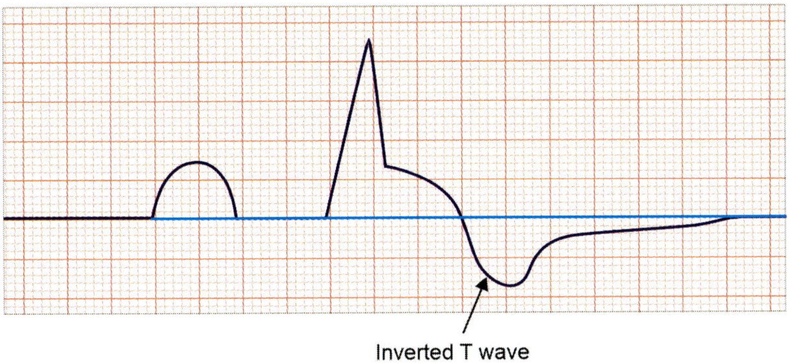

10. QT interval (0.33–0.43 sec)

- Normal QT interval is half of preceding RR interval.
- Corrected (Bazett formula) $QT_c = QT/\sqrt{RR}$

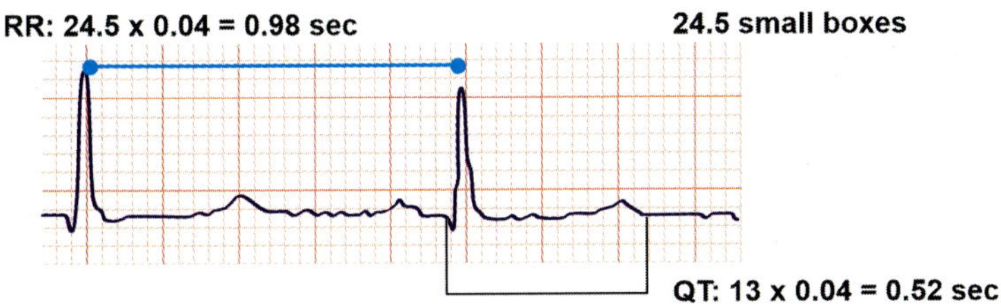

$$QTc = \frac{QT}{\sqrt{RR}} = \frac{0.52}{\sqrt{0.98}} = \frac{0.52}{0.989} = 0.525 \text{ or } 0.53 \text{ sec}$$

QT interval is inversely proportionate to serum calcium level

- Prolong QT interval QT_c >0.45 sec—hypocalcaemia, MI
- Narrow QT interval QT_c <0.33 sec—hypercalcaemia, digitalis effect

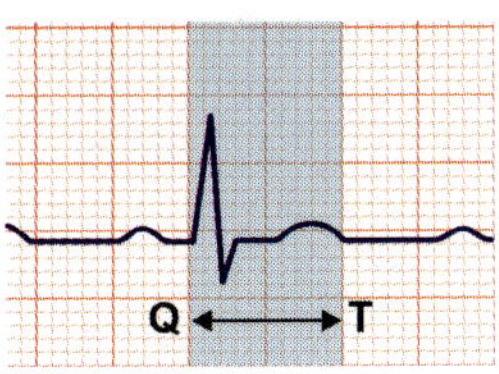

Normal QT interval

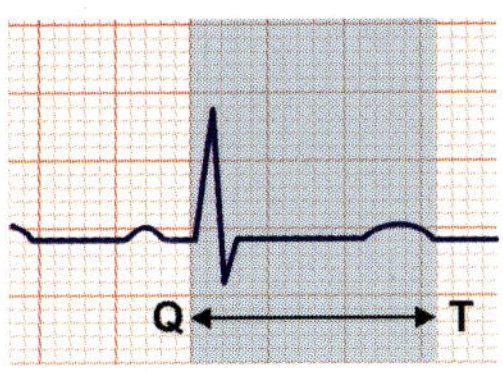

Long QT interval

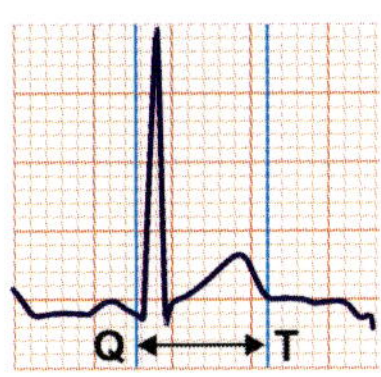

Short Q-wave

Sokolow-Lyon Criteria for Heart Chamber Hypertrophy

For LVH

- Add deepest S wave in V_1 or V_2 + tallest R wave in V_5 or V_6 If >35 mm s/o LVH
- LAD

For RVH

- RAD
- R wave in V_1 >7 mm
- R/S >1 in V_1 or <1 in V_5, V_6

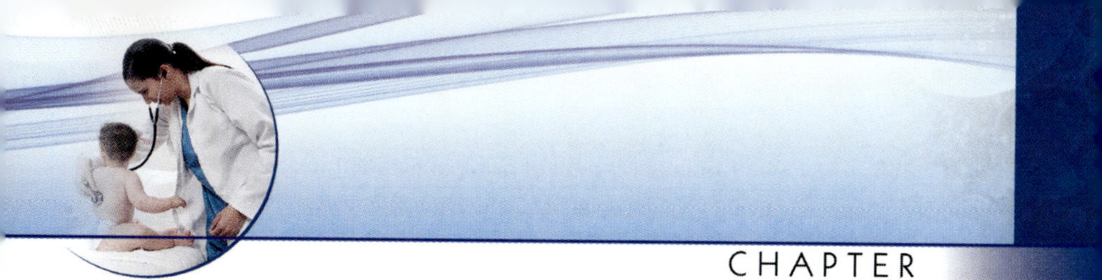

CHAPTER

24

Growth Charts

HEAD CIRCUMFERENCE FOR AGE (GIRLS)

Birth to 5 years (Z-scores)

World Health Organization

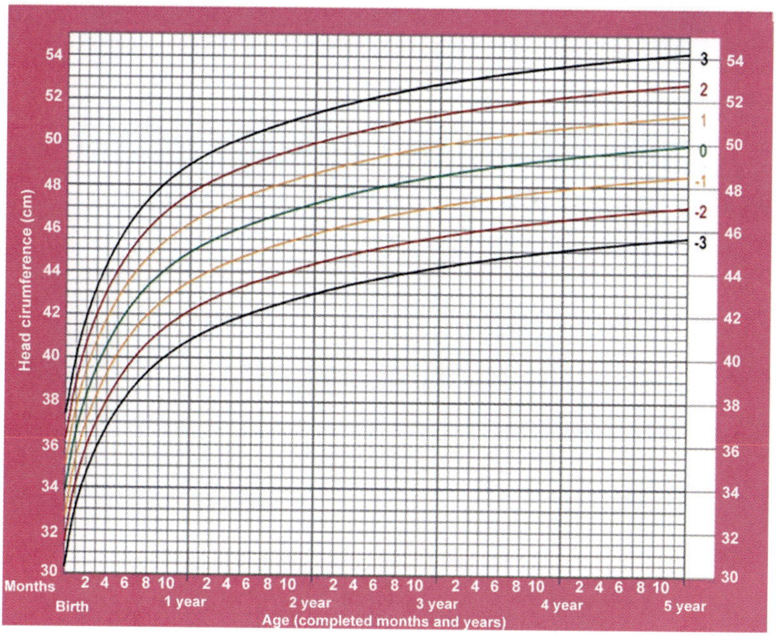

HEAD CIRCUMFERENCE FOR AGE (BOYS)

Birth to 5 years (Z-scores)

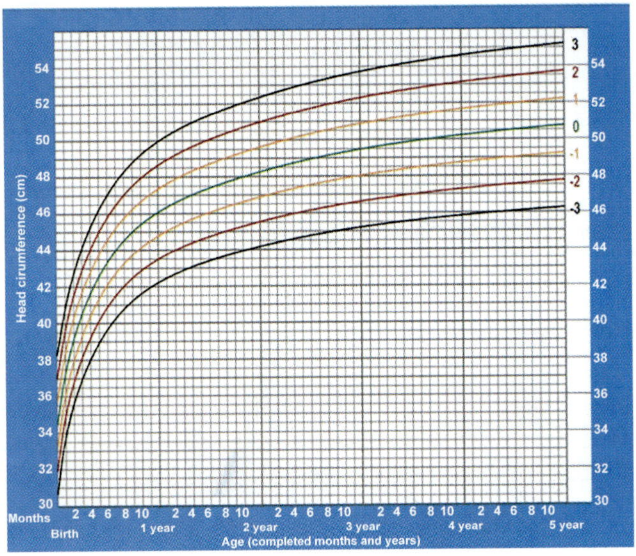

WEIGHT FOR AGE (GIRLS)

Birth to 5 years (z-scores)

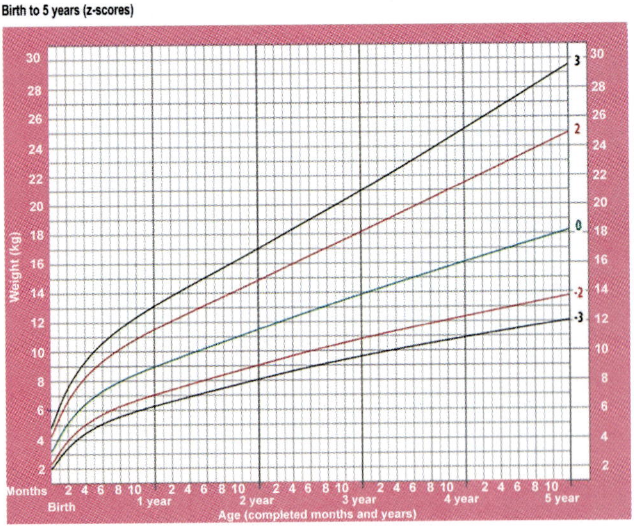

WEIGHT FOR AGE (BOYS)

Birth to 5 years (z-scores)

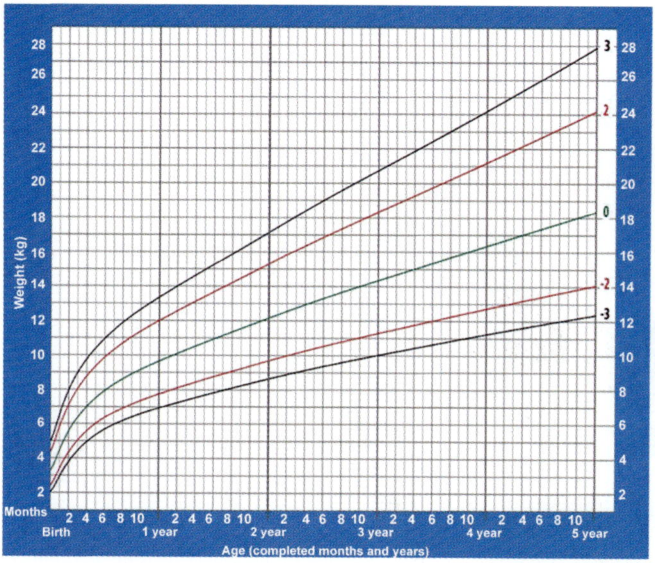

LENGTH/HEIGHT FOR AGE (GIRLS)

Birth to 5 years (z-scores)

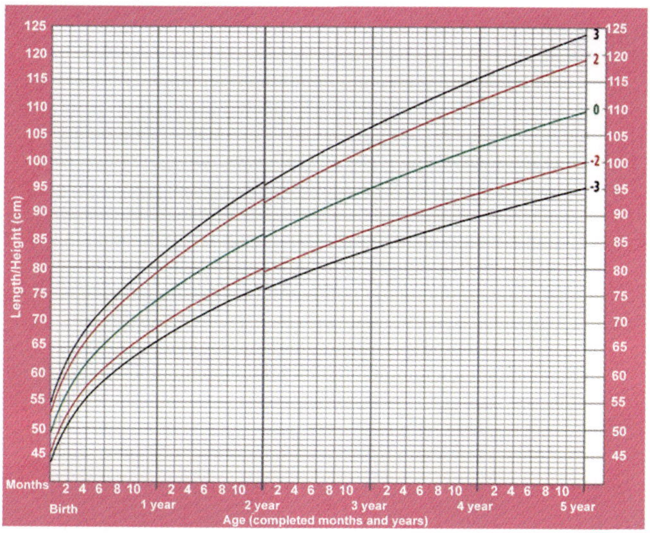

LENGTH/HEIGHT FOR AGE (BOYS)

Birth to 5 years (z-scores)

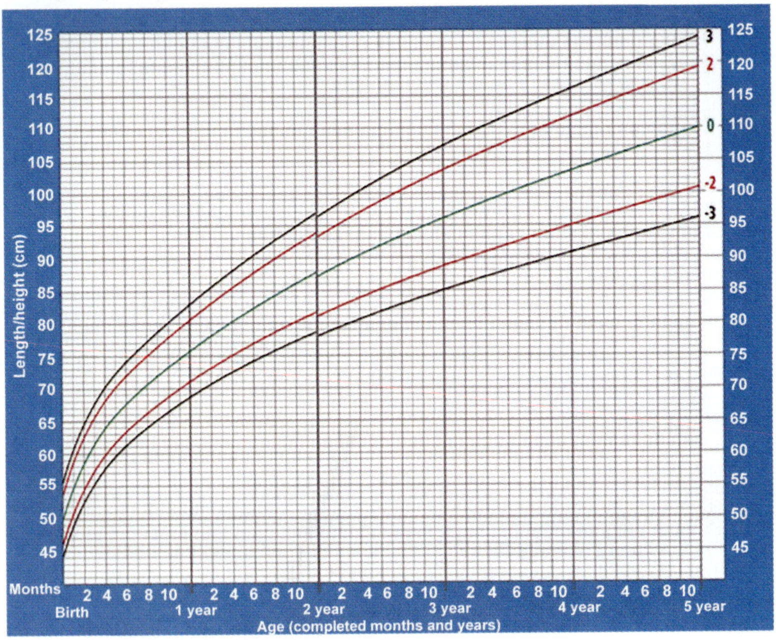

IAP BMI CHART FOR BOYS

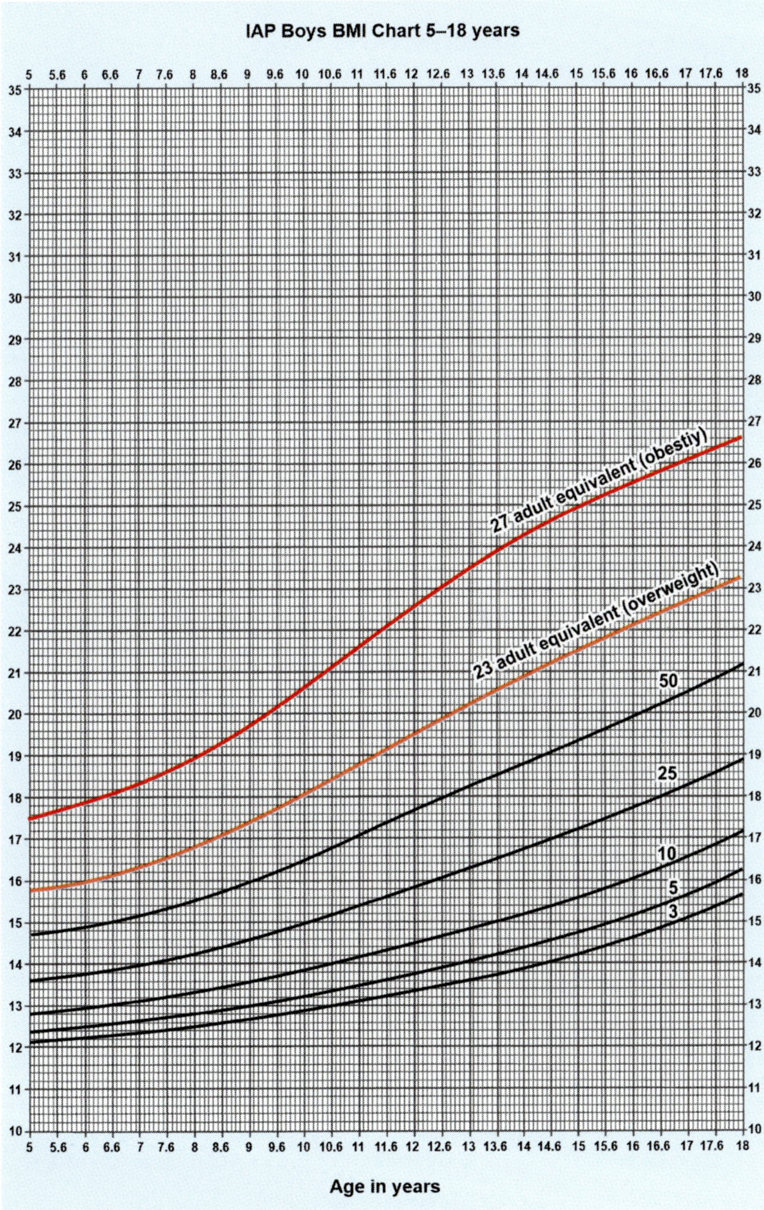

IAP BMI CHART FOR GIRLS

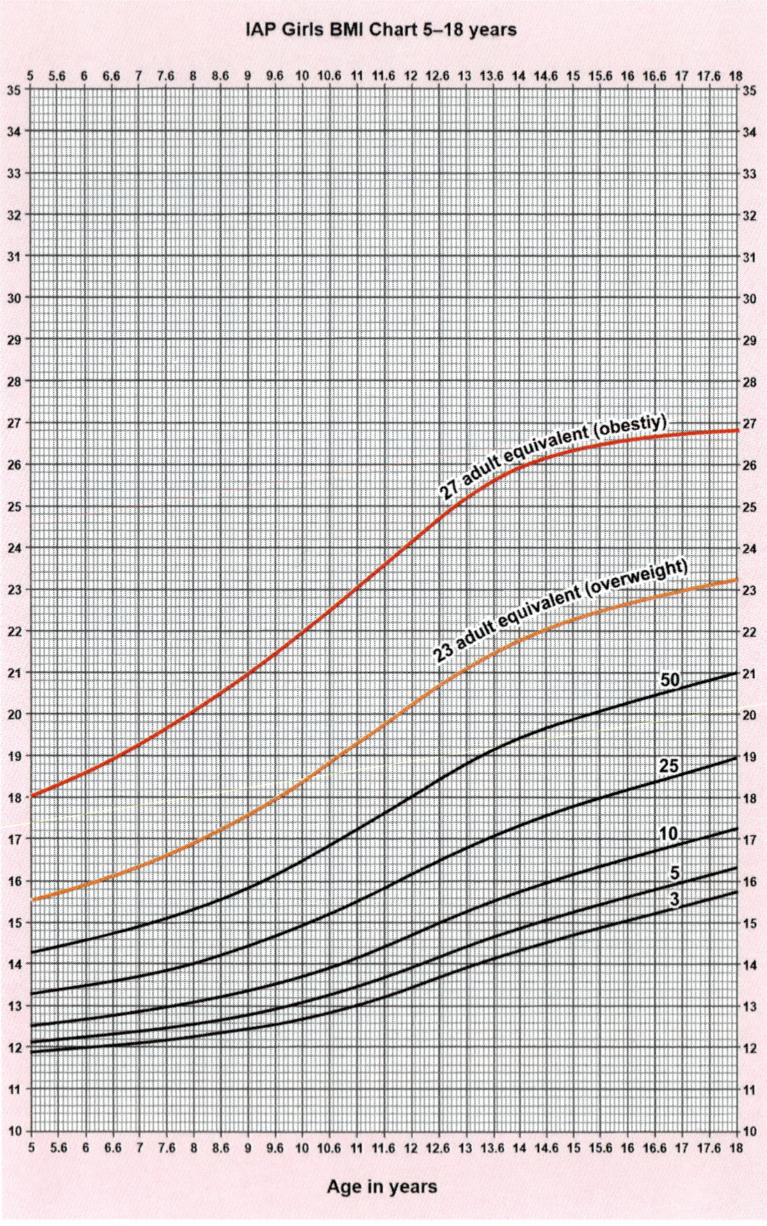

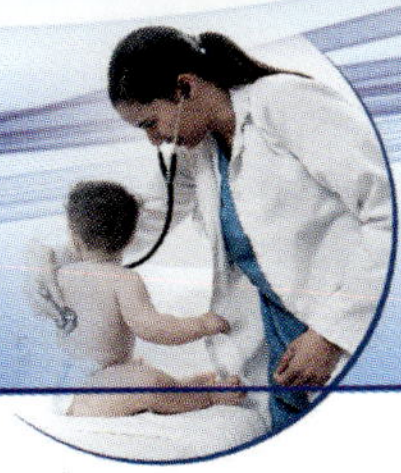

CHAPTER

25

Miscellaneous

NORMAL VALUES (Children)	
S. sodium	135–150 mEq/L
S. potassium	3.5–5.5 mEq/L
S. calcium	8.5–11 mg/dl
S. phosphorus	4.5–5.5 mg/dl
S. creatinine	0.3–1 mg/dl
BUN	5–18 mg/dl
S. uric acid	2–5.5 mg/dl
S. proteins	5.5–7.5 g/dl
S. albumin	3.5–5 g/dl
S. bilirubin	0.2–1 mg/dl
S. ALP	150–550 U/L
S. amylase	<100 U/ml >1000 is suggestive of pancreatitis
S. ammonia	<75 mmol/L
S. glucose	50–100 mg/dl
TSH	0.7–6.4 mIU/L
ALT (SGPT), AST (SGOT)	5–40 U/L
CPK	<200 U/L
ASO	<200 Todd units /ml
S. osmolality	275–295 mOsm/kg water
Total count (WBC)	4500–11000/mm^3
Platelet	1.5–4 lac/mm^3
Hb	11.5–14.5 g/dl or g%

ABG—NORMAL VALUES

pH	7.38–7.42
$PaCO_2$	35–45 mm Hg
PaO_2	80–100 mm Hg
HCO_3	22–28 mEq/L
O_2 saturation	95–100%

Note:

- Hyperventilation (increase RR) leads to CO_2 washout—Acidosis
- Normal value of CVP (central venous pressure)—6–10 cm of water

Urine output (ml/kg/hour)	Significance
>1	Normal
>4	Polyuria
<1	Oliguria
<0.5	Anuria

Urine protein:

- Normal—150 mg/day or
- <4 mg/m^2/hour

Nephrotic range proteinuria:

- >40 mg/m^2/hour or
- >1 g/m^2/day

WHO Cutoff of Anaemia

6 months–6 years	<11 g%
6 years–14 years	<12 g%
Adult male	<13 g%
Adult female	<12 g%

MNEMONICS TO REMEMBER

Aedes mosquito **DAC R yellow**	Dengue, chikungunya, yellow fever, Rift valley fever
Culex mosquito **West C JET**	West Nile fever, Japanese Encephalitis, Tularaemia
Anopheles mosquito MA	Malaria
Fanconi anaemia— **CASHH**	Chromosomal breakage, Aplastic anaemia, Short stature, Hyperpigmentation, Hypoplasia of thumb/radial side.
CCF treatment **(4Ds)**	Dilators-vasodilators Digoxin Diuretics Dopamine/dobutamine
Fever with rash **Very sick patient must take double tablets**	Day of appearance of rash in a febrile patient Varicella (day 1) Scarlet fever (day 2) Pox (day 3) Measles (day 4) Typhus (day 5) Dengue (day 6) Typhoid (day 7)
Intrauterine infection **STORCH**	Syphilis Toxoplasmosis Rubella CMV Herpes/HIV
Fallot's Triology—PRA Tetralogy—PRVO Pentalogy—PRVOA	 PRA—pulmonary stenosis, RVH, ASD PRVO—pulmonary stenosis, RVH, VSD Overriding of aorta PRVOA—TOF + ASD or PDA
Nephrotic syndrome complication **NEPHROTIC**	Na retention Edema Proteinuria Hypertension Thrombotic Infection Hypercoagulable state

Contd.

Congenital adrenal Hyperplasia (CAH)- CAH	**C**ongenital **A**mbiguous genitalia **H**yperpigmentation **H**yponatraemia **H**ypoglycaemia **H**ypotension
Autosomal dominant **DOMINANT**	**D**ystrophic Myotonia **O**steogenesis Imperfecta **M**arfan syndrome **I**ntermittent Porphyria **N**oonan syndrome, **A**chondroplasia **N**eurofibromatosis, **T**uberous sclerosis
Congenital Hypothyroidism- THYROID	**T**one (hypotonia) Tongue (large), **H**ypothermia/Hernia (umbilical), **H**oarse voice, **Y**ellow jaundice, **R**ough skin (coarse facies), **O**pen Fontanelle, **I**ntellectual disability, **D**evelopmental delay
Unconjugated Hyperbilirubinaemia GUN	**G**ilberts' syndrome, Crigler–Najjar syndrome
HODGKIN'S Lymphoma chemotherapy **COPP, ABVD Cycle**	COPP- **C**yclophosphamide, **O**ncovin (Vincristine), Procarbazine, **P**rednisolone ABVD: **A**driamycin (Doxorubicin), Bleomycin, **V**inblastine, **D**acarbazine
Acute lymphoblastic leukaemia (ALL) chemotherapy **VAAP** (Induction)	**V**incristine **A**driamycin **A**sparaginase-L **P**rednisolone
Treatment of hypoxic spell (TET spell) in TOF-BP OK	**B**icarbonate **P**ropranolol and Phenylepherine **O**xygen **K**etamine

Contd.

OP poisoning- **SLUDGE**	Small pupil **S**weating **S**alivation **L**acrimation **U**rination **D**efaecation **G**I upset **E**mesis
ALF (acute liver failure) **Causes:** 1. Acute hepatitis 2. Metabolic-**G2-WATCH** 3. Hepatotoxic drugs	**G2-WATCH** Glycogen storage disorder, Galctosaemia, Wilsons's disease, Alpha-1-antitrypsin deficiency, Tyrosinaemia, Cystic fibrosis, Hereditary fructose intolerance
WAGR syndrome	**W**ilms' tumour **A**niridia **G**ential abnormalities **M**ental retardation
VACTERL syndrome	**V**ertebral anomalies **A**norectal malformation **C**ardiac anomaly **T**racheoesophageal fistula **E**xomphalos (aka omphalocele) **R**enal anomalies **L**imb anomalies
Down syndrome **DOWNS** **CHILD** **HAS** **PROBLEM**	**D**ysplastic ears/dysplastic pelvis (seen on X-ray) **O**cciput is flat **W**idely spaced 1st and 2nd toes and a high-arched palate/weak/floppy baby **N**eck skin abundant **S**hort, broad hands with single palmar crease/slanting eyes/speckled iris (Brushfield's spots) • CHD, hypothyroidism, increased gap between 1st and 2nd toe, leukemia risk, duodenal atresia • Hirschsprung disease, Alzheimer disease, short neck • Protruding tongue, round flat face, oblique eye fissure, Brushfield spot, law nasal bridge, epicanthal fold, MR

Contd.

Life-threatening attack of Asthma **CHEST**	**C**yanosis/confusion/coma **H**ypotension **E**xhaustion **S**ilent chest **T**hreatening PEFR <33% predicted in those above 5 years old
Chronic diarrhoea **5 Cs**	**C**rohn's disease **C**olitis ulcerative **C**ystic fibrosis **C**eliac disease **C**ow's milk intolerance
Brain tumours/SOL **BAN HENS**	**B**lurred vision **A**taxia (clumsiness) **N**ystagmus **H**eadache **E**ndocrine dysfunction **N**ausea and vomiting **S**quint (6th nerve palsy)
Celiac disease not to eat- **BROB**	**W**heat **O**at **R**ye **B**arley
Hypothalamus controls **SEAT**	**S**ex, **S**leep **E**ndocrine, **E**motions **A**utonomic NS, **A**ppetite **T**hirst, **T**emperature

Some Triads to Remember

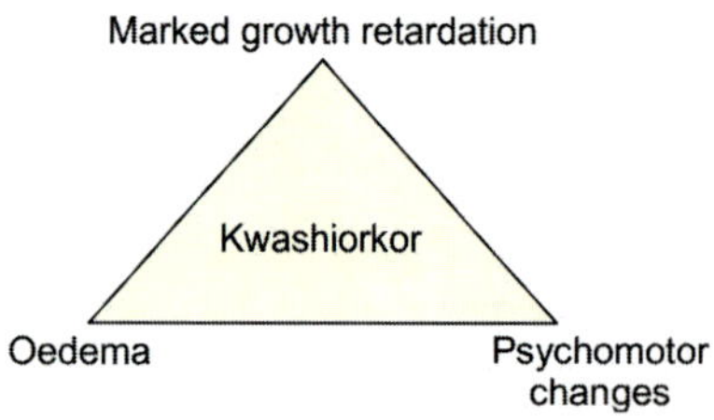

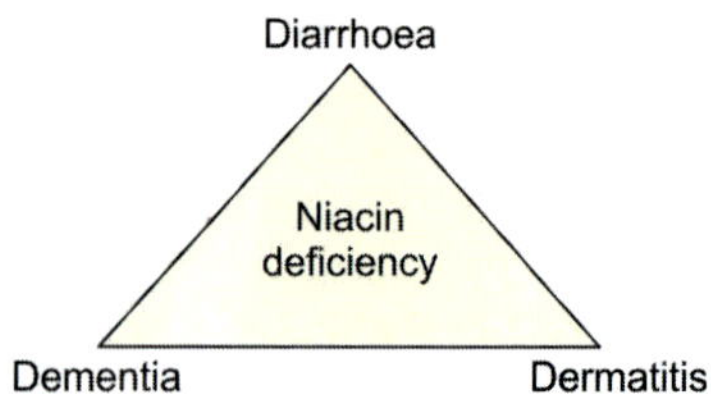

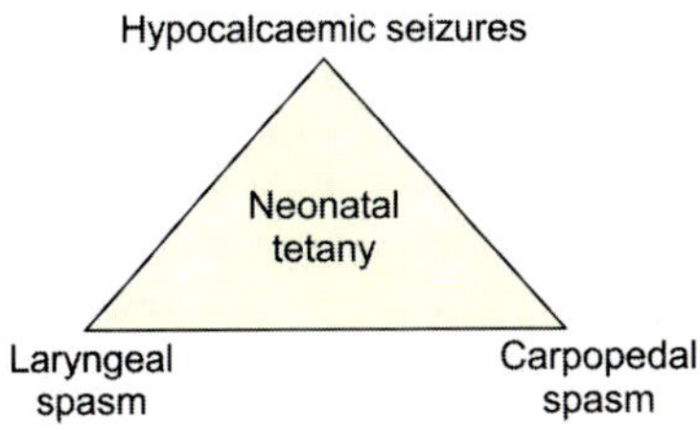
Hypocalcaemic seizures
Neonatal tetany
Laryngeal spasm
Carpopedal spasm

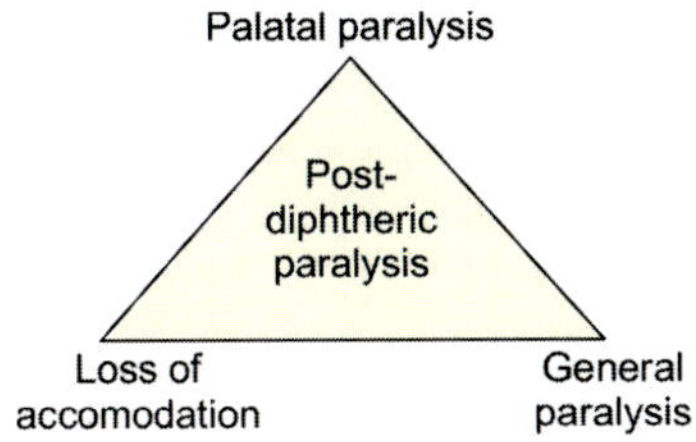
Palatal paralysis
Post-diphtheric paralysis
Loss of accomodation
General paralysis

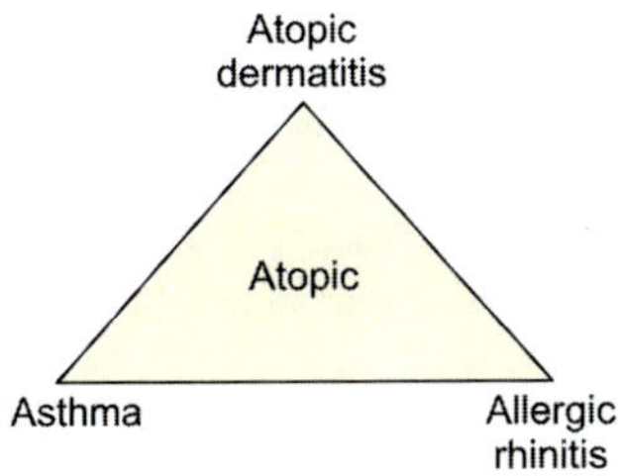
Atopic dermatitis
Atopic
Asthma
Allergic rhinitis

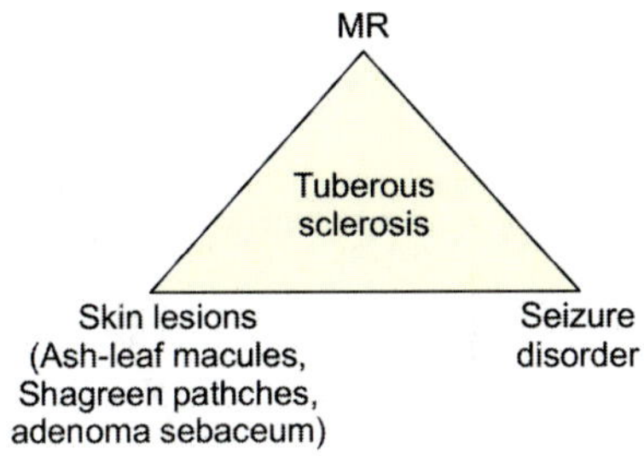
MR
Tuberous sclerosis
Skin lesions (Ash-leaf macules, Shagreen pathches, adenoma sebaceum)
Seizure disorder

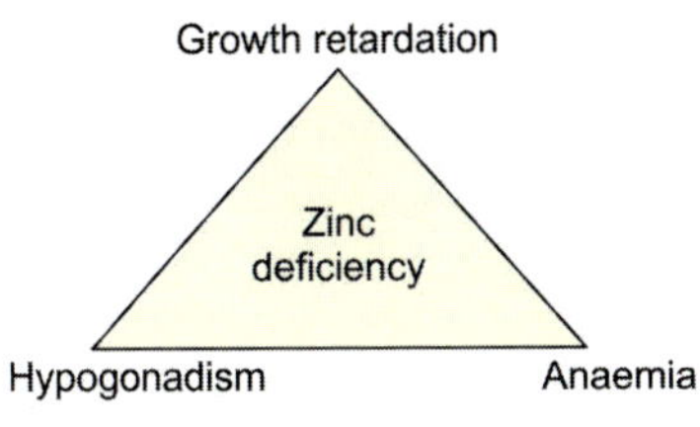
Growth retardation
Zinc deficiency
Hypogonadism
Anaemia

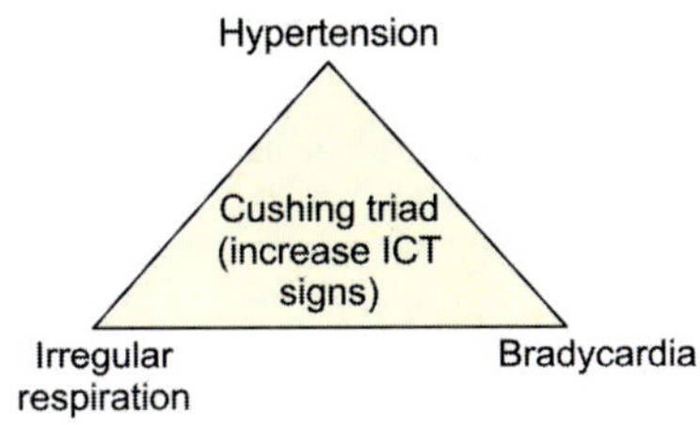
Hypertension
Cushing triad (increase ICT signs)
Irregular respiration
Bradycardia

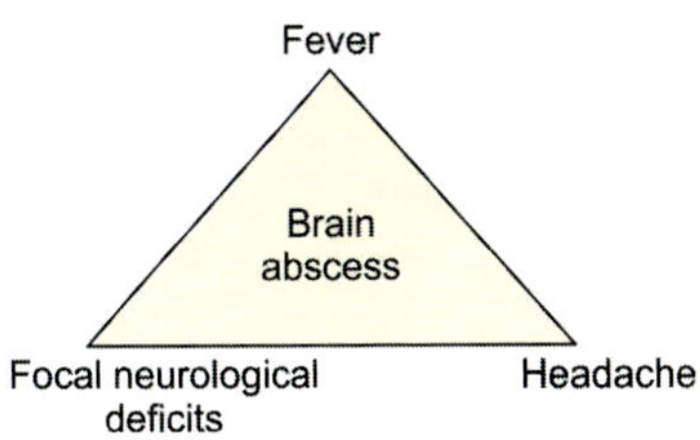
Fever
Brain abscess
Focal neurological deficits
Headache

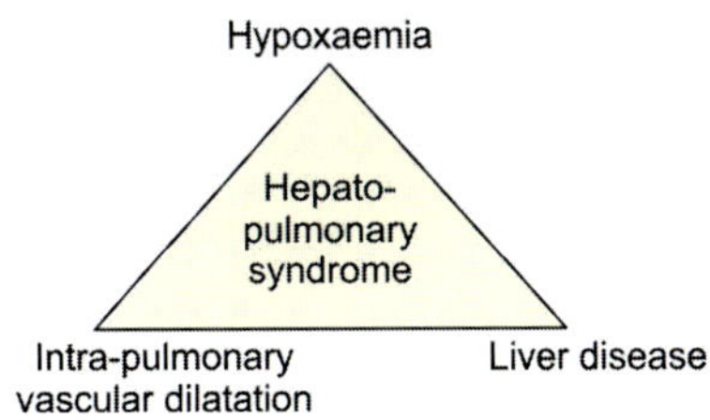
Hypoxaemia
Hepato-pulmonary syndrome
Intra-pulmonary vascular dilatation
Liver disease

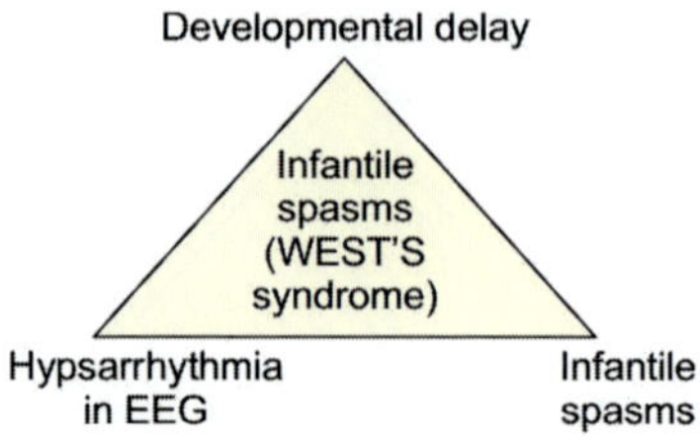
Developmental delay
Infantile spasms (WEST'S syndrome)
Hypsarrhythmia in EEG
Infantile spasms

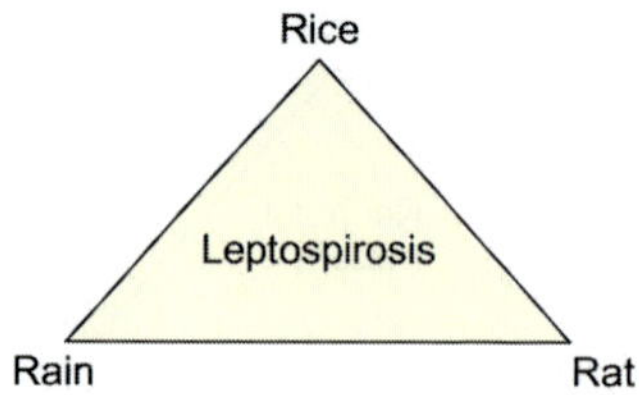
Rice
Leptospirosis
Rain
Rat

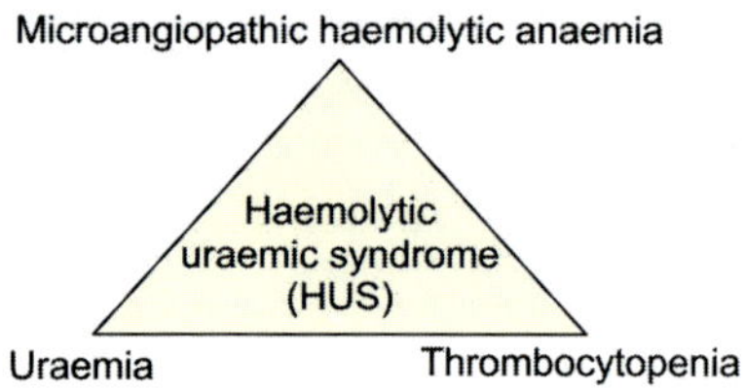
Microangiopathic haemolytic anaemia
Haemolytic uraemic syndrome (HUS)
Uraemia
Thrombocytopenia

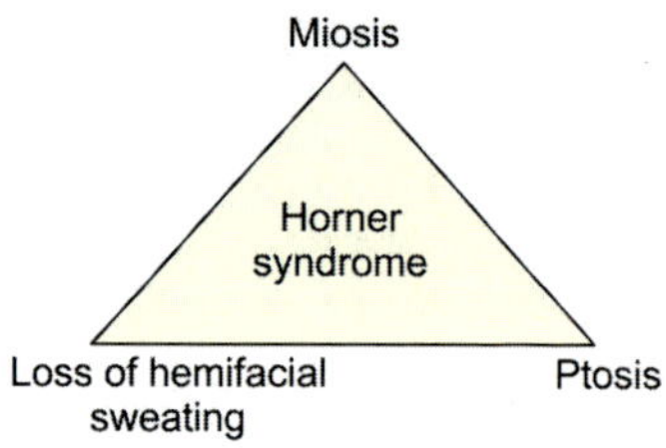
Miosis
Horner syndrome
Loss of hemifacial sweating
Ptosis

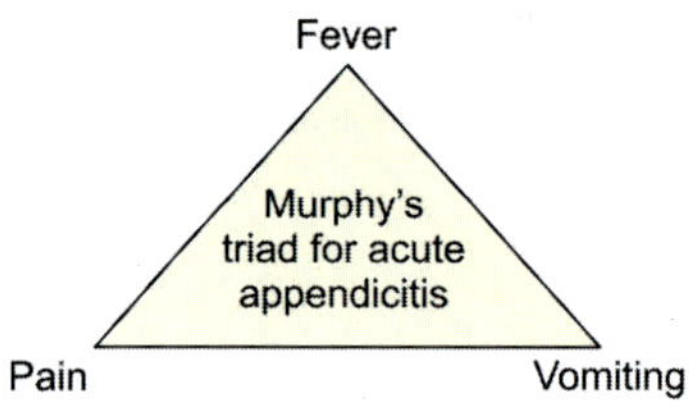
Fever
Murphy's triad for acute appendicitis
Pain
Vomiting

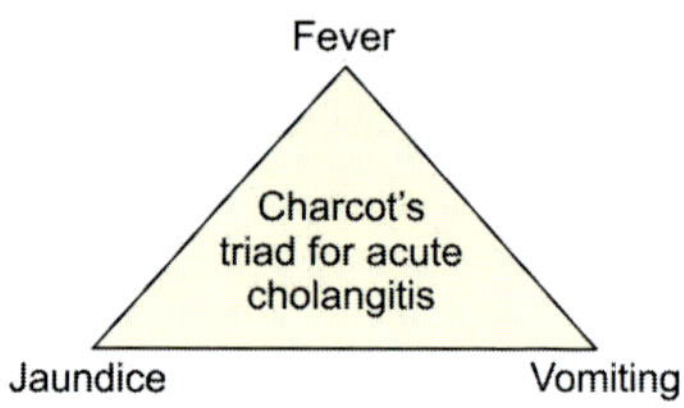
Fever
Charcot's triad for acute cholangitis
Jaundice
Vomiting

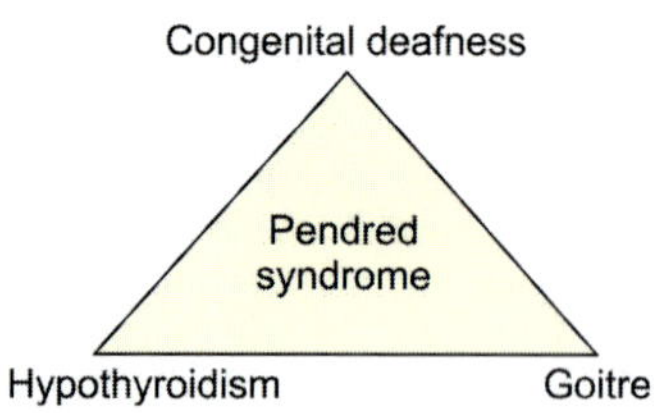
Congenital deafness
Pendred syndrome
Hypothyroidism
Goitre

Index

2-deoxy glucose 100
2% Ketoconazole shampoo 185
2nd left ICS pulsation 106
2nd sexual character 77
2024 theme 177

A

Abdominal 136
  aortic aneurysm 121
Abducents (VI) 126
ABG 262
AC: Air conduction 128
ACE inhibitor 188
Acetaminophen 204
Acetyl salicylic acid 181
Acrodermatitis enteropathica 63
Acuity of vision 125
Acute
  encephalitis syndrome (AES) 143
  flaccid paralysis 143
  lymphoblastic leukaemia (ALL) 264
  respiratory infection (ARI) control programme 90
Acyanotic CHD 105
Acyclovir 185
Addison's disease 115
Adenoid 64
Adenosine 198
Addison's disease 115
ADHD (attention deficit hyperactive disorder) 12
Adjuvant 20
Adolescent 11
Adrenaline/epinephrine 198
Advanced bone age 47
Advanced US/LS 51
Aedes mosquito 263
Aegophony 85
AETCOM 205
AGA 159
Air conduction 128
Albendazole (zentel, bendex) 185
ALF (acute liver failure) 265
Alfred DE Musset's sign 114
ALT (SGPT) 261
ALT (SGPT), AST (SGOT) 261
Amikacin 182
Amiodarone 198
Amitriptyline 203
Amlodipine 188
Amoxicillin 182
Amphetamines 204
Amphotericin B (Liposomal) 185
Amyl nitrite 204
Anaemia (megaloblastic) 62
Anal 136
Analgesic 181
Angular stomatitis 115
Aniridia 69
Ankle jerk 131
Anopheles mosquito 263
Anophthalamia 70
Anotia 69
Antacids 182
Anterior fontanelle 67
Anterolateral spinothalamic tract column sensation 137
Anthropometry 44
Antibiotics 18, 182
Antibody tests 98
Anti-diarrhoeal 190
Anti-epileptics 187
Antifungal 185
Antihistaminics 186
Antihypertensive 188
Anti-mongoloid slant 65
Antiparasitic 185
Antipyretic 181
Antiretroviral therapy—ART 193
Antisnake venom 203
Antispasmodic 187
Antiviral 185
Ant wall MI 252
Anuria 262
Aortic area 108
Apex beat 106
APGAR score 170
Apical impulse 109
Apraxia 138
AP view 233
  wrist X-ray 240
ARBs 188
ARC 22
Areas of lung 83
Arm span 52
Arsenic 204
Artemisinin combination therapy (ACT) 192
ART regimen in children 193
ASO 261
Aspart 199
Aspirin 181
Assessment of asthma severity 90
Assessment of intelligence 11
AST (SGOT) 261
Asymmetrical TNR 171
Ataxic gait 139
Atomoxetin 190
Atomoxetin (Axepta) 190
Atrial
  depolarization 241
  repolarization 245
Atrioventricular node 241
Atropine 198, 203
  /belladona poisoning 204
  pralidoxime 204
Attention deficit hyperactive disorder 12
Attitude 130
  ethics and communication Module (AETCOM) 205
Augmented leads 242
Aural atresia 69
Auscultation 89
Autism 12
Auto-antibodies 145
Automated external defibrillator (AED) 198
Autonomic nervous system 140
  parasympathetic 140
  sympathetic 140
Autosomal dominant 264
AV node 241
Avomin 188
Axepta 190
Axillary hairs 77
Axis calculation 248
Azithromycin 184

B

Baby-friendly hospital initiative (BFHI) 174
Bacillus-Calmette Guerin (BCG) vaccine 21
Baclofen 190
Bag and mask 160
  ventilation 163
BAL 204
Balanced diet 16
Barlow manoeuvre 151
Bayley's scale of infant development 11
BCG scar 2
Bell's phenomenon 127
Benzodiazepines 204
Beta blocker 189
Bharat biotech 30
Biceps jerk 131
Bidextrous grasp 7
Bilious vomiting 121
Binocular vision 9
BIOVAC-A 27

Biphasic P wave 249
Birth history 1
Bisyllables 8
Bitot's spot 63
Blood group incomptability 179
Blood pressure 40
  BP in children 41
  korotkoff sounds 41
  respiratory rate 41
  tachypnoea 42
Blood tranfusion 202
Blue
  light phototherapy 179
  sclera 68
Bobbling of head 92
Body
  mass index (BMI) 51
  surface area (BSA) 53
Bone
  age 47
  age estimation 77
  conduction 128
  marrow aspiration 227
  marrow needles 228
  marrow transplant 21
Bossing of skull 50
BP
  centile char 40
  in Children 41
Brainstem 125
Brain tumours 266
Breast
  development 75
  engorgement 173
Breastfeeding: benefits 175
Breath holding spells 12
Breathing 161
Bronchophony 85
Broncho-vascular marking 235
Brucellosis 38
Brudzinski's leg sign 140
Bruit 120
Brush field 70
Bruxism 12
Budesonide 91
Bulbar conjunctiva 54
Bulk 130
Bullae 78
BUN 261
Bundle of His 241
Burn 200
Burrows 79
Buttoning/unbuttoning 7

C

Calcium 63
  channel blocker 188
  Gluconate (10%) 198
Calculation of drops/minute 194
Calculation of maintenance IV fluids 194
Calorie requirement 13
Canine 10
Captopril 188
Caput succedaneum 177
Carbamazepine 187
Carbon
  dioxide detector 167
  monoxide 204
Cardiomegaly 234
Cardiopulmonary failure 195
Cardio-thoracic ratio 234
Cardiovascular system 104
Carnitine 190
Carotid-pulsation 106
Carpopedal spasms 63
Cartridge based nucleic acid test 93
Case sheet 1
Casting/object permanence (constancy) 7
Cavity in right upper lobe in pulmonary TB 236
CCF treatment 263
CD4 22
Cefaclor 182
Cefixime 183
Cefoperazone with sulbactum sodium 182
Cefotaxime 182
Cefpodoxime 183
Ceftazidime 183
Ceftriaxone 183
Celiac disease 266
Cellular immune response 20
Central
  cyanosis 113
  nervous system 123
  venous pressure 262
Cephalexin (sporidex) 183
Cephalhaematoma 177
Cephalocaudal 6
Cephalosporin antibiotics 182
Cerebellar
  dysfunction 141
  signs 139
Cerebral palsy 142
Cervarix 28
Cervavac 28
Cervical
  cancer 28
  lymph nodes 57, 61
Cetrizine 186
Charactor of murmurs 110
Check list 209
Cheilitis 115
Chemotherapy 21, 264
Chest 233
  circumference (CC) 51
  compression (CC) 165
  leads 242
Cheyne–Stokes 42
Child
  labour 221
  neglect 221
  nutrition programs 214
Chloroquine 192
  resistant 192
Chlorpromazine 204
Cholera vaccine 27
Chronic
  abdominal pain 122
  diarrhoea 266
Chronological age (CA) 47
Ciprofloxacin 183
Circulation and drugs 161
Clasp knife 136
Classification of rickets 154
Clinodactyly 4
Clobazam 188
Clonus, 132
Clotrimazole 185
Cloxacillin 183
Clubbing 55, 60
Club foot 154
  talipes equinovarus 152
CMV (continuous mandatory ventilation) 202
CO_2 monitor 160
Cobra 203
Cog-wheel 136
Coin test 85
Cold
  chain 21
  intolerance 63
Colistin 184
Collapse 234
Colostrum 176
Colour blindness 145
Combination vaccine 34
Complete protein 16
Complete urinary examination 219
Computed tomography scan 144
Confidentiality 212, 221
Confrontation method 125
Congenital
  adrenal hyperplasia 77, 264
  diaphragmatic hernia 234
  hypothyroidism 264
  talipus equino varus (club foot) CTEV 153
Conjugated vaccines 25
Constipation 122
Constitutional growth delay 47
Continuous
  fever 38
  mandatory ventilation 202
  positive airway pressure 202
Cooked rice 14
Coordination of movements 130
Corbevax 31

Cord
  clamping 170
  milking 170
Corneal reflex 136
Coronary dilatation 148
Coronavirus
  disease 94
  vaccines 30
Cortical sensation 137
Costochondral beading 155
Costophrenic angles 235
Co-trimoxazole (septran) 183
Counselling a parents 206
Covaxin 30
Cover uncover test 71, 127
COVID-19 94
Covishield 30
COVOVAX 30
Cow milk protein allergy 218
Cow's milk 176
CPAP (continuous positive airway pressure) 202
CPK 261
Cradle cap 173
Cranial nerves 125
Craniosacral outflow 140
Craniotabes 50
Crawling 9
Crawls 6
Creatinine kinase 146
Cremasteric reflex 136
Crepitation 85
Cretinoid 64, 66
Crigler–Najjar syndrome 264
Crude touch 137
Cruising 6
Cruising around furniture 6
Cryoprecipitate 202
CSF Values 225
CT
  abdomen/KUB 221
  severity score 100
Cubitus
  valgus 153
  varus 153
Culex mosquito 26, 263
Cushingnoid 64
Cyanide 204
Cyanosis 55, 60
Cyanotic CHD 105
Cyproheptadine 190
Cystic hygroma 68

D

DAC R yellow 263
Datura poisoning 203
Decubitus films 233
Deep reflexes 131
Deferiprone (Kelfer) 189
Defibrillation 198
Degludec 199
Delayed
  bone age 47
  closure of anterior fontanelle 68
  cord clamping 170
  dentition 10
  puberty 77
Dengue 38
Denver development screening test 11
Depth of respiration 42
Dermatomes 138
Desferoxamine 189, 204
Desmopressin (DDAVP) 189
Detemir 199
Developmental dysplasia of the hip (DDH) 151
Development history 6
Development observation chart 11
Deworming 218
Dexamethasone 186
Dextromethorphan 189
Diabetic ketoacidosis 42, 200
Diagnostic criteria for diabetes mellitus type 1 199
Diagnostic criteria MIS-C 102
Diaphragmatic hernia 167
Diazepam 187, 199, 204
Diclofenac 181
Dicyclomine 187
Didanosine (DDI) 193
Di-ethyl-carbamazine citrate (DEC) 186
Dietic history 13
Diet rich in iron 218
Digitalis effect 253
Digoxin 189, 204
Digoxin specific antibody fragments 204
Diphtheria toxoid 23
Dipping method 117
Disorders of sex development (DSD) 77
Disproportionate short stature 47
Dissociation 6
Distal weakness 123
  muscle 148
Distant vision 125
DMARDs 147
DMSA scan (dimercaptosuccinic acid scan) 221
DNA plasmid-based COVID-19 vaccine 31
DNS 194
Dobutamine 198
Doll's eye phenomenon 70
Domestic rodent 29
Domperidone (Domstal) 188
Domstal 188
Dopamine 198
Dorsal column sensation 137
Dorsum of tongue 54
DOTS 191
Downe score 173
Down syndrome 72, 265
Doxycycline 184
DPT vaccine 23
Draw a MAN test 11
Drugs
  contraindicated during breast feeding 176
  /formulary 181
Drumstick appearance 55
Dry
  beriberi 62, 64
  by day 8
  by night 8
  powder inhaler (DPI) 231
DTPA scan (diethylenetriamine pentaacetate scan) 221
Duchenne muscular dystrophy 145
Dullness of renal angle 119
Dysarthria 139
Dyscalculia 12
Dysdiadochokinesia 139
Dyslexia 12
Dysmenorrhoea 181
Dysmetria 139
Dyspnoea 87
Dyssynergia 139

E

Ear examination 82
Early
  closure of anterior fontanelle 68
  neonatal period 158
Ebstein's anomaly 105
Ecchymosis 78
ECG 241
  paper 244
Ectropion 68
EDT 204
EDTA 204
Efavirenz (EFV) 193
Eisenmenger syndrome 105
EKG 241
  monitor 163
ELBW 159
Electrical conduction of heart 241
Electrocardiogram 241
Electrodes 242
Electroencephalogram (EEG) 144
Electronic vaccine intelligence network (eVIN) 34
Embryo 10
Emergency drugs 198
Emergency paediatrics 195
Emeset 188
EMG 146
Enalapril 188
Enanthem 78

Encopresis 12
Endemic 103
Endotracheal
intubation 167
tubes 160
Energy 16
Enophthalamos 70
Enough sachets 190
Enterohepatic circulation 178
Entropion 68
Enuresis 12
Epidemic 103
Epigastric pulsation 106
Epigastrium 115
Epiglottitis 25
Epinephrine 168
Epstein pearl 173
palatal/prepucial 173
Equine RIG 30
Erosion 78
Erythema
marginatum 149
toxicum 173
Erythromycin 182
Essential
amino acid 15
fatty acids 15
tremors 139
Ethambutal (E) 191
Ethanol 204
Ethylene glycol 204
Examination
axillary lymph node 57
epitrochlear lymph node 58
Exanthem 78
Exchange transfusion 179
Exotropia 71
Expected weight 13, 44
Expressionless face 64, 66
Extended spectrum beta -lactamase producing microorganisms 184
External markers of kidney disease 220
Extinction 138
Extrapyramidal 136
Extrapyramidal dysfunction 141
Exudates ascites fluid 121
Exudates pleuraL effusion 92

F

Facial (VII) nerve 127
Facies associated with diseases 64
Fallot's tetralogy 263
Familial 47
short stature 47
Family
history 37
income per month (in Rs) 36
Fanconi anaemia 263
Fasciculation/tremors 133
Fast acting (insulin analogue) 199
Fasting blood glucose FBS 199
Fat 16
Febrile seizure prophylaxis 188
Feeding toddler 16
Ferrous sulfate 218
Fever 38
graph 39
of unknown origin 39
with rash 263
Fexofenadine 186
FiO_2: Fractional oxygen 202
Field of vision 125
Fine motors 7
Fissure 78
Flanks 116
Flapping tremors 117
Fluconazole 185
Fluid thrill 119
Flumazenil 204
Fluoride 63, 65
Fluoroquinolones 183
antibiotics 183
Fluticasone 91
Foetus 10
Folic acid 62
Follow my finger test 127
Food mix 17
Forced
expiratory volume (FEV_1) 88
vital capacity (FVC) 88
Foreign body
aspiration 237
suspected 202
Foremilk 177
Formoterol 91
Fractional
doses of IPV (fIPV) 23
oxygen 202
Fragility test 114
Fresh frozen plasma 202
Friction test 85
Frisium 188
Fructo/galacto/oligosaccharides 61
Fukuda step test 128
Functional age 9
Functional residual capacity 88
Fundus 125
Furosemide 189
Future vaccines 34
cancer vaccine 34
dengue virus vaccine 34
HCV vaccine 34
HIV vaccine 34
malaria vaccine 34

G

Gag reflex 128
Gait 135, 143
ataxic/drunken gait 143
circumduction gait 143
diplegic/spastic gait 143
high stepping gait 143
parkinsonian gait 143
waddling gait 143
GARDASIL-9 28
Gargoylism 64
Gastrointestinal system 115
Gemcovac 19
General examination 54
Generalized L/N 58
Genitourinary tract 219
Gentamicin inj 182
Genu-valgum 4
Genu valgus/knock knees 150
Genu varus 151
Gilberts' syndrome 264
Gingivitis 115
Glargine 199
Glassgow coma scale (GCS) 142
Global development delay 9
Glosso-pharyngeal (IX) 128
Glycemic index 213
Grade the power 133
Grading of
ascites 120
DTR 132
hepatomegaly 117
murmur 112
parasternal heave 112
splenomegaly 118
Graphaesthesia 138
Great vessels 235
Grimace 170
Gross
motor 6
vision 125
Grower sign 146
Growth
charts 255
spurt 77
Grunt 86
Gynecomastia 77, 117

H

Haemangioma 120
Haematemesis 121
Haematochezia 120
Haemoglobin A1c 200
Haemogram 217
Haemolytic 64, 66
Haemophilia 145
Haemoptysis 121
Hairs 3
Hamate 77
Hand and foot desquamation 148
Handedness 7
Hand washing steps 216
Harrison's sulcus 155
Havrix 27
Hb 261

HBsAg positive 24, 25
HCO_3 262
HDN 170
Head circumference 49
  for age (boys) 256
  for age (girls) 255
Head-to-toe examination 3
Hearing 8
Heart
  chamber hypertrophy 254
  murmurs 109
  sounds 109
  variation 109
Heaving apex beat 106
Height 45
  age 47
  for-age 48
Heimlich manoeuvre 202
Hemophilus influenzae type B 25
Henoch-Schönlein purpura (HSP) 147
Heparin 204
Hepatitis-
  A vaccine 27
  B 24
  B vaccine 24
Hepatoma 120
Hepatosplenomegaly 118
Herd immunity 22
Hernial orifices 117
Heterologous booster 31
Hg lead 204
Hib conjugated vaccines 25
High-arched palate 66, 68
Higher mental function 124
  B/L vocal cord palsy 125
  broca speech 124
  bulbar palsy 125
  cerebellar lesion 125
  delirium 124
  emotional lability 124
  hallucination 124
  illusion 124
  intelligence 124
  level of consciousness—drowsy 124
  memory 124
  obtundation 124
  orientation to time/place/person 125
  pseudobulbar palsy 125
  speech 124
  stupor 124
  U/L vocal cord palsy 125
  Wernicke speech 125
High risk area for resistance 192
Hind milk 177
History of presenting illness 1
HIV treatment 193
Hodgkin's lymphoma 264
Holliday and Segar formula 13
Hooking method 117
Ht for age 48
Human
  diploid cell vaccine 29
  milk vs cow's milk 176
  papillomavirus (HPV) vaccines 28
Hydrocortisone 187
Hydroxyzine (atarax) 186
Hymenal tags 173
Hyoscine (buscopan) 187
hyperbilirubinaemia 179
Hyperdynamic apex beat 106
Hyperinflated lung 234
Hyperinflation 234
Hyperkalaemia 252
Hyperplasia 77, 264
Hyperpnoea 86
Hyperpyrexia 38
Hypertelorism 65, 66
Hypertension 40
Hypertonia 136
Hypertrophic pulmonary osteoarthopathy 55
Hypertrophic pulmonary osteoarthopathy (HPOA) 55
Hyperventilation 262
Hypervitaminosis A 64
Hypogamma-globulinaemia 22
Hypogastrium 116
Hypoglossal (XII) 129
Hypogonadism 63
Hypokalaemia 252
Hypopnoea 86
Hypotelorism 66, 67
Hypothalamus 266
Hypotonia 136
Hypovolemic shock 194
Hypoxic-ischemic encephalopthy 179
Hypoxic spell (TET spell) 264

I

IAP
  BMI chart for boys 259
  BMI chart for girls 260
  classifiaction of malnutrition 44
  immunization time table 32
Ibuprofen 181
ICS: Inhaled corticosteroids 91
Icterus 54, 60
I/D (intradermal) 21
Illiterate "E" chart 9
Imipenem/cilastatin 184
Imipramine 190, 203
Immune system 18
Immunization 18
Immunoglobulin 21
IMNCI guidelines 210
IMV: intermittent mandatory ventilation 202
  synchronized 202
Inactivated influenza vaccines 24
Incisors 10
Incovacc 30
Incubation period 94
Indian Council of Medical Research (ICMR 30
Indicators of child health 214
Indinavir, ritonavir 193
Infancy 11, 159
Infant feeding tube 225
Infantile US/LS 51
Infantometer 45
Infective
  endocarditis 113, 114
  period 94
Inferior wall MI 252
Influenza vaccines 24
Informed consent 211
Inhaled corticosteroids 91
Inner
  canthal distance 65
  papillary distance 65
Innocent murmers 112
Inspiratory/expiratory film 234
Inspiratory
  film 234
  time 202
Insulin 199
  injection 232
Inteellectual disability 11
Intelligence quotient 11
Intensified mission indradhanush 34
Intermediate acting 199
Intermittent fever 38
  quartan 38
  quotidian 38
  tertian 38
Intermittent mandatory ventilation 202
Intestinal
  obstruction 238
  perforation 238
Intraosseous cannulation 168
Intratracheal dose 168
Intrauterine infection 263
Intubation 160
Intussusceptions 27
Inverted P wave 249
Involuntary movements 133
  athetoid movement 143
  ballismus 143
  TICS 143
  tremors 143
Involuntary movements 143
Iodine 63, 65
IPV 22
IQ 11

IRIS coloboma 70
Iron 63, 65, 204
  chelating agent 189
  deficiency anaemia 217
  panel 217
Ishihara test 125
Isolation 103
Isolyte-p 194
Isoniazid 191, 204
Isophane (NPH) 199
IV drug abusers 113
Ivermectin 186
IV fluids 194
IVIG 148

J

Jaeger's chart 125
Japanese B encephalitis vaccine 26
Jaundice in the newborns 178
Jaw jerk 126, 132
JEEV 26
Jendrassik manoeuvre , 132
JENVAC 26
Jet injector 31
Joint sense 137
Jones criteria for rheumatic fever 149
Jugular venous pressure (JVP) 3
Juvenile
  idiopathic arthritis 146
  rheumatoid arthritis 146
Rheumatoid arthritis or JIA 145
JVP measurement 104

K

Kangaroo mother care 177
Karyotype 71
Kawasaki disease 148
Kayexalate 190
Keratomalacia 63
Kernicterus 179
Kernig's sign 140
KF ring 70
Klinefelter syndrome 73
Klippel–Feil syndrome 47
Knee jerk 131
Koilonychia 63
Korotkoff sounds 41
Krait 203
Kramer's scale 179
Kuppuswamy's socioeconomic status scale 35
Kussmaul's breathing 42
Kwashiorkor 49
Kyphosis 4

L

LABA: long-acting beta agonists 91
Lactobacillus 61
Lactulose 190
Lagophthalamus 70
Lamivudine (3TC) 193
Landau reflex 171
Language delay 8
Language–receptive/expressive 8
Laryngeal mask airway 167
Laryngoscope 160
Lasix 189
Late neonatal period 158
Lateral
  column sensation 137
  neck X-ray 238
  wall MI 252
Laws of development 6
LBW 44, 159
Lead 204
  pipe 136
Leads 242
Leflunomide 147
Left
  heart border 107
  hypochondrium 115
  Iliac region 116
  lumbar region 116
  parasternal heave 106
  to right shunt 105
Length/height
  for age (boys) 258
  for age (girls) 257
Lente 199
Level of consciousness 124
Levetiracetam 188
LF units 23
LGA 159
Lice 186
Lidocaine 198
Life-threatening attack of asthma 266
Light's criteria 92
Light touch 137
Limb leads 242
Linezolid 184
LISCH nodules 70
Lispro 199
Live
  attenuated bacterial 19
  attenuated viral 19
  biopsy needle 226, 227
  span 119
Localized L/N 58
Long acting 199
  beta agonists 91
Longest acting 199
Lordosis 4
Losartan 188
Lovibond angle 55, 60
Lower GIT 115
  epigastrium 115
  hypochondriac region 115
  hypogastrium 115
  iliac region 115
  lumbar region 115
  umbilical area 115
Lower
  GIT region 116
  motor neuron lesion 141
  palpebral conjunctiva 54
  respiratory tract 82
Low
  glycemic index 213
  hair line 66, 67
  risk papulations 149
  set ears 66, 67
Lumbar puncture 223
  needles 224
Lunate 77
Lung fields 234
Lung/pulmonary function test 87
LVH 254
Lymphadenopathy 56, 61
Lymphangioma 68
Lyon hypothesis 145

M

Macrocephaly 50
Macrolides antibiotic 182
Macrostomia 70
Macule 78
Maculosquamous dermatitis 62
MAG-3 scan (mercaptoacetyltri-glycine scan) 221
Magnetic resonance imaging (MRI) 144
Maintenance fluids 194
Malaena 120
Mammalian bites 29
Mammary 83
Management
  of a newborn of a HIV-infect-ed mother 193
  of bronchial asthma 91
  of rabid animal bite 29
  plan for IDA 218
Mantoux
  positive 22
  test 232
Marasmic kwashiorkor 49
Marasmus 49
Marfan syndrome 53, 68
Mask and spacer 229
Mass immunization 23
Mature milk 177
Mean
  arterial pressure (MAP) 104
  corpuscular hemoglobin concentration 217
  corpus-cular volume 217
Measles 24
  vaccine 24
Mebendazole 186

Mechanical ventilation 202
Meconium-stained liquor 171
Mediastinal shadows 234
Medical research council scale 133
Medical waste—colour coding 215
Mefenamic acid 181
Megalocornea 66
Melaena 120
Memory B cell 21
Menarche 77
Menghini technique 226
Meningeal signs 140
  Brudzinski's 140
  Brudzinski's leg sign 140
  kernig's sign 140
  neck rigidity 140
  straight leg 140
Meningococcal vaccine 33, 28
Meningoencephalitis 124
Mental trauma 101
Menveo vaccine 33
Meropenem 184
Metered dose inhaler (MDI) 229
Metformin 199
Methanol 204
Methemoglobinemia 204
Methotrexate 147
Methylene blue 204
Metronidazole 184
Microcephaly 50
Microcornea 66
Micropenis 77
Microscopic haematuria 113
Microscopy 220
Microstomia 70
Microtia 69
Micturating cystourethrography (MCU) 221
Mid arm circumference (MAC) 50
Midazolam 199
Mid
  inspiratory films 234
  parental height 47
Midriasis 202, 203
Mid upper arm circumference (MuAC) 50
Migratory polyarthritis 147
Milestones 10
Milia 173
Miliary TB 21
Milroy syndrome 59
Mimicking 8
Miosis 70, 202
Mission Indradhanush (MI) 34
Mitral area 107
Mixed infection 193
MMR (measles/mumps/rubella) vaccine 24
Mnemonics to remember 263
Moderate acute malnutrition (MAM) 45
Moderna 19
Modes of ventilation 202
Modified
  Duke criteria for infective endocarditis 113
  Jones criteria 149
  Kuppuswamy's socioeconomic status scale 35
  Sarnat and Sarnat 179
Molar 10
Molecular genetics 146
Mongolian spot 173
Mongoloid 64, 66
  slant 64, 65, 66, 70
Monocular fixation 9
Monosyllables 8
Montelukast 190
Moro reflex 171
Morphine 204
Motion sickness 188
Motor 125
  system 130
Mouthing 7
MPH (mid parental height) 47
MR (Measles + Rubella) 24
mRNA based 19
MRSA 184
MR vaccine 24
Multisystem inflammatory syndrome in children (MIS-C) 101
Murmur based on timing 111
  early diastolic murmur 111
  ejection systolic murmur 111
  late systolic murmur 111
  mid diastolic murmur 111
  pansystolic murmur 111
Muscle
  biopsy 146
  bones, joints and rheumatic disorders 145
Mydriasis 70, 202
Myocardial infarction 252
Myopathy 149

N

N-acetyl cysteine 204
Nada's criteria 105
$NaHCO_3$ 198
Naloxone 168, 198, 204
Naproxen 147, 181
Nasal
  cannula 159
  covaxin vaccine 30
  prongs 159
Nasogastric tube 225
Natal teeth 173
National
  Immunization Schedule 31
  Institute of Virology (NIV) 30
  Malaria Eradication Programme 192
  Programs in India 214
  Tuberculosis Elimination Program 191
NCV 146
Near vision 125
Nebulisers 228
Neck holding/head control 6
Neck length 66, 68
Neck rigidity 140
Neonatal case sheet 156
  congenital anomalies 157
  gestational Age 156
  IIIrd trimester (41 weeks) 156
  IInd trimester (28 weeks) 156
  Ist trimester (12 weeks) 156
  mode of delivery 156
  POG (period of gestation) 156
  rupture of membrane 156
  umbilical cord 157
Neonatal reflexes 171
  asymmetrical TNR 171
  Landau 171
  Moro 171
  palmar grasp 171
  parachute 171
  plantar 171
  rooting 171
  symmetrical TNR 171
Neonatal
  resuscitation 159
  thyroid screening 180
Neonate/newborn 158
Neonates
  of unknown HIV 22
  with HIV infection 22
Neonatology 156
Nephrotic 263
  range proteinuria 262
  syndrome 263
  syndrome complication 263
Nervus
  intermedius 129
  terminalis 129
Neurocutaneous markers 4
Neurofibromatosis 4
Neuropathy 149
Neurosonogram (NSG) 144
Nevirapine (NVP) 193
New ballard scoring system 157
Newborn 11
New York Heart Association grading (NYHA) 105
Niclosamide 186
Night blindness 63
Nocturnal enuresis 190
No dehydration 61
Nodule 78

Non-consanguineous marriage 37
Non
nucleoside reverse transcriptase inhibitors (NNRTI) 193
pitting oedema 59
thrombocytopenic purpura 147
Nonvigorous baby 171
Noonan syndromes 66
No pneumonia 90
Normal
CSF values 224
liver span 119
sinus rhythm 247
variations in newborn 173
NRP flow diagram 169
NS 194
NSAIDs 181
NSTEMI 252
NTEP guideline for tberculosis
first line drugs 191
second line drugs 192
Nucleoside reverse transcriptase inhibitors (NRTI) 193
Nystagmus 71

O

O_2 saturation 262
Obesity 51
Objective structured clinical examination 205
Observed stations 206
Oculo-cephalic reflex 70
Oculomotor
(III) 126
(III), trochlear (IV) 126
Oedema 58, 62
Ofloxacin 183
Oka strain 27
Olfactory 125
Oligaemic lung fields 234
Oliguria 262
Ondansetron (Emeset) 188
Opacities 234
OP poisoning 204, 265
Optic (II) 125
Oral
hypoglycaemic agents 199
iron, chelating agent 189
iron therapy 218
Orchidometer 76
Organophosphorus poisoning 203
Orthopnoea 87
Ortolani manoeuvre 152
OSCE 205
Osmolality 200
Ossification centres 77
Osteomyelitis 25
Outer canthal distance 65
Overexposed film 233
Overweight 51
Ovum 10
Oxcarbazepine 187
Oxygen 204
Oxygen cylinders 159

P

Pacemaker cells 241
Packed cell volume 202
$PaCO_2$ 262
Pad size 198
Paediatric
assessment triangle (PAT) 195
case sheet 1
drugs 181
Paediatrics/ALS algorithm 197
Pallor 54, 60
Palmar
erythema 117
grasp 171
Palpable sound 107
Palpate
liver 117
spleen 117
Palpebral conjunctiva 54
Pandemic 103
Pantoprazole 182
PaO_2 262
Papule 78
Paracetamol 181
Parachute reflex 171
Paradoxical breathing 43
Parallelism 6
Parameters 44
Parenteral iron therapy 218
Parkland formulas 201
Parotid swelling 117
Paroxysmal nocturnal dyspnoea (PND) 87
Partial TPN 204
Parts of nebuliser 229
Passive immunization 21
Past history 1
Pathological jaundice 179
blood group incompatibility 179
blue light phototherapy 179
exchange transfusion 179
kernicterus 179
PDA closure 181
Peak
expiratory flow rate (PEFR) 88, 231
inspiratory pressure 202
Pectus
carinatum 4
excavatum 4
Pediatric
basic life support algorithm 196
respiratory severity score 92
Pedigree chart 37
Peeling of skin 173
PEEP (positive end expiratory pressure) 202
Pelebstein fever 38
Pendular knee jerk 139
Penicillin G benzathine (penidure) 184
Penidure 184
Penis 75
Pentalogy 263
Pentavalent 31
PEP 29
PEP measure 29
Percussion note 89
Performance liquid chromatography (HPLC)/hemoglobin electrophoresis 219
Pericardial effusion 107
Pericardial rub 107
Pericarditis 252
Perimetry 125
Perinatal period 11, 158
Period of growth 10
Peripheral
cyanosis 113
pulses 40
Peripheral smear 217
Peritonsillar abscess quinsy 82
Persistent
diarrhoea 120
L/N 58
Personal social 7
Pertussis 23
PES
cavus (claw foot) 153
planus (flat foot) 153
Pet dog 29
Petechiae 78
Peutz–Jeghers syndrome 115
P. falciparum 192
Pfizer 19
pH 262
Phases of breast milk 176
colostrum 176
foremilk 177
hind milk 177
mature milk 177
transitional milk 176
Phenobarbitone 187
Phenytoin 187
Phosphorus 63, 65
Physical abuse 221
Physiological phimosis 173
Physostigmine 204
Pica 12
Pincer grasp 7
Pioglitazone 199
Piperacillin with tazobactam 184
PIP: Peak inspiratory pressure 202

Pisiform 77
Pitch/frequency 110
Pitting 58
Pivoting 9
Plantar reflex 171, 136
Platelet 261
  conc 202
Platypnoea 87
Plethoric lung fields 234
Pleural rub 85
Pleximeter 86
Plexor 86
P. malariae 38
P. mitrale 249
Pneumococcal
  polysaccharide vaccine 25
  vaccine 25
Pneumonia 90
Pneumosil 25
Pneumothorax 235
Pointing 8
Points of good latching 175
Poisoning 202
Polio
  free 23
  vaccine 22
Polyarthralgia 147
Polydactyly 4, 68
Polymorphous exanthema 148
Polyuria 262
Ponderal Index 47
Position sense (proprioception) 137
Positive end expiratory pressure 202
Positive grower sign 146
Posterior
  fontanelle 4
  or dorsal column tract sensation (PCT) 137
Post
  -exposure prophylaxis 33
    for healthcare personal 193
  prandial blood glucose (PPBS) 200
  -term 159
Potassium exchange resin 190
Potter 64, 66
Power 133
PPD 232
PP (pulse pressure) 104
P. pulmonale 249
Pralidoxime 203
Prazosin 190, 204
Precocious puberty 77
Predicted adult height 47
Prednisolone 187
Preductal saturation 163
Premature babies 21
Premolar 10
Preschool 11
Pressure sense 137
Preterm 159
  infants 167
Prevenar 25
Primaquine 192
Primary dentition 10
Principle of nebulisation 229
PR interval 246, 249
Probiotics 61
Progressive neurological disease 23
Projectile vomiting 121
Prolactin 175
Promethazine theoclate 188
Propanolol 189
Proportionate short stature 47
Proprioception 137
Proptosis 68
Protamine sulfate 204
Protease inhibitors 193
Protein 16
Protein requirements 13
Provisional diagnosis 5
Provocative testing 232
Proximal
  muscle weakness 148
  weakness 123
PR segment 246
Pseudoclubbing 56, 60
Pseudohypertrophy 146
Pseudomonas aeruginosa 183
Pseudo-paralysis 62
Pseudotumor cerebri 64
Ptosis 68
Pubarche 77
Pubic hair 74
Puddle sign 119
Pulmonary area 108
Pulmonary function test 87
  forced expiratory volume (FEV_1) 88
  forced vital capacity (FVC) 88
  functional residual capacity (FRC) 88
  peak expiratory flow rate (PEFR) 88
  residual volume (RV) 88
  tidal volume 87
  total lung capacity 88
  vital capacity (VC) 87
Pulse
  oximetry 163
  polio 23
  pressure 104
  rate 40
PUO 39
Pupillary/accommodation 125
Purified chick embryo cell 29
Purified vero cell vaccine 29
Purkinje fibres 241
Purpura 78
Pustule 78
P. vivax/falciparum 38
P wave 245, 248
Pyloric stenosis 121
Pyogenic meningitis 225
Pyrazinamide (Z) 191
Pyrexia/fever of unknown origin 39
Pyridoxin 204
Pyrimethamine 192

Q

QRS complex 245, 251
QT interval 245, 253
Quarantine 102
Quartan 38
Quotidian 38
Q wave 250

R

Rabid animal bite 29
Rabies
  immunoglobulin 30
  immunoglobulin/monoclonal antibody 29
  vaccines 29
Rabipur 29
Rabisheild 30
Rabisheild, serum institute of India 30
Rabishield 33
Rabivax 29
Racecadotril 190
Rachitic rosary 155
Radiation of murmur 111
Radio-
  femoral delay 40
  femoral delay—COA (coarctation of aorta) 40
  radial delay 40
Random blood glucose 199
Ranitidine 182
Rapid
  antigen detection test 98
  weight loss 49
Rate 248
rDNA techniques 24
Ready to use therapeutic food 45
Real-time reverse transcription-polymerase chain reaction (RT-PCR) 98
Rebound phenomenon 139
Receptive language 8
Recombinant
  DNA technology 28
  nanoparticle vaccine 30
Rectal examination 118
Red
  cell distribution width 217
  flag signs 10
Reduced Hb 114
Re-exposure 30

Referral 221
Reflux oesophagitis 188
Regular insulin 199
Regularly irregular 247
Remittent fever 38
Renal
  artery stenosis 120
  lump 121
Residual volume (RV) 88
Respiratory
  devices 228
  failure 195
  rate 41
  system 81
Resuscitation 159, 161
  fluid 194
Resuscitators 167
Revised National Tuberculosis Control Program 191
Rheumatic
  arthritis 150
  carditis 114
  fever 149
Rheumatoid arthritis 150
RHMAB (rabies monoclonal antibody cocktail) 30
Rhythm 246
  strip 246
Rickets 63, 154
Rifampacin (R) 191
Right
  heart border 107
  hypochondrium 115
  Iliac region 116
  lumbar region 116
  middle lobe pneumonia 236
  to Left Shunt 105
Rigidity 136
RIG (rabies immunoglobulin) 30
Rinne's test 128
Risus sardonicus 64, 66
RMNCH + A 214
RNTCP 191
Role playing 8
Romberg's sign 128, 137
Rooting reflex 171
Rotarix 26
Rotasil 27
Rotateq 27
Rotavac 27
Rotavirus vaccine 26
Rule of
  nines 200
  percussion 86
  17 (seventeen) 129
Rupture of membrane 156
RVH 254

S

S_2 splitting 109
SA 14-14-2 vaccine 26
SABA: short-acting beta agonists 91
Saddle back fever (biphasic fever) 38
S. albumin 261
Salbutamol 91, 229
Salmeterol 91
S. ALP 261
S. ammonia 261
S. amylase 261
Sanitation 35
SA node 241
SARS-CoV-2 (RNA) 94
S. bilirubin 261
Scabies disease 79
  bullae 78
  burrows 79
  ecchymosis 78
  enanthem 78
  erosion 78
  erythema nodosum 79
  exanthem 78
  fissure 78
  macule 78
  nodule 78
  papule 78
  pediculosis 80
  petechiae 78
  purpura 78
  pustule 78
  scabies 79
  sinus 78
  telangiectasia 78
  ulcer 78
  vesicle 78
  wheal 78
S. calcium 261
Scanning speech 139
Scaphoid 77
Scar 21
Scarf sign 136
  /heel to ear 136
Schamroth's sign 55, 60
Schirmer's test 127
School age 11
Scoliosis 4
Scorbutic beads 62
Scorpion
  bite 190, 204
  sting 203
S. creatinine 261
Screening of development 11
Scribbling 7
Scrotum/testicular volume 75
Scurvy 62
Sea snake 203
Secondary dentition 10
Secretomotor 127
Seizures 124
Self-inflating bag 163
Semi-essential AA 15
Sensory
  inattention 137
  system 137
Septran 183
Serositis 146
Serum institute of India (SII) 30
Severe acute malnutrition 45
Severe pneumonia 90
Sexual
  abuse 221
  maturity rating 74
S. ferritin 217
SGA 159
S. glucose 261
Shadow pandemic 101
Shakir tape 50
Shifting dullness 119
Short
  acting beta agonists 91
  acting (soluble, regular) 199
  neck 66, 67
  stature 46
Sickle cell anemia 219
Significant L/N 58
Signs of
  correct tube position 167
  dehydration 59
  liver failure 117
Silhouette sign 234
Simple febrile seizure 142
SIMV: synchronized intermittent mandatory ventilation 202
Sino atrial node 241
Sinus 4, 78
S. iron 217
Site of murmurs 111
Skin
  dimples/sinuses 173
  diseases 78
  lesions 78
  to-skin contact 161
  turgor/pinch test 59
Skull 3
  and spine 140
SMR 74
  female 74
  male 75
Snakes 203
Snellen's
  chart 125
  test 126
Social smile 7
Socioeconomic
  class 36
  history 35
  status scale 35
Sokolow-Lyon criteria 254
Some dehydration 61
S. osmolality 261
Spasticity 136

Specific learning disorders 12
Speech delay 8
Spermarche 77
S. phosphorus 261
Spinal accessory (XI) 129
Splenomegaly 121
S. potassium 261
Spring-powered jet injector 31
S. proteins 261
Squint 70
S. sodium 261
Stadiometer 46
Straight leg raising test 140
Status epilepticus 199
Steeple sign 238
STEMI 252
Steps of hand washing 216
Step up and step down approach 91
Stereognosis 137
Steroid myopathy 148
Steroids 186
Stillbirth 158
Stork bites 173
Strabismus 70
Stranger anxiety 7
Strawberry tongue 148
Streptomycin 191
Streptomycin (S) 191
Stridor 87
ST segment 245
Subacute combined degeneration 62
Subconjunctival haemorrhages 173
Subcutaneous
  emphysema 234
  nodules 149
Succussion splash 85
Suction catheter 159, 160
Sulphadoxine 192
Sulphasalazine 147
Superficial reflexes 136, 139
Supinator jerk 131
Suprasternal pulsation 106
Supraventricular tachycardia 198
S. uric acid 261
Symmetrical TNR 171
Sympathetic 140
Symptoms and sings of genitourinary tract disease 219
Synbiotics 61
Synchronized intermittent mandatory ventilation 202
Syndactyly 4
Synflorix 25
Systemic lupus erythematosus (SLE) 145, 147

T

Tablespoon 16
Tachycardia 40
Tachypnoea 42
Tactile
  discrimination 137
  localisation 137
  stimulation 162
Tandem walking 139
Tanner staging 74
Taste sensation 127
TB treatment 191
Td 23
Tdap 23
Teaspoon 16
Telangiectasia 78
Telemedicine 103
Temperature 38
  biphasic fever 38
  continuous fever 38
  fever 38
  hyperpyrexia 38
  hypothermia 38
  intermittent fever 38
  pelebstein fever 38
  remittent fever 38
  saddle back fever 38
  undulant fever 38
Tenesmus 120
Terbutaline 91
Term 158
Tertian 38
Test
  doses 232
  for assessment of intelligence 11
  for screening of development 11
  to diagnose tuberculosis 93
Testicular
  atrophy 117
  volume 75
Tetanus toxoid 23
Tetralogy 263
Texas children's hospital, texas 31
Thalassemia 219
Thelarche 77
Thelarche–pubarche–menarche 77
Thermoregulation 161
Thoracolumbar outflow 140
Thrill 106
Thumb
  print sign 238
  sign 68
Thyroglossal cysts 69
Thyroid myopathy 148
Thyroxin 191
Tidal
  percussion 84
  volume (6–10 ml/kg) 202
  volume (VT) 87
Ti: Inspiratory time 202
Titmus fly test 9
Toddler 11
Toilet training 8
Tone 136
Tongue 8
  depressor 232
  tie 8
Tonic neck reflex 171
Torsades de pointes 251
Total
  count (WBC) 261
  iron binding capacity 217
  lung capacity 88
  serumbilirubin (TSB) 178
Toxin 19
T piece resuscitator 164
Trace mineral deficiency (micronutrients) 63, 65
Tracheal shift 88
  bronchiectasis 88
  collapse 88
  consolidation 88
  emphysema 88
  empyema 88
  fibrosis 88
  hydropneumothorax 88
  pleural effusion 88
  pneumothorax 88
Tracheo-oesophageal fistula 237
Tranexamic acid 190
Transferrin saturation 217
Transitional milk 176
Transjugular liver biopsy 226
Transudates 92
Transudates and exudates ascites fluid 121
Transverse colon obstruction 121
Transverse myeliitis 143
Trapezium 77
Trapezoid 77
Traube's space 84
Traumatic LP 224
Traumatic neuritis 143
Treatment history 1
Treatment of hypoxic spell (TET spell) 264
Treatment of malaria 192
Tremor intention 139
Tricep jerk 131
Trichotillomania 12
Triclofos (pediclory) 190
Tricuspid area 107
Tricyclic antidepressants overdose 203
Trigeminal (V) 126
Triology 263
Triquetral 77
Trisomy 21 72
Trivandrum development screening 11
Trochlear (IV) nerve 126

Tropical eosinophilia 186
Trucut liver biopsy 226
Truncus arteriosus 105
TSH 261
TT 23
Tubercular meningitis 21
Tuberculin syringe 21
Tuberculin syringe 232
Tuberculosis 93
Tuberculous meningitis 225
Tuberous sclerosis 4
Tuning fork 137
Turner syndrome 73
T wave 245, 252
Twinrab 33
Two-point discrimination 137
Type of respiration 42
Typhoid 38, 183
  conjugate vaccine 26
  vaccine 26

U

Ulcer 78
Ultralente 199
Umbilical
  area 115
  catheter 160
  cord 157
Umbilicus 116
UMN lesion 128
Unconjugated
  hyperbilirubenimia 264
  pneumococcal polysaccharide vaccine 26
Uncooked
  cereals 15
  dal 14
  pulses 15
Under nutrition 49
Undescended/ectopic testes 122
Undulant fever 38
Unidextrous grasp 7
Unilateral clubbing 56
Upper bulbar conjunctiva 54
Upper GIT 115
Upper respiratory tract 81
  cottle test 81
  DNS 81
  ethmoid sinus 82
  frontal sinus 81
  maxillary sinus 82
  paranasal sinuses 81
  peritonsillar abscess 82
  PND 82
  throat 82
Upper segment: lower segment ratio 51
Urine
  output 262
  protein 262
Ursodeoxy cholic acid (UDCA) 190
USG-KUB 221
Uvula (X) 128
U wave 245

V

Vaccines 18, 19
  for high-risk children 33
  under special circumstances 33
  vial monitor 22
VACTERL syndrome 265
Vaginal bleeding/discharge 173
Vagus (X) 128
Valley sign 146
Valproate 188
Vancomycin 184
Variation of
  murmurs with posture 112
  murmur with respiration 111
Varicella/chickenpox vaccine 27
Vascular phenomena 113
Vasculitis 145
V. cholera 28
Vegetation 113
Venous hum 106, 120
Ventilation 35
Ventricular
  depolarization 242
  repolarization 245
Verorab 29
Vertigo 128
Very severe pneumonia 90
Vesicle 78
  herpes 115
Vestibulo-cochlear (VIII) nerve 128
Vestibulo-ocular reflex 128
Vibration 137
Viper 203
Vi PS-capsular polysaccharide unconjugated vaccine 26
Viral encephalitis (AES) 225
Virus like particles (VLP) 28
Vision 9
Vit A 32
Vital capacity (VC) 87
Vitals 3, 38
Vitamin A 62
Vitamin A deficiency 63
Vitamin B_1 (Thiamine) 62
Vitamin B_2 (Riboflavin) 62
Vitamin B_3 (Niacin) 62
Vitamin B_6 (Pyridoxine) 62
Vitamin B_{12} (Cobalamine) 62
Vitamin C 62
Vitamin D 63, 65
Vitamin E 63, 65
Vitamin K 63, 65, 170, 204
VLBW 159
Vocal fremitus 83
Vocal fremitus 89
Vocal resonance 89
Volume expanders 170
Voluntary consent 212
VT: Tidal volume 202
VVM (vaccine vial monitor) 22

W

WAGR syndrome 265
Waist hip ratio 51
Warfarin 204
Wasting 48
Watch test 128
Waterlow classification 48
  malnutrition 48
Weaning/complementary feeding 16
Weber's test 128
Weight 44
  bands 191
  for age (boys) 257
  for age (girls) 256
  for-height 48
Wet-beriberi 62, 64
Wheal 78
Wheeze 87
Whispering pectoriloquy 85
WHO
  classification of HIV-associated clinical disease 193
  classification of malnutrition 48
  classification of pneumonia 90
  cutoff of anaemia 262
  ORS 61
Widely spaced nipple 66, 68
Wolf-Parkinson-White (WPW) syndrome 249
World breastfeeding week 177
World TB day 21
Wrist sign 68
Wt for ht 48

X

Xerophthalmic fundus 63
X-linked dominant familial hypophosphataemic rickets 63
X-ray 233
  abdomen 238
  bones 239

Y

Yellow fever vaccine 33

Z

Zidovudine (AZT) 193
Zinc 63, 65
ZyCoV-D 31